Neurointensive Care

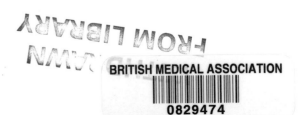

Katja E. Wartenberg • Khalid Shukri
Tamer Abdelhak

Editors

Neurointensive Care

A Clinical Guide to Patient Safety

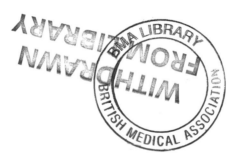

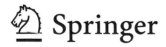 Springer

Editors
Katja E. Wartenberg
Neurological Intensive Care Unit
Martin Luther University Halle-Wittenberg
Halle (Saale)
Sachsen-Anhalt
Germany

Tamer Abdelhak
Department of Neurology
Southern Illinois University School
of Medicine
Springfield, IL
USA

Khalid Shukri
Department of Critical Care
Medinah National Hospital
Medinah Munnawarah
Saudi Arabia

ISBN 978-3-319-17292-7   ISBN 978-3-319-17293-4   (eBook)
DOI 10.1007/978-3-319-17293-4

Library of Congress Control Number: 2015943707

Springer Cham Heidelberg New York Dordrecht London
© Springer International Publishing Switzerland 2015

Printed on acid-free paper

Springer International Publishing AG Switzerland is part of Springer Science+Business Media
(www.springer.com)

Preface

Neurocritical care is a rapidly developing specialty worldwide with participation of multiprofessional health-care workers and the aim to provide high-quality care and to improve outcomes of patients with life-threatening neurological diseases. At the same time, in the midst of increasingly available high-end monitoring techniques and invasive technologies, the focus has shifted toward patient safety and quality of patient care. With accumulating economic pressure, the rising number of patients in our aging population, fast turnover, and expanding application of technology and measurements, the patient's safety and well-being may be at risk.

This book is an effort of international multidisciplinary health-care providers with a focus on neurocritical care to draw the attention back to treating patients in a neurointensive care unit with a safe environment, with secure management protocols and algorithms according to various disease and intensive care categories. After an introduction of quality measures and safety in patient care, risks of patient safety and safety barriers will be discussed in general and case based for a wide range of neurological diseases requiring critical care and intensive care management principles. At the end of each chapter, treatment protocols and the "dos and don'ts" in management of the particular neurological disease or intensive care measure will be summarized. The international representation of authors was essential to reflect the practice of neurocritical care worldwide so that evidence-based materials presented can be applied in different parts of the world.

Neurointensive Care: A Clinical Guide to Patient Safety will present the world of a neurocritical care unit in the light of high-quality and safe patient care and may help with development of protocols, algorithms, and structured plans even in the absence of countless resources.

Halle (Saale), Germany   Katja E. Wartenberg, MD, PhD
Medinah Munnawarah, Saudi Arabia   Khalid Shukri, MD, FCCM
Springfield, IL, USA   Tamer Abdelhak, MD

Contents

1   **Patient Safety Standards in the Neuro-ICU** 1
Susan Yeager and Sarah Livesay

2   **Airway Safety in the Neurocritical Care Unit** 19
Venkatakrishna Rajajee

3   **Mechanical Ventilation in the Neuro-ICU** 43
Sang-Beom Jeon and Younsuck Koh

4   **Nutrition in Neuro-ICU** 57
Sandeep Kantor, Maher J. Albahrani, and Sadanandan Prakash

5   **Monitoring in the Neurocritical Care Unit** 73
Said Hachimi-Idrissi

6   **Intracranial Pressure Monitoring** 87
Othman Solaiman and Faisal Al-Otaibi

7   **Postoperative Care in Neurooncology** 95
Konstantin A. Popugaev and Andrew Yu Lubnin

8   **Subarachnoid Hemorrhage** 125
Edgar Avalos Herrera and Corina Puppo

9   **Intracerebral Hemorrhage** 145
Moon Ku Han

10 **Patient Safety in Acute Ischemic Stroke** 157
Ivan Rocha Ferreira da Silva and Bernardo Liberato

11 **Cerebral Venous Thrombosis** 171
Liping Liu and Ruijun Ji

12 **Bacterial Meningitis** 185
Yasser B. Abulhasan and Pravin Amin

13   **Brain Abscess**   201
     Bijen Nazliel

14   **Seizures and Status Epilepticus in the Intensive Care Units**   209
     Johnny Lokin

15   **Traumatic Brain Injury.**   219
     Tamer Abdelhak and Guadalupe Castillo Abrego

16   **Patient Safety in Guillain–Barré Syndrome and Acute
     Neuromuscular Disorders**   249
     Maxwell S. Damian

17   **Acute Spinal Disorders**   257
     Regunath Kandasamy, Wan Mohd Nazaruddin Wan Hassan,
     Zamzuri Idris, and Jafri Malin Abdullah

18   **Care for Complications After Catastrophic Brain Injury**   279
     Vera Spatenkova and Nehad Nabeel Mohamed AL-Shirawi

19   **Neuroimaging in the Neuro-ICU**   299
     Sharon Casilda Theophilus, Regunath Kandasamy,
     Khatijah Abu Bakar, and Jafri Malin Abdullah

20   **Brain Death.**   313
     Michael A. Kuiper, Gea Drost, and J. Gert van Dijk

21   **Ethics in the Neuro-ICU**   327
     Ludo J. Vanopdenbosch and Fred Rincon

Index   337

Contributors

Tamer Abdelhak, MD Department of Neurology, Southern Illinois University School of Medicine, Springfield, IL, USA

Jafri Malin Abdullah, FASC, MD, PhD, DSCN, FRCS Center for Neuroscience Services and Research, Universiti Sains Malaysia, Kota Bharu, Kelantan, Malaysia

Guadalupe Castillo Abrego, MD Critical Care Department, Caja de Seguro Social Hospital, Panama City, Panama

Yasser B. Abulhasan, MB, ChB, FRCPC Faculty of Medicine, Health Sciences Center, Kuwait University, Safat, Kuwait

Maher J. Albahrani, MBChB Department of Anesthesia and Critical Care, Royal Hospital, Muscat, Oman

Faisal Al-Otaibi, MD Division of Neurological Surgery, Department of Neuroscience, King Faisal Specialist Hospital and Research Centre, Riyadh, Saudi Arabia

Nehad Nabeel Mohamed AL-Shirawi, MRCP King Abdulla Medical City, Makka, Kingdom of Saudi Arabia

Pravin Amin, MD, FCCM Department of Critical Care Medicine, Bombay Hospital Institute of Medical Sciences, Mumbai, Maharashtra, India

Khatijah Abu Bakar, MD (UKM), MMed Radiology (UM) Department of Radiology, Sultanah Aminah Johor Bahru, Johor Bahru, Johor, Malaysia

Maxwell Simon Damian, MD, PhD Department of Neurology, Cambridge University Hospitals, Cambridge, UK

Ivan Rocha Ferreira da Silva, MD Department of Neurocritical Care, Hospital Copa D'Or, Rio de Janeiro, Brazil

Gea Drost, MD, PhD Department of Neurology, University Medical Center Groningen, Groningen, The Netherlands

Said Hachimi-Idrissi, MD, PhD, FCCM, FAAP Critical Care Department and Cerebral Resuscitation Research Group, Universiteit Ziekenhuis, Ghent, Belgium

Moon Ku Han, MD, PhD Department of Neurology, Seoul National University Bundang Hospital, Seongnam, South Korea

Wan Mohd Nazaruddin Wan Hassan, MD, Master in Medicine Departments of Anaesthesiology and Intensive Care, Hospital Universiti Sains Malaysia, Kota Bharu, Kelantan, Malaysia

Edgar Avalos Herrera, MD, MsC Department of Neurology and Neurophysiology, Hospital General San Juan de Dios, Guatemala City, Guatemala

Zamzuri Idris, MBBch, MS Neurosurgery Center for Neuroscience Services and Research, Universiti Sains Malaysia, Kota Bharu, Kelantan, Malaysia

Sang-Beom Jeon, MD, PhD Department of Neurology, Asan Medical Center, Seoul, Republic of Korea

Ruijun Ji, MD, PhD Neurology and Stroke Center, Beijing Tiantan Hospital, Beijing, China

Regunath Kandasamy, MBBS, MRCS, MS Neurosurgery Center for Neuroscience Services and Research, Universiti Sains Malaysia, Kota Bharu, Kelantan, Malaysia

Sandeep Kantor, MBBS, DA, MD, FCCP, FCCM Department of Anesthesia and Critical Care, Royal Hospital, Muscat, Oman

Younsuck Koh, MD, PhD, FCCM Department of Pulmonary and Critical Care Medicine, Asan Medical Center, Seoul, Republic of Korea

Michael Kuiper, MD, PhD Intensive Care Department, Medical Center Leeuwarden, Leeuwarden, The Netherlands

Bernardo Liberato, MD Department of Neurology, Hospital Copa D'Or, Rio de Janeiro, Brazil

Liping Liu, MD, PhD Neurology and Stroke Center, Beijing Tiantan Hospital, Beijing, China

Sarah Livesay, DNP, RN, ACNP-BC, ACNS-BC College of Nursing, Rush University, Chicago, IL, USA

Johnny Lokin, MD Neuro-Intensive Care Unit, Chinese General Hospital and Medical Center/University of Santo Tomas Hospital, Manila, Philippines

Andrew Yu Lubnin, MD, PhD Department of Neuroanesthesia, Burdenko Neurosurgical Research Institute, Moscow, Russia

Bijen Nazliel, MD Neurology-Neurointensive Care Unit, Gazi University Faculty of Medicine, Ankara, Turkey

Konstantin A. Popugaev, MD, PhD Department of Neurocritical Care, Burdenko Neurosurgical Research Institute, Moscow, Russia

Sadanandan Prakash, MBBS, DA, MD, FFARCS (I), EDIC Department of Anesthesia and Critical Care, Royal Hospital, Muscat, Oman

Corina Puppo, MD Department of Emergency and Critical Care, Clinics Hospital, Universidad de la República School of Medicine, Montevideo, Uruguay

Venkatakrishna Rajajee, MBBS Department of Neurosurgery, University of Michigan – Ann Arbor, Ann Arbor, MI, USA

Fred Rincon, MD, MSc, MB Ethics, FCCM, FNCS Department of Neurosurgery, Thomas Jefferson University Hospital, Philadelphia, PA, USA

Othman Solaiman, MD, SB-IM, AB-IM Department of Critical Care Medicine, King Faisal Specialist Hospital and Research Centre, Riyadh, Saudi Arabia

Vera Spatenkova, MD, PhD Neurointensive Care Unit, Neurocenter, Liberec, Czech Republic

Sharon Casilda Theophilus, MD (USU), MS Neurosurgery (USM) Department of Neurosurgery, Sultanah Aminah Johor Bahru, Johor Bahru, Johor, Malaysia

J. Gert van Dijk, MD, PhD Department of Neurology, Leiden University Medical Center, Leiden, The Netherlands

Ludo J. Vanopdenbosch, MD, FAAN Department of Neurology, AZ Sint Jan Brugge Oostende, Brugge, Belgium

Susan Yeager, MS, RN, CCRN, ACNP, FNCS Department of Neurocritical Care, The Ohio State University Wexner Medical Center, Columbus, OH, USA

Chapter 1
Patient Safety Standards in the Neuro-ICU

Susan Yeager and Sarah Livesay

Historical Perspective

The origins of the current healthcare quality and safety movement can be traced back centuries [1]. Early pioneers include Florence Nightingale, Ernest Codman, and Avedis Donabedian. Nightingale, a nurse, utilized statistical principles to correlate illness to poor sanitary conditions. She then utilized the findings to create interventions aimed at improving sanitation [1]. Codman, a US surgeon, introduced the concept of an *end results card*, meant to measure outcomes following surgery [1]. Donabedian, a physician, founded the model of care where healthcare quality focused on structure, process, and outcome of service [2].

Despite these early efforts, global changes to healthcare quality and safety are still evolving. The *Report to the Carnegie Foundation* published in 1910, first detailed the lack of standards to guide physician training and hospital care [2]. As a result of this work, five minimum standards were recommended to improve hospital care which include: hospital medical staff organization; medical staff membership limited to those with quality education, competency demonstration, and appropriate licensure and certification; regular staff meeting and clinical review establishment; medical record development and maintenance; and supervised diagnostic and treatment facility creation [2]. This publication led to the initial establishment of a compliance review process where representatives from a number of professional societies, such as the Canadian Medical Association, the American College of Physicians, the American Medical Association, and the American College of Surgeons, visited hospitals to

S. Yeager, MS, RN, CCRN, ACNP, FNCS (✉)
Department of Neurocritical Care, The Ohio State University
Wexner Medical Center, Columbus, OH, USA
e-mail: syeager@columbus.rr.com

S. Livesay, DNP, RN, ACNP-BC, ACNS-BC
College of Nursing, Rush University, Chicago, IL, USA

© Springer International Publishing Switzerland 2015   1
K.E. Wartenberg et al. (eds.), *Neurointensive Care: A Clinical Guide
to Patient Safety*, DOI 10.1007/978-3-319-17293-4_1

Table 1.1 Performance standards for healthcare clinicians and organizations	Care is based on continuous healing relationships
	Care is customized according to patient needs and values
	The patient is the source of control
	Knowledge is shared and information flows freely
	Decision making is evidence based
	Safety is a system property
	Transparency is necessary
	Needs are anticipated
	Waste is continuously decreased
	Cooperation among clinicians is a priority

ensure compliance with minimum standards [2]. In 1952, members from each of the organizations formally united to form the Joint Commission on Accreditation of Hospitals [2].

The most recent pivotal developments to guide healthcare quality and safety movements are the seminal publications from the Institute of Medicine, *To Err is Human: Building a Safer Health System* [3], and *Crossing the Quality Chasm: a New Health System for the 21st Century* [4], published in 1999 and 2001 respectively. These reports synthesized several decades of research, outlining the staggering number of deaths attributed to health care-related error. *To Err is Human* demonstrated that US healthcare errors are responsible for anywhere from 44,000 to 98,000 deaths annually translating to 1.7 medical errors daily [5]. In response to these findings, the IOM created a document, *"Crossing the Quality Chasm"* which outlined ten key initiatives to fundamentally change the quality and safety breakdown in healthcare [4] (See Table 1.1).

Further articles from other countries confirmed that deficiencies and reduced quality of care are not confined to the United States [6–9]. While the veracity of numbers and applicability in other countries may be debated, the fact that a large number of human errors occur in healthcare cannot be denied [5]. As a result of both foundational and recent work, a call to action to urgently redesign global care systems to enhance quality and improve patient safety has become a priority.

Measures of Quality and Safety Measures

While quality programs are both defined and measured by certifying agencies and professional associations, no clear definition of quality specific to Neurocritical care currently exists. Therefore, a culmination of quality recommendations and research findings from both general and Neurocritical care arenas will be presented. Utilizing Donabedian's healthcare quality model, quality measures may be classified as structure measures, process measures, or outcome measures. A structure measure may include the presence or absence of key infrastructure components. Examples may include physician or nurse caregivers with specific competency and education, or physiologic monitoring equipment that provides care to a specific patient population. Process measures are care elements known to be associated with improved outcomes. For example, the early administration of antithrombotics in the setting of acute ischemic stroke is associated with a reduction in subsequent stroke events. Therefore, a measure of healthcare process might include patients who with ischemic stroke appropriately received an antithrombotic as indicated by the medical research. Outcome measures that are patient focused may include morbidity or mortality measures, readmission or reoccurrence rates, or other measures of patient or population health or illness. The following will be an overview of these measures as they relate to the Neurocritical care unit.

Structure Measures

Specialized Neurocritical Care Units

The polio outbreak first highlighted the need for neurologic specialty care. Despite this early notion, modern development and implementation of specialized Neurocritical care units (NCCU) remains a relatively new phenomenon [10]. The recent NCCU development has occurred due to private hospital growth, economic increases, and expansion of medical subspecialty caregivers into Neurocritical care [11]. Further driving support for NCCUs are research findings which highlight the types of patients and care providers that can be utilized to improve patient care. Creating the research foundation for which patients should receive care in a NCCU, Zacharia noted that typical diagnoses who may benefit from specialty care were post-cardiac arrest, ischemic and hemorrhagic strokes, postoperative spine and brain diseases, traumatic injuries, seizures, and neuromuscular diseases [12–14].

Literature evaluating where and by whom neurologic critically ill patients should receive care is evolving. Multiple research studies have attempted to answer questions to determine if a physical unit, the presence of a specialized team, or combination of both is responsible for improved patient outcomes. Supporting the creation of a dedicated NCCU are studies that have noted improved outcomes in the form of reduced mortality, reduced ICU and hospital length of stay, improved resource utilization, decreased sedation usage, increased nutritional support, and increased fiscal benefits [15–23]. The majority of studies to date suggest experienced and specialized Neurocritical care units likely provide better outcomes due to focused and consistent attention to neurologic details [15]. If a dedicated NCCU is not possible, several creative solutions have been presented and evaluated. One creative approach to location of care was described in a Canadian based study. In this work, the creation of a virtual Neurocritical care unit within a mixed ICU was evaluated by looking at the implementation of this care without a dedicated NCCU. Changes in patient allocation, physician staffing, and care protocols were developed to support this effort. The program created multiple tools to overcome barriers of inconsistent care inherent in a virtual unit including team education, rounding protocols, and patient triage algorithms that were then implemented by a collaborative team of clinicians [24]. The study demonstrated the model is feasible. Another creative solution was presented by Burns. This study evaluated the impact of a Neurocritical care service line without a dedicated NCCU. Improvement was noted in hypertensive control and dysphagia screening but results also indicated an associated trend toward a longer length of stay in intracranial hemorrhage (ICH) patients [25]. Despite some positive finding in the latter studies, both authors emphasized that the ideal care model goal should still be a specialized, dedicated NCCU [24].

System Support

While support for dedicated Neurocritical care units is growing, research regarding the impact of systemic integration is largely lacking. Although healthcare providers exert influence at the point of care, very often system failures are the proximal cause of error [25]. According to Tourgeman-Baskin, 95 % of near healthcare misses were attributable to work environment and system factors [25]. Therefore, system factors and work environments need to be optimized to prevent error or mitigate consequences should an error occur [26].

The ideal institutional design supports interdepartmental integration. In a study conducted in the United Kingdom, researchers noted increased survival of critically ill neurologic patients when system integration occurred between critical care unit, emergency department, and step down unit [27]. National certifying bodies also acknowledge the importance of system integration. For example, integrated team-based care from admission to discharge is required for any organization seeking Comprehensive Stroke Certification by The Joint Commission.

Team

Role modeling of positive unit culture is frequently set by institutional and unit leadership but ultimately supported by a team. Specific team interactions and behaviors identified as having a positive impact on care include: humor, personal sharing, and inclusion of all levels of staff in key decision making. These behaviors were found to improve information flow and team relations which translated to enhanced patient safety. Flat hierarchies and clear role expectation policies were also noted as potential ways to improve care. In a study by Suarez, care delivered by a specialized neurologic critical care team was noted to be associated with reduced in-hospital mortality and LOS without changes in readmission rates or long-term mortality [28]. The Brain Attack Coalition consensus statement also reiterates the positive impact of a dedicated neurologic team. These recommendations include the mandatory presence of dedicated, neurologic expert staff and licensed independent care providers 24 h a day, 7 days a week.

Unit Leaders

According to the American Association of Critical Care Nurses, a healthy work environment consists of several key factors including authentic leaders [29]. In 2000, France utilized a multidisciplinary safety attitudes survey and found that a positive safety climate was impacted by the staff's perception of management [30, 31]. In a study of 32 Australian general ICUs, collaboration with competent and respectful medical staff and nursing unit management were cited as key to a safe care environment [32, 33]. Therefore, unit leadership is necessary to role model and impact behavior that supports a positive unit culture. Formally and informally identified team leaders can be found among a variety of NCCU healthcare professionals. Included among this group are intensivists, advanced practice providers, managers, bedside nurses, pharmacists, and specialized therapy professionals.

Intensivists

Evidence to guide the necessary personnel included in the Neurocritical Care team is mixed. Several studies reflect that there may be no benefit to subspecialty ICUs [34, 35] and question the benefit of the intensivist-led team model [36]. However, other studies have found positive outcomes attributed to the introduction of an intensivist. These include the decreased number of complications, reduced LOS, higher home or rehab discharges, and improved documentation [20, 36–41]. In a study by Pronovost, 17 studies evaluated intensivist staffing levels and hospital mortality. Sixteen of those reflected lower in-hospital mortality with the mandatory presence of an intensivist [42]. Given these results, both the Society of Critical Care Medicine and the Leapfrog Group implemented guidelines supporting the need for a dedicated "intensivist" to staff all ICUs [42–47]. While this recommendation does not specifically outline the presence of a specialty trained neurointensivist, a study by Markandaya indicates that 70 % of practitioners believe neurointensivists are important for quality care of the neurologically critically ill [34].

Adequate staffing levels have also been identified as a factor affecting patient safety. A statement from the Society of Critical Care Medicine Taskforce was created to address Intensivist/patient ratios in a general closed ICU. Literature is present to support that in academic medical ICUs; ratios greater than 1:14 had negative impacts on education, staff well-being, and patient care [48]. While specific intensivist number recommendations could not be established for all institutional types, realistic markers were suggested. High staff turnover or decreases in quality indicators may be overload markers. While 24 h a day, 7 days per week physician staffing is recommended by a Society of Critical Care Medicine guideline, a Canadian study of general adult and pediatric ICUs reflected compliance variability due to financial or resource unavailability [49]. Solutions listed as useful solutions to suboptimal intensivist staffing includes the utilization of non-intensivist medical staff, such as advanced practice professionals (Nurse Practitioners and Physician Assistants), and telemedicine [48].

Advanced Practice Providers

As Neurocritical Care (NCC) is a relatively new and evolving subspecialty, the evidence to specify practitioner skill mix is also being formed [34]. Despite this gap in research regarding types of providers, that a division of labor for these complex patients would enable practitioners to subspecialize their focus with concomitant outcome improvement [34]. In a variety of critical care units are an emerging group of clinicians. Non-physician providers, midlevel practitioner, and advanced practice providers (APP) are all terms utilized to refer to advanced level practitioners including nurse practitioners (NPs), physician assistants (PAs), and clinical nurse specialists (CNSs).

NPs and PAs are the most commonly used advanced practice direct care providers in the ICU. The utilization of NP and PA practice providers has been catalyzed by the National Health Service Management Executive group secondary to the decrease in available resident/junior medical staff [50]. Physician manpower issues have occurred due to resident work hour restrictions and intensivist caregiver shortfalls. According to the Society of Critical Care Medicine, these shortfalls are projected to continue due to the anticipated lack of trainees [51, 52]. NPs and PAs have been identified as a growing group of healthcare providers of critical care providers to meet the gap in ICU coverage. The Leapfrog staffing group recognizes that NPs and PAs that reach ICU patients in less than 5 min, along with an intensivist response by pager, can help to promote quality ICU staffing coverage [51, 53]. General ICU studies that have examined care outcomes from NP and PA providers have included positive results in ventilator weaning [51], length of stay, readmission rates, mortality, costs, discharge instructions, radiograph interpretation, and physician time savings [51]. While actualization and education of NP and PA roles vary, general roles and responsibilities include patient assessment, history and physical examinations, rounding with multidisciplinary teams, admissions, discharges, routine care, medication administration, ordering/reviewing/interpreting diagnostic and laboratory tests, updating families, coordinating care, and insertion of invasive procedures such as arterial lines, central lines, lumbar punctures, suturing, first assist, and cranial monitoring devices [51, 54–56]. In a study by Van Rhee, PA care for acute stroke among other diagnosis found that fewer laboratory resources for stroke patients were noted with the implementation of PA providers [51, 57]. Shorter lengths of stay, lower rates of UTI and skin breakdown, shorter time to Foley discontinuation, and time to mobility were noted in a study that specifically evaluated NP care for neuroscience ICU patients [51, 54]. In this study, the shorter length of stay totaled 2,306 fewer days which translated to $2,467,328 worth of savings [54]. Finally, in a study by Robinson, NP's and PA's care was associated with higher scores in safety, improved ability to promote a team environment, ability to address patient or staff concerns, enhanced communication, and most importantly, the ability to anticipate or prevent a neurological deterioration [58].

The role of the Clinical Nurse Specialist varies by country. Regardless of the exact actualization of this role, common attributes include the need for: advanced assessment skills, experience in the field of practice, postgraduate qualifications, role autonomy, and contributions to both education and research within their specialty. In a 15-hospital study, improved stroke evidence-based practice application occurred when driven by a CNS. Improved outcomes of smoking cessation, dysphagia screening, national institutes of health stroke scale use, and documentation of reasons for the lack of tissue plasminogen activator (t-PA) utilization were noted [59]. Jahnke also noted improved emergency room door to exam by physicians; order and completion of head CAT scans; t-Pa utilization; and pathway use and compliance when driven by a CNS-created process improvement effort [60].

While limited positive research regarding NCCU specific CNSs, NPs, and PAs exists, the complete impact of these providers in the NCCU setting is yet to be determined. Despite these research gaps, the utilization of these providers appears to enhance patient outcomes and should be considered when creating NCCU core staff.

Nursing Management

Literature is scarce to address whether outcomes are improved through the support of a NCCU specific manager. In a 2004 Suarez study, the hiring of a neurologic specific nurse manager along with specialty trained 24 h/day bedside nursing staff was associated with reduced Neurocritical care and hospital length of stay and in-hospital mortality [28]. In another study, essential skills for an effective nurse manager included trust, motivation, excellent communication, and problem-solving skills [61]. Having someone with these skills present, to specifically advocate for this subspecialty and oversee the staff and care given, intuitively translates to adherence of patient quality and safety initiatives.

Direct Care Nursing Staff

As the largest proportion of healthcare workers, nurses remain integral to the provision of quality care. In an international study, the presence of specialty-trained nurses with the ability to perform skilled neurologic exams was noted to be paramount to optimal neurologic critical care [34]. Despite the limited evidence, it is intuitive that having a 24 hours per day, 7 days per week staff with specialty training to assist with the early identification of subtle changes in neurologic critical care patients is imperative to patient safety. Therefore, obtainment of neurologic specific training should occur to enable preemptive, rather than reactive, care.

In addition to proper education, adequate nurse staffing is necessary to support optimal patient care. In a multinational study, errors on medication administration were attributed to excessive workload, extended working hours, fatigue, and sleep deprivation [25]. Workload also impacted the risk of iatrogenic infection rates [25]. In a study evaluating the effect of workload on infection risk, higher nurse staffing equated to a 30 % reduction in infection [25]. In a study by Beckmann, drug administration/documentation problems, lack of patient supervision, ventilator or equipment set up errors, accidental extubations, patient/family dissatisfaction, and physical injury had an inverse relationship with staffing [62]. Therefore, ICU managers and administrators need to optimize schedule design to ensure appropriate staffing levels [25]. That said, what equates to adequate bedside nurse staffing remains allusive. A consensus driven method was created in Australia in an attempt to define formulas to determine the required number of nurses to staff critical care units [63]. The American Association of Critical Care Nurses states that adequate staffing matches the skillset of the provider with the needs of the patients [64, 65]. A more literal translation adopted by most American and Canadian critical care units as the unofficial staffing guideline is one to two patients per nurse with some states mandating this ratio [64, 66, 67]. Australia, New Zealand, Europe, and the United Kingdom all recommend at least one RN to one patient however with the RN workforce shortage; practical application of these ratios may at times be unachievable [64].

Multidisciplinary Providers

In addition to specialty trained physician, APP, management, and nursing staff, optimal NCC should be further supplemented with the incorporation of a variety of specialty staff. Specialty focused pharmacists have been identified as providing safe and effective use of medications in a NCCU [6]. Physical therapists, occupational therapists, dieticians, and speech therapists with neurologic expertise also enhance care and should be considered when establishing a critical care team.

Education

A highly trained workforce with adequate resources for education is required to support optimal patient care [25]. Since the inception of critical care units, practice standards outlining nursing educational preparation have been developed along with fundamental critical care training [32, 64]. Results of several studies in general critical care environments suggest that support of knowledgeable and educated nurses is crucial and may translate to improved outcomes [64]. Increased education has been found in nursing research to promote more assertiveness in practice which leads to greater confidence and job satisfaction. Additionally, hospitals with a greater proportion of Bachelor's prepared critical care nurses were noted to experience a lower odds of death [67]. The Australian College of Critical Care Nurses, European Federation of Critical Care Nursing associations, World Federation of Critical Care Nurses, and New Zealand Nurse's Organization Critical Care Nurses Section adopted the position statement that critical care nurses should have postgraduate qualification in critical care nursing [64]. Despite this consensus, debate continues on whether all nurses, or just a percentage of nurses within these critical care units, require all these qualifications and the content of critical care course curriculum remain [64].

In addition to formalized academic training, certification has been noted to increase critical care and neurologic nursing knowledge. Results show that in addition to having a larger percentage of baccalaureate trained nurses, units with a larger numbers of nurses with additional certification training had lower 30-day mortality and failure to rescue rates [68]. Neuroscience Registered Nurses, Stroke Certified Registered Nurses, and Critical Care Registered Nurses are three certification exams that focus on the enhancement of neurological, stroke, and critical care nursing expertise and should be considered to support improvement in care safety and quality.

Advanced practice provider education requirements for CNSs, NPs, and PAs either already require or are evolving to standardize masters level education as the minimum expected educational foundation. In 2013, an APP nursing consensus document was released and determined that advanced education must match the needs of the patient for whom care is being provided. Only acute care trained practitioners have been educated and trained to manage critically ill patients in an ICU setting [51]. Therefore, acute care, not primary or family care education and certification, should be the foundation for APP nursing providers working within the NCC environment.

In a study of 980 physicians, 57 % of those that responded indicated that neurology residency training should offer a separate training track for those that desire NCC as a career path [34]. Neurosurgeons also recommended neurologic intensive care training to be important to neurosurgical resident education [15]. The United Council of Neurological Subspecialties is a nonprofit organization that is committed to the development of neurological fellowship training programs. To that end, the UCNS formally granted Neurocritical care acceptance as a medical subspecialty opening the door for specialty training and certification exams [34]. In Germany, 6 months in a neurosurgical intensive care is required to sit for board certification. Post board certification requires an additional 2 years plus completion of a catalogue specifying interventions given [15]. Two years of NCC fellowship training is required in the United States. Neurosurgery, anesthesiology, internal medicine, and emergency medicine residency were also supported as background specialties into NCC entry [34]. This variation reflects the need for training standardization to support NCC specialty training.

Process Outcomes

Culture

Organizations with a culture of safety are more likely to have less adverse events, decreased mortality, and staff that are more likely to report errors or near misses than organizations without this culture [69]. The impact of organizational culture on safety has been studied widely throughout various inpatient settings. A recent systematic review identified 33 culture of safety studies that evaluated the impact of interventions. In an organization with a culture of safety, leadership plans programs that acknowledge that delivering healthcare is a high-risk endeavor. Organizations with a culture of safety prioritize team-based care, high-quality communication, family involvement in decision making, and utilization of evidence-based practice, including protocols and other means to standardize care to reduce variation [4, 70]. The presence and involvement of the patient and family in patient care rounds and ongoing decision making is a best practice established in several studies in pediatric and general medical ICUs [71]. No research to date has evaluated organizational patient safety initiatives or culture of safety characteristics related specifically to a NCC program but it stands to reason that the global concepts also apply to the NCC population [6].

Quality and Safety

As the field of NCC grows and develops, defining quality and safety in NCC programs will likely incorporate existing measures from general critical care and other fields of neurology such as stroke. These global measures can then be used in combination or to focus developing measures unique to the NCC population. Within the field of general critical care, national organizations such as the Society of Critical Care Medicine, The Leapfrog Group, and the National Quality Form (NQF) and Centers for Medicare and Medicaid Services (CMS) contribute a number of quality and safety measures. Included in these measures are physician staffing models, infection rates including blood stream infection rates, ventilator associated pneumonia, and catheter associated urinary tract infections, sepsis rates and resuscitation, and overall ICU mortality. These measures are certainly relevant to a Neurocritical care program, and should be used as a means to benchmark the care in the NCC unit to other critical care units throughout the nation.

Additionally, stroke certification programs offered through The Joint Commission and Det Norske Veritas (DNV) publish standards and quality metrics that the stroke program must meet. Many of these standards and metrics relate specifically to NCC. For example, the standards for Comprehensive Stroke Certification with TJC require a model of NCC, and an organized approach to disease management within the NCC unit. Several of the TJC proposed quality metrics also relate to processes occurring in the NCCU unit. Examples of these metrics include: infection rates and complication monitoring associated with external ventricular drains, craniectomy, and neurointerventional procedures; procoagulant reversal in the setting of intracerebral hemorrhage; and interdisciplinary peer review process creation to address any complications occurring in a patient with the diagnosis of ischemic stroke, intracerebral hemorrhage, and subarachnoid hemorrhage. However, these standards are stroke specific and do not address the varied diagnoses routinely seen in a NCC program. Therefore, a high-quality NCC program could reasonably be expected to develop and utilize protocols or standard operating procedures to guide care of both routine and high-risk patient care situations including; placement and maintenance of an external ventricular drain, management of elevated ICP and herniation syndromes, and disease processes such as ischemic stroke, ICH, SAH, meningitis/encephalitis, status epilepticus, and other common diseases.

While protocols and standard operating procedures help standardize care, formal and informal communication mechanisms are required to assist with communication of the care given. The importance of team communication is highlighted in a number of publications dating back to the IOM safety series published in 2000 and 2001. Handoff between providers, hospital locations, and inpatient and outpatient organizations represents an area of recent interest and concern as it relates to patient safety and quality outcomes. Studies suggest that poor handoff between care team providers as well as between unit or hospital locations is associated with a number of safety risks, including errors and omissions in care [72]. Electronic health records (EHRs) are one potential solution. There is evidence that EHRs minimize errors in some regards while increasing the risk for error and miscommunication in other areas [73]. EHRs decrease errors related to transcription, incomplete and or incomprehensible medical records, but may place practitioners at risk for errors of omission related to unmet data display needs, insufficient interaction with software or hardware content, and lack of attention to matching EHR process to typical workflow processes in patient care [73]. However, EHRs may improve data capture, allowing for quality monitoring and intervention that was traditionally manually collected when paper documentation was prevalent. Best practice in provider-to-provider handoff is also being researched. Evaluation of verbal versus verbal accompanied by written shift-to-shift handoff as well as other initiatives is currently underway to define and measure best practice in this area but has yet to be established [74].

Outcome Measures

Managing Error and Quality Improvement

With the rapid expansion of technology and knowledge, there is a gap between what providers know should be done and what is actually done [75, 76]. To bridge this gap, practitioners should understand the basics of healthcare process improvement [75].

As critically ill patients require a higher intensity of care, they are at a greater risk of iatrogenic harm. Given the increase in illness severity and likely comorbid states, resiliency to combat the error is less likely [77]. Therefore, ways to eliminate or minimize the occurrence of these errors is imperative. Before errors can be addressed, they have to be recognized. Two studies noted enhanced error recognition and reporting when a paper-based reporting system was utilized [5]. Anonymous reporting has also been found to increase the likelihood of reporting errors or near misses. Cultures that embrace formal sharing through morbidity and mortality and review of outcome data were also found to create cultures where care could be enhanced through the evaluation of errors and identification of trends. The creation of a data repository in a study by O'Connor noted a threefold improvement in efficiency and accuracy of care when reports from this data were utilized [78]. Therefore, communication cultures should be established that support error reporting and trending of patient outcomes.

Patient Outcomes

Reduction in hospital acquired infections is a priority for worldwide healthcare. Higher mortality, longer hospital stays, and additional cost are all associated with infected patients. Between 15 and 30 % of hospital-acquired infections are felt to be preventable [78–81]. Variability in care and outcomes, and a growing evidence base makes critical care a prime target for improvement efforts. Despite the growing evidence base, implementation of best practices has either been delayed or incomplete [79]. Routine procedures are therefore a starting point for systematic patient improvement efforts [25]. One routine practice that has major implications related to infection is better hand washing. Despite being an easy first step, healthcare provider compliance with hand washing remains poor with compliance largely overestimated by physicians. Quality outcomes were also found to be enhanced through education and protocol bundle implementation for line insertion and maintenance. Through these efforts, central line associated bloodstream infections were noted to decrease [25].

Adverse events related to medications have also been reported to be among the most prevalent types of error [6]. Electronic prescriptions or pharmacist involvement to guide clinical decision making support for correct dosing, drug/lab value check and drug/drug interaction, have been reported to decrease error [6]. Improving interdisciplinary communication during bedside rounds is also associated with medication error decrease [6]. Factors adversely effecting medication events include attention deficit, elevated workload, communication failure, time pressure, and insufficient staffing [6]. Therefore, efforts to reduce the incidence of these triggers should occur. Solution examples might include providing quiet areas that limit disruption, enhancing cultures of communication and safety, and providing adequate staffing.

QI Programs Based on Total Quality Management Principles Quality/Safety Reporting

Incorporating new guidelines or best practice is difficult to achieve due to the need to change clinical routine and the organization of care. Changing practice routines requires a systematic, well-planned approach that considers practitioner, system, and patient relevant factors. Engaging practitioners in both the development of the innovation as well as the implementation of the plan will not only aide in identifying issues but also with addressing potential system barriers. Attempts to change clinical practice should be accompanied by ongoing monitoring to follow progress or adjust plans. There are a variety of process improvement methodologies that can be utilized to support efforts. Examples of these methods include six-sigma, plan-do-study-act (PDSA) and lean. Each methodology has similar techniques [75]. Six-Sigma uses a rigorous statistical measurement methodology to decrease process variation. It is achieved through a series of steps: define, measure, analyze, improve, and control [75]. PDSA is the most common approach for rapid cycle improvement. This involves a trial and learning approach. In this method, a hypothesis or suggested change is tested on a smaller group before implementing within the whole system. Detailed improvement plans, assigned tasks, and expectations are created. Measures of improvement are then selected and trended during the implementation phase. If deviations from the plan occur, these are analyzed and adjustments are made and implemented in the next test cycle [75].

Lean methodology is driven by the identified needs of the customer and aims to improve processes by removing non-value-added activities (NVAA). NVAA do nothing to add to the business margin or the customer's experience. Value stream mapping is the tool that graphically displays the process using inputs, throughputs, and outputs. Using this process, areas of opportunity are highlighted allowing staff to generate ideas for improvement [75]. To identify waste lean experts will frequently use the 5 "S" strategy: Sort: sort items in the immediate work area and keep only those that are needed frequently, Shine: clean and inspect equipment for abnormal wear, Straighten: set work items in order of workflow efficiency, Systemize: standardize workflow processes, and Sustain: sustaining gains made in the first four steps [75]. Focusing on processes that are either high frequency or at increased potential for harm is most effective [25]. No matter the process used, commitment by formal and informal unit leaders is necessary to support all levels of quality innovation and change.

Possible NCCU specific measures of quality may include the use and availability of EEG monitoring for seizure or status epilepticus, timeliness of recognition and care in acute meningitis or encephalitis, as well as procedure related processes for neurosurgery or neurointervention. Measures of outcome may include overall unit morbidity and mortality measures as well as specific disease processes and procedures. The morbidity and mortality measures should be compared to other programs using national databases such as Premier, University Hospital Consortium (UHC), or other national/international databases.

Conclusions

Despite historical evidence reflecting the need for specific neurologic care, NCCUs are in their infancy. Building upon general intensive care data, NCCU quality and safety practices can be extrapolated and then enhanced to focus on the unique needs of the neurological critically ill patient. To ensure the safe passage of these vulnerable patients, systems, units, providers, and processes need to be determined and established. The specifics of what constitutes quality within the NCCU continue to require further study.

References

1. Marjoua Y, Bozic KJ. Brief history of quality movement in US healthcare. Curr Rev Musculoskelet Med. 2012;5(4):265–73. doi:10.1007/s12178-012-9137-8.
2. Luce JM, Bindman AB, Lee PR. A brief history of health care quality assessment and improvement in the United States. West J Med. 1994;160(3):263–8.
3. Kohn LT, Corrigan JM, Donaldson MS. To err is human: building a safer health system. Washington, DC: National Academies Press; 1999.
4. Hurtado MP, Corrigan JM. Crossing the quality chiasm: a new health system for the 21st century. Washington, DC: National Academies Press; 2001.
5. Rossi P, Edmiston CE. Patient safety in the critical care environment. Surg Clin North Am. 2012;92:1369–86.
6. Pagnamenta A, Rabito G, Arosio A, Perren A, et al. Adverse event reporting in adult intensive care units and the impact of a multifaceted intervention on drug-related adverse events. Ann Intens Care. 2012;2:47. http://www.annalsofintensivecare.com/content/2/1/47.
7. Wilson RM, Runciman WB, Gibberd RW, Harrison B. The quality in Australian care study. Med J Aust. 1995;163:458–71.
8. Vincent C, Neale G, Woloshynowych M. Adverse events in British hospitals: preliminary retrospective record review. BMJ. 2001;322:517–9.
9. Sheldon T. Dutch study shows that 40 % of adverse incidents in hospitals are avoidable. BMJ. 2007;334:925.
10. Ricon F, Mayer SA. NeuroCritical care: a distinct discipline? Curr Opin Crit Care. 2007;13(2):115–21.
11. Mateen F. NeuroCritical care in developing countries. Neurocrit Care. 2011;15:593–8. doi:10.1007/s12028-011-9623-7.
12. Zacharia BE, Vaughan KA, Bruce SS, et al. Epidemiological trends in the neurologic intensive care unit from 2000–2008. J Clin Neurosci. 2012;19:1668–72.
13. Martini C, Massei R, Lusenti F, et al. Pathology requiring admission t the neurosurgical intensive care. Minerva Anestesiol. 1993;59:659–66.
14. Park SK, Chun HJ, Kim DW, et al. Acute physiology and chronic health evaluation II and simplified acute physiology score II in predicting hospital mortality of neurosurgical intensive care unit patients. J Korean Med Sci. 2009;24:420–6.
15. Lang JM, Meixensberger J, Unterberg AW, Tecklenburg A, Krauss JK. Neurosurgical intensive care unit-essential for good outcomes in neurosurgery? Langenbecks Arch Surg. 2011;396:447–51. doi:10.1007/s00423-011-0764-0.
16. Pronovost PJ, Angus DC, Dorman T, Robinson KA, Dremsizov KA, Young TL. Physician staffing patterns and clinical outcomes in critically ill patients. A systemic review. JAMA. 2002;288:2151–62.

17. Bershad EM, Feen ES, Hernandez OH, Suri MF, Suzrez JI. Impact of a specialized neurointensive care team on outcomes of critically ill acute ischemic stroke patients. Neurocrit Care. 2008;9:287–92.
18. Varelas PN, Schultz L, Conti M, Spanaki M, Genarrelli T, Haccein-Bey L. The impact of a neuro-intensivist on patients with stroke admitted to a neurosciences intensive care unit. Neurocrit Care. 2008;9:293–9.
19. Josephson SA, Douglas VC, Lawton MT, English JD, Smith WS, Ko NU. Improvement in intensive care unit outcomes in patients with subarachnoid hemorrhage after initiation of neurointensivist co-management. J Neurosurg. 2010;112(3):626–30.
20. Mirski MA, Chang WJ, Cowan R. Impact of a neuroscience intensive care unit on neurosurgical patient outcomes and cost of care: evidence-based support for an intensivist-directed specialty ICU model of care. J Neurosurg Anesthesiol. 2001;13:83–92.
21. Varelas PN, Eastwood D, Yun HJ, Spanaki MV, Bey LH, Kessaris C, Gennarelli TA. Impact of a neurointensivist on outcomes in patients with head trauma treated in a neurosciences intensive care unit. J Neurosurg. 2006;104:713–9.
22. Varelas PN, Abdelhak T, Wellwood J, Benczarski D, Elias S, Rosenblum M. The appointment of neurointensivists is financially beneficial to the employer. Neurocrit Care. 2010;13:228–32. doi:10.1007/s12028-010-9371-0.
23. Bleck TP. The impact of specialized NeuroCritical care. J Neurosurg. 2006;104:709–10.
24. Botting MJ, Phan N, Rubenfeld GD, Speke AK, Chapman MG. Using barriers analysis to refine a novel model of NeuroCritical care. Neurocrit Care. 2014;20:5–14. doi:10.1007/s12028-013-9905-3.
25. Burns J, Green DM, Lau H, et al. The effect of a NeuroCritical care service without a dedicated neuro-ICU on quality of care in intracerebral hemorrhage. Neurocrit Care. 2013;18:305–12. doi:10.1007/s12028-013-9818-1. Valentin A. The importance of risk reduction in critically ill patients. Current Opin Crit Care. 2010;16:482–6. doi:10.1097/MCC.0b013e32833cb861.
26. Tourgeman-Baskin O, Shinar D, Smora E. Causes of near misses in critical care neuronates and children. Acta Paediatr. 2008;97:299–303.
27. Damian MS, Ben-Shlomo Y, Howard R, Bellotti T, Harrison D, Griggs K, Rowan K. The effect of secular trends and specialist NeuroCritical care on mortality for patients with intracranial haemorrhage, myasthenia gravis and Guillian-Barre syndrome admitted to crtical care: an analysis of the Intensive Care National Audit & Research Centre (ICNARC) national United Kingdom database. Intensive Care Med. 2013;39(8):1405–12. doi:10.1007/s00134-013-2960-6.
28. Suarez J, Zaidat O, Suri J, et al. Length of stay and mortality in neurocrically ill patients: impact of a specialized NeuroCritical care team. Crit Care Med. 2004;32(11):2311–7. doi:10.1097/01.CCM.0000146132.29042.4C.
29. AACN Standards for Establishing and Sustaining Healthy Work Environments: executive Summary. http://www.aacn.org. Copyright 2007. Downloaded 29 Nov 2013.
30. France D, Greevy R, Liu X, et al. Measuring and comparing safety climate in intensive care units. Med Care. 2010;48(3):279–84.
31. Sexton JB, Helmreich RL, Neilands TB, et al. The safety attitudes questionnaire: psychometric properties, benchmarking data, and emerging research. BMC Health Serv Res. 2006;6:44.
32. Storesund A, McMurray A. Quality of practice in an intensive care unit (ICU): a mini-ethnographic case study. Intensive Crit Care Nurs. 2009;25:120–7. doi:10.1016/j.iccn.2009.02.001.
33. Darvas JA, Hawkins LG. What makes a good intensive care unit: a nursing perspective. Aust Crit Care. 2002;15(2):77–82.
34. Markandaya J, Thomas KP, Jahromi B, et al. The role of NeuroCritical care: a brief report of the survey results of neuroscience and critical care specialists. Neurocrit Care. 2012;16:72–81. doi:10.1007/s12028-011-9628-2.
35. Lott JP, Iwashyna TJ, Christie JD, Asch DA, Kramer AA, Kahn JM. Critical illness outcomes in specialty versus general intensive care units. Am J Respir Crit Care Med. 2009;179(8):676–83.

36. Levy MM, Rapoport J, Lemeshow S, Chalfin DB, Phillips G, Danis M. Association between critical care physician management and patient mortality in the intensive care unit. Ann Intern Med. 2008;148(11):801–9.
37. Diringer MN, Edwards DF. Admission to the neurolic/neurosurgical intensive care unit is associated with reduced mortality rate after intracerebral hemorrhage. Crit Care Med. 2001;29(3):635–40.
38. Webb DJ, Fayad PB, Wilbur C, et al. Effects of a specialized team on stroke care: the firs two years of the Yale Stroke Program. Stroke. 1998;27:1353–7.
39. Wentworth DA, Atkinson RP. Implementation of an acute stroke program decreases hospitalization costs and length of stay. Stroke. 1998;27:1040–3.
40. Varelas PN, Conti MM, Spanaki MV, et al. The impact of a neurointensivist-led team on a semiclosed neurosciences intensive care unit. Crit Care Med. 2004;32(11):2191–8.
41. Varelas PN, Spanaki MV, Hacein-Bey L. Documentation in medical records improves after a neurointensivist's appointment. Neurocrit Care. 2005;3(3):234–6.
42. Samuels O, Webb A, Culler S, Martin K, Barrow D. Impact of a dedicated NeuroCritical care team in treating patients with aneurismal subarachnoid hemorrhage. Neurocrit Care. 2011;14:334–40.
43. Brown JJ, Sullivan G. Effect on ICU mortality of a full-time crtical care specialist. Chest. 1989;96(1):127–9.
44. Li TC, Phillips MC, Shaw L, Cook EF, Natanson C, Goldman L. On-site physician staffing in a community hospital intensive care unit. JAMA. 1984;252(15):2023–7.
45. Manthous CA, Amoateng-Adjepong U, al-Kharrat T, et al. Effects of a medical intensivist on patient care in a community teaching hospital. Mayo Clin Proc. 1997;72(5):391–9.
46. Hanson CW, Deutschman CS, Anderson HL, et al. Effects of an organized crtical care service on outcomes and resource utilization: a cohort study. Crit Care Med. 1999;27(2):270–4.
47. Milstein A, Galvin RS, Delbanco SF, Salber P, Buck CR. Improving the safety of health care: the leapfrog initiative. Eff Clin Pract. 2000;3(6):313–6.
48. Ward NS, Afessa B, Kleinpell R, Tisherman S, Ries M, Howell M, Halpern N, Kahn J, Members of Society of Critical Care Medicine Taskforce on ICU Staffing. Intensivist/patient ratios in closed ICUs: a statement from the Society of Critical Care Medicine Taskforce on ICU staffing. Crit Care Med. 2013;41(2):638–45. doi:10.1097/CCM.0b013e3182741478.
49. Parshuram CS, Kirpalani H, Mehta S, Granton J, Cook D, Canadian Critical Care Trials Group. In-house, overnight physician staffing: a cross-sectional survey of Canadian adult and pediatric intensive care units. Crit Care Med. 2006;34(6):1674–8.
50. Harris D, Chaboyer W. The expanded role of the critical care nurse: a review of the current position. Aust Crit Care. 2002;15(4):133–7.
51. Kleinpell R, Ely W, Grabenkort R. Nurse practitioners and physician assistants in the intensive care unit: an evidenced-based review. Crit Care Med. 2008;36(10):2888–97.
52. Gordon CR, Axelrad A, Alexander JB, et al. Care of the critically ill surgical patients using the 80 h Accreditation Council of Graduate Medical Education work-week guidelines: a survey of current strategies. Am Surg. 2006;72:497–9.
53. Angus DC, Shorr AF, White A, et al. Critical care delivery in the United States: distribution of services and compliance with leapfrog recommendations. Crit Care Med. 2006;34:1016–24.
54. Russell D, VorderBrueegge M, Burns SM. Effect of an outcomes-managed approach to care of neuroscience patients by acute care nurse practitioners. Am J Crit Care. 2002;11:353–64.
55. Kaups KL, Parks SN, Morris CL. Intracranial pressure monitor placement by midlevel practitioners. J Trauma. 1998;45:884–6.
56. Sarkissian S, Wennberg R. Effects of the acute care nurse practitioner role on epilepsy monitoring outcomes. Outcomes Manag Nurs Pract. 1999;3:161–6.
57. Kirton OC, Folcik MA, Ivy ME, et al. Midlevel practitioner workforce analysis at a university-affiliated teaching hospital. Arch Surg. 2007;142:336–41.
58. Robinson J, Clark S, Greer D. NeuroCritical care clinicians's perceptions of nurse practitioners and physician assistants in the intensive care unit. J Neurosci Nurs. 2014;46(2):E3–7. doi:10.1097/JNN.0000000000000040.

59. Stoeckle-Roberts S, Reeves M, Jacobs B, Maddox K, Choate L, Wehner S, Mullard A. Closing gaps between evidence-based stroke care guidelines and practices with a collaborative quality improvement project. Jt Comm J Qual Patient Saf. 2006;32:517–27.
60. Jahnke H, Zadrozny D, Garrity T, Hopkins S, Frey J, Christopher M. Stroke teams and acute stroke pathways: one emergency departments's two year experience. J Emerg Nurs. 2003;29:133–9.
61. Mullarkey M, Duffy A, Timmins F. Trust between nursing management and staff in critical care: a literature review. Nurs Crit Care. 2011;16(2):85–91.
62. Beckmann U, Baldwin I, Durie M, Morrison A, Shaw L. Problems associated with nursing staff shortage: an analysis of the first 3600 incident reports submitted to the Australian Incident Monitoring Study (AIMS-ICU). Anaesth Intensive Care. 1998;26(4):396–400.
63. Williams G, Clarke T. A consensus driven method to measure the required number of intensive care nurses in Australia. Aust Crit Care. 2001;14(3):106–15.
64. Gill F, Leslie G, Grech C. A review of critical care nursing staffing, education, and practice standards. Aust Crit Care. 2012;25:224–37.
65. Hartigan C. The synergy model in practice establishing criteria for 1:1 staffing ratios. Crit Care Nurse. 2000;20(2):112–6.
66. Rose L, Goldsworthy S, O'Brien-Pallas L, Nelson S. Critical care nursing education and practice in Canada and Australia: a comparison review. Int J Nurs Stud. 2008;45(7):1103–9.
67. Kelly DM, Kutney-Lee A, McHugh MD, Sloane DM, Aiken LH. Impact of critical care nursing on 30-day mortality of mechanically ventilated older adults. Crit Care Med. 2014;42(5):1089–95. doi:10.1097/CCM.0000000000000127.
68. Blegen MA. Does certification of staff nurses improve patient outcomes? Evid Based Nurs. 2012;15(2):54–5.
69. Weaver SJ, Lubomkski LH, Wilson RF, Pfoh ER, Martinez KA, Dy SM. Promoting a culture of safety as a patient safety strategy: a systematic review. Ann Intern Med. 2013;158(5 Pt 2):369–74. doi:10.7326/0003-4819-158-5-201303051-00002.
70. Sammer CE, Lykens K, Singh KP, Mains DA, Lackan NA. What is patient safety culture? A review of literature. J Nurs Scholarsh. 2010;42(2):156–65. doi:10.1111/j.1547-5069.2009.01330.x.
71. Garrouste-Orgeas M, Willems V, Timsit JF, Diaw F, Brochon S, Vesin A, Philippart F, Tabah A, Coquet I, Bruel C, Moulard ML, Carlet J, Misset B. Opinions of families, staff, and patients about family participation in care in intensive care units. J Crit Care. 2010;25(4):634–40. doi:10.1016/j.jcrc.2010.03.001.
72. Cohen MD, Hilligoss PB. The published literature on handoffs in hospitals: deficiencies identified in an extensive review. Qual Saf Health Care. 2010;19(6):493–7. doi:10.1136/qshc.2009.033480.
73. Meeks DW, Smith MW, Taylor L, Sittig DF, Scott JM, Singh H. An analysis of electronic health record-related patient safety concerns. J Am Med Inform Assoc. 2014. doi:10.1136/amiajnl-2013-002578.
74. Wohlauer M. Fragmented care in the era of limited work hours: a plea for an explicit handover curriculum. BMJ Qual Saf. 2012;21 Suppl 1:i16–8. doi:10.1136/bmjqs-2012-001218.
75. Varkey P, Reller K, Resar R. Basics of quality improvement in health care. Mayo Clin Proc. 2007;82(6):735–9.
76. National Committee for Quality Assurance. The State of Health Care Quality: 2004. Available at: www.ncqa.org/communications/SOMC/SOHC2004.pdf. Accessed 28 Nov 2013.
77. Latif A, Rawat N, Pustavoitau A, Pronovost PJ, Pham JC. National study on the distribution, causes, and consequences of voluntary reported medication errors between the ICU and non-ICU settings. Crit Care Med. 2013;41(2):389–98. doi:10.1097/CCM.0b013e318274156a.
78. O'Connor S, Ayres A, Cortellini L, Rosand J, Rosenthal E, Kimberly WT. Process improvement methods increase the efficiency, accuracy, and utility of a NeuroCritical care research repository. Neurocrit Care. 2012;17(1):90–6. doi:10.1007/s12028-012-9689-x.
79. O'Brien JM, Kumar A, Metersky ML. Does value-based purchasing enhance quality of care and patient outcomes in the ICU? Crit Care Clin. 2013;29:91–112.

80. Pronovost P, Needham D, Berenholtz S, et al. An intervention to decrease catheter-related bloodstream infections in the ICU. N Engl J Med. 2006;355(26):2725–32.
81. Berenholtz SM, Pham JC, Thompson DA, et al. Collaborative cohort study of an intervention to reduce ventilator-associated pneumonia in the intensive care unit. Infect Control Hosp Epidemiol. 2011;32(4):305–14.

Chapter 2
Airway Safety in the Neurocritical Care Unit

Venkatakrishna Rajajee

Introduction

A substantive understanding of issues related to airway management and safety is essential for the neurointensivist. In the United States, "death or serious disability associated with airway management" has been classified as a level I adverse patient safety event [1]. Many "airway disasters" are a result of a failure to anticipate problems and inadequate preparation. This chapter will provide an overview of several important safety concerns related to the management of the airway in the neurocritical care unit.

The Decision to Intubate

Case 1

A 62-year-old hypertensive diabetic male is admitted to the ICU with a 45 mL right-sided intracerebral hemorrhage. Repeat imaging 6 h following the initial scan demonstrates mild hematoma expansion. His Glasgow Coma Scale (GCS) is 7; he localizes to pain. He has sonorous respiration and there is audible pooling of secretions. He has a gag reflex and a weak cough. A decision is made not to intubate the patient in order to preserve the neurological examination. Overnight, he has a large emesis and is seen to aspirate,

V. Rajajee, MBBS
Department of Neurosurgery, University of Michigan – Ann Arbor,
Ann Arbor, MI, USA
e-mail: vrajajee@yahoo.com

© Springer International Publishing Switzerland 2015
K.E. Wartenberg et al. (eds.), *Neurointensive Care: A Clinical Guide
to Patient Safety*, DOI 10.1007/978-3-319-17293-4_2

requiring emergent intubation. He subsequently develops the acute respiratory distress syndrome (ARDS) and requires tracheostomy. He is discharged to a long-term acute care facility and requires ventilator support for a month following admission.

Risks to Patient Safety

Inability to Protect the Airway

With very few exceptions—such as the need for emergent defibrillation or the initiation of chest compressions following cardiac arrest—protection of the airway is the first essential step in the resuscitation of the unstable patient. An important safety concern in the neuroICU is the patient with acute neurological injury with the unrecognized need to establish an airway. Obstruction of the airway in a poorly responsive patient by the tongue and the soft tissue of the upper airway can be recognized by the presence of ineffective respiratory effort and abdominal movement without corresponding chest expansion. This is often preceded or accompanied by snoring and audible intermittent opening of the upper airway. This form of airway compromise can typically be immediately managed with a head-tilt/chin lift or a jaw thrust, while preparation to establish a definitive airway is underway. The example above describes a patient with poor airway protective reflexes in whom securing the airway was likely inordinately delayed, with the consequences of increased morbidity, length of stay, and time on the ventilator. A GCS ≤ 8 strongly predicts the need for subsequent intubation [2, 3] and a patient with a level of alertness below this level should likely be intubated unless rapid improvement is expected— such as the patient who has just had a generalized tonic–clonic seizure. It is important to note though, that other factors may be more important in determining the adequacy of the airway. A poor cough and audible pooling of secretions, as were evident in the patient described, are important indicators of inadequate airway protection [4, 5]. Inadequate airway protective reflexes may result in aspiration of gastric contents, which may then result in serious pulmonary injury, including ARDS. Aspiration in patients with diminished alertness is associated with an increased risk of cardiac arrest, time on the ventilator, and length of ICU stay [6]. Of note, the presence of a gag reflex cannot be used to reliably determine the need for intubation [2].

Anticipating the Need for Intubation

An important safety consideration is the identification of patients with the ability to maintain airway patency and adequate respiratory function at the time of admission who are, however, at high risk for catastrophic decline in the near future. Performing an intubation while the patient is relatively stable and not in respiratory failure may be a safer alternative to attempting intubation in a "crashing" patient. This is particularly true when a difficult airway is anticipated—options available to the relatively stable patient, such as an awake fiberoptic intubation, may not be available to the severely hypoxic or apneic patient. Patients with a large intracerebral hemorrhage or severe traumatic brain injury can be expected to clinically decline from worsening cerebral edema in the 48–72 h period following the event and are likely only to worsen in terms of their ability to protect their airway. The patient with the low cervical spinal cord injury (C5–7) can also appear deceptively stable, with the only warning sign of future severe respiratory failure frequently being transient episodes of desaturation related to a poor cough and mucus plugging.

Neck Hematoma

A specific airway crisis encountered in the neuroICU is the patient with a neck hematoma following carotid endarterectomy, cervical spine surgery, or other neck-related surgery. A growing hematoma in the neck represents a critical threat to the patient's airway. In this situation, severe displacement of the trachea can result with difficult or impossible direct laryngoscopy and orotracheal intubation. Although an "awake look" under mild sedation with a direct or video laryngoscope to determine the likelihood of successful rapid sequence intubation (RSI) is reasonable, immediate treatment should consist of opening the surgical wound at the bedside with release of the hematoma followed by orotracheal intubation at the bedside with preparation for surgical airway if necessary. Transport to the Operating Room for intubation may be preferable if the patient's condition permits.

Safety Barriers and Risk–Benefit Assessment

A frequently cited reason to defer intubation in the patient with acute brain injury is the need to closely follow the clinical examination in order to determine the need for surgical or other intervention. Intubation and mechanical ventilation, with the frequent need for subsequent sedation to permit synchrony, frequently does impair the ability to monitor the patient's neurological exam. A risk–benefit assessment must therefore frequently be performed, with an objective assessment of the timing and benefit of surgical or other intervention for the specific disease in question versus the potentially disastrous consequences of aspiration or respiratory arrest from an obstructed airway. A patient with traumatic brain injury, 3 mm midline shift and a large contusion with preserved airway reflexes and a GCS of 8 or 9 who is following commands may benefit from close observation in the ICU without intubation to determine the need for hematoma evacuation and decompressive craniectomy. On the other hand, the patient described in the case above, with intracerebral hemorrhage, a poor cough, audible pooling of secretions, and a GCS of 7, should likely be intubated.

Performing Intubation Safely

> **Case 2**
> A 52-year-old man with a large and aggressive glioblastoma multiforme, admitted to the ICU following debulking initially has a GCS of 14 but declines to 6 (withdrawal only) the night of postoperative day 1, pupils remain 3 mm and reactive bilaterally. A rapid sequence intubation is performed using etomidate and rocuronium. Emergent repeat imaging reveals a 1 cm midline shift and effacement of basal cisterns. One hour following return to the ICU there is no response to pain. The right pupil is 6 mm and dilated and the left 3 mm. Emergent surgical decompression is performed, however, subsequent imaging reveals ischemic injury including bilateral infarction in the posterior cerebral artery territory likely caused by cerebral herniation. Care is withdrawn on postoperative day 7.

Risks to Patient Safety

While endotracheal intubation can be a life-saving measure, few procedures are associated with such immediate risk to life when problems arise. There are several risks to patient safety associated with intubation, several of which are specific to the neuroICU.

The Difficult Airway

Possibly the most important safety consideration prior to intubation of the neuro-critical care patient is the anticipation of and preparation for the difficult airway. Certain factors that increase the difficulty of intubation, such as immobilization of the cervical spine, are particularly common in the neuroICU. Recognizing the difficult airway permits appropriate preparation and selection of the appropriate technique. The mnemonic LEMON has been demonstrated to accurately predict difficult intubation [7, 8].

L: Look externally—This provides a general impression, based on obvious external features related to anatomy, body habitus, facial features, or trauma, that the airway will be difficult.

E: Evaluation with the 3-3-2 finger rule—The ability to fit 3 of the patient's fingers between the incisors (estimates mouth opening), 3 fingers between the chin (mentum) and the hyoid bone, and 2 fingers between the hyoid and the superior notch of the thyroid cartilage. An inadequacy of any of these spaces may predict difficulty with visualization of the glottis opening with direct laryngoscopy.

M: Malampatti score—The patient is asked to open the mouth to permit assessment of the oropharyngeal space [9]. The ability to use this score is often limited because many neuroICU patients who require intubation are unable to cooperate with adequate mouth opening.

O: Obstruction/Obesity—Is there redundant tissue (obesity), mass, infection, blood, or other likely source of upper airway obstruction that may limit visualization of and access to the glottis inlet?

N: Neck—The ability to extend the neck, or attain a "sniffing" position, to obtain an adequate laryngoscopic view. This is a common problem in the neuroICU, because of patients with traumatic injury or spine surgery with immobilization of the cervical spine. This is also a problem with rheumatoid arthritis or elderly patients with degenerative disease in whom the ability to passively extend the neck may be limited.

The provider must review prior intubation records, often from prior surgeries, for every ICU admission. The quality of the laryngoscopic view is typically documented with the Cormack–Lehane grading system [10].

Grade 1: Full view of the glottis inlet.
Grade 2: Partial view of the glottis.

  2a: All but the most anterior part of the glottis is visible.
  2b: Only the arytenoids or most posterior part of the glottis inlet is visible.

Grade 3: Only epiglottis is visible.
Grade 4: Neither epiglottis nor glottis is visible.

Any patient found to have a difficult airway on intubation must be labeled as such, using a "Difficult Airway" sign in the room and with a detailed notation in the medical record detailing the ease of bag-mask ventilation, type of laryngoscope and blade used (direct vs video laryngoscope, Mac vs Miller blade with size), Cormack–Lehane grade, airway maneuvers used during intubation (cricoid pressure, BURP maneuver, RAMP positioning), accessory equipment used (bougie), and the level at which the endotracheal tube was secured. At our institution, a colored tape labeled "Difficult Airway" is also affixed to the endotracheal tube.

Difficult Bag-Mask Ventilation

The mnemonic MOANS has been suggested as a means to identify patients with validated risk factors for difficult bag-mask ventilation [11]:

M: Difficult to apply a mask, because of facial hair, blood or other external impediment.

O: Obstruction of the upper airway, caused by severe obesity, edema, mass, blood, or other agent.

A: Age—Older patients may be harder to bag-mask ventilate because of a loss of elasticity of facial tissue.

N: No teeth—Teeth provide adequate support for the mash and edentulous patient may be harder to bag-mask ventilate.

S: Stiffness—from any cause of increased pulmonary airway pressures, including restrictive disease, mucus plugging, pneumothorax, ARDS, and pulmonary edema.

Cerebral Herniation

The case described above (Case 2) describes a patient with likely raised intracranial pressure (ICP) who suffered cerebral herniation during intubation with consequent devastating ischemic injury. Manipulation of the airway during direct laryngoscopy results in a reflex sympathetic response with a rise in heart rate and blood pressure with resultant cerebral hyperperfusion and increase in ICP [12]. There is also thought to be a reflex increase in ICP following laryngeal stimulation independent of the reflex sympathetic response. In a patient with a mass lesion or high ICP from any other cause, this reflex increase in ICP during laryngoscopy can result in cerebral herniation. The patient may also suffer a sharp elevation in pCO_2 following induction of apnea, resulting in a surge in ICP. Patients with elevated ICP requiring intubation should ideally undergo rapid sequence intubation (RSI), which is the virtually simultaneous administration of a sedative and a neuromuscular blocking agent to render a patient rapidly unconscious and flaccid in order to facilitate emergent endotracheal intubation and to minimize the risk of aspiration. The use of propofol or thiopental as an induction agent might be particularly beneficial in terms of a reduction in cerebral metabolic demand and cerebral blood volume with a consequent reduction in ICP, although these agents are also most likely to cause hypotension and a reduction in cerebral perfusion pressure (CPP). The risk of cerebral herniation during laryngoscopy might reasonably be mitigated by initiation of measures to emergently decrease ICP parallel to preparation for intubation, such as a 30–60 mL bolus of 23.4 % NaCl, to minimize the risk of hypovolemia. Mannitol (0.25–0.5 g/kg in the patient with elevated ICP and 1–1.5 g/kg in the patient with cerebral herniation) is a reasonable alternative in the patient with adequate hemodynamic and volume reserve. Several pharmacological agents may be used in conjunction with RSI to minimize the reflex increase in ICP. These include the following:

(a) *Lidocaine*: An intravenous dose of 1.5 mg/kg of lidocaine administered 60–90 s prior to intubation may blunt the direct laryngeal reflex; however, there is conflicting evidence of its benefit during intubation of the patient with elevated ICP [13, 14].
(b) *Fentanyl*: A dose of 2–3 mcg/kg administered over about 30–60 s may blunt the reflex sympathetic response while minimizing the risk of hypotension [15].

Certain pharmacological agents may cause an increase in ICP. Succinylcholine is associated with a brief elevation in ICP during the fasciculating phase. This elevation is of very short duration (several seconds), however, and in view of the benefits of succinylcholine (short duration of action, ability to achieve adequate intubating conditions), elevated ICP alone is not considered a contraindication to the use of succinylcholine. Ketamine, an effective induction agent, has traditionally been thought to increase ICP [16]. More recent research suggests ketamine may in fact be relatively safe in the patient with elevated ICP [17].

In addition to pharmacological intervention, several simple measures should be taken to prevent devastating injury from cerebral herniation during intubation. The head of the bed should be elevated to 30° rather than kept flat during intubation to minimize ICP elevation, while the head is maintained in extension or the sniffing position. Every effort should be made to maintain minimum minute ventilation, since a sudden elevation in CO2 following RSI might result in a sharp increase in ICP and herniation. This might require the provision of 6–8 manual breaths during the apneic period, and attention to adequate manual ventilation following insertion of the endotracheal tube. Following intubation, the immediate use of end-tidal CO2 (ETCO2) monitoring can facilitate avoidance of hypo- and hyperventilation. Lastly, it is essential to perform frequent pupillary checks immediately prior to and following intubation, to rapidly detect and correct herniation when it does occur. Emergent steps to correct cerebral herniation include hyperventilation to an ETCO2 of 25–30 mmHg, raising the head of bed to the highest level that the patient's hemodynamic status will permit and administration of 30–60 mL of 23.4 % NaCl or 1–1.5 g/kg of mannitol. Appropriate emergent management can result in reversal of herniation and good long term outcomes following subsequent definitive therapy, such as surgical evacuation of hematoma [18, 19]. Figure 2.1 depicts a flowchart for intubating the patient with raised intracranial pressure [20].

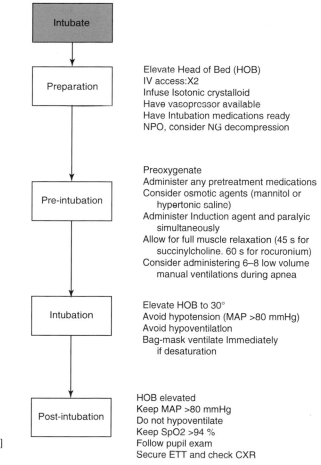

Fig. 2.1 Flowchart for intubation in patients with raised intracranial pressure (From Seder and Mayer [20] with permission)

Cerebral Ischemia

Endotracheal intubation may also be complicated by the development of cerebral ischemia, particularly in the patient with critically compromised cerebral perfusion prior to intubation, such as the patient with acute cerebrovascular thromboembolic occlusion or delayed ischemia following cerebrovascular hemorrhage. The patient with high ICP, as described in Case 2, is also at significant risk of cerebral ischemia through a fall in the mean arterial pressure (MAP) and therefore the cerebral perfusion pressure (CPP=MAP- ICP). Attention must be paid specifically to the CPP, rather than the MAP alone, while intubating. A CPP >50–60 mmHg should be maintained, with vasopressors used as required to meet CPP goals. The agents used for RSI, particularly agents such as propofol and barbiturates are particularly likely to cause hypotension, the effect of which may be somewhat mitigated through a reduction in cerebral metabolic demand and ICP. For the patient at high risk for hemodynamic compromise, etomidate or ketamine may be good options for induction. While the immediate impact of etomidate on the patient's hemodynamics is minimal, adrenal suppression and a more delayed fall in blood pressure may occur. Ketamine may be particularly useful in the hypotensive patient. Inadvertent iatrogenic hyperventilation following intubation may result in cerebral ischemia and has been associated with worsened outcomes following traumatic brain injury [21]. The use of ETCO2 following intubation may be useful in avoiding inadvertent hyperventilation (pCO2 < 25 mmHg) [22].

Succinylcholine and the Risk of Hyperkalemia

Succinylcholine typically causes a transient mild increase in serum potassium. Life-threatening hyperkalemia can occur, however, in the susceptible individual, resulting in bradycardia and asystolic cardiac arrest. Patients with periods of paralysis >48–72 h, caused by stroke or other central nervous system injury may undergo upregulation of extra-junctional acetylcholine receptors, placing the patient at increased risk for release of intracellular potassium and hyperkalemia. Patients with denervation from lower motor neuron disease, such as with Amyotrophic Lateral Sclerosis, may be at particularly high risk. Therefore, while succinylcholine is likely safe to use in the first several hours following acute brain or spinal cord injury of any cause, it should probably be avoided in any patient with significant paralysis for more than 48–72 h, a very common situation in the neuroICU.

Worsening of Cervical Spine Injury

Although primarily encountered in the emergency department, unrecognized cervical spine injury may occur following trauma. Extension of the head during intubation may therefore worsen compression of the cervical spine cord. In the patient with a history of trauma sufficiently severe to produce cervical spine injury, therefore, the cervical spine should be immobilized. This is performed using manual in-line stabilization (MILS), with an assistant standing at the bedside immobilizing the head in the neutral position with a hand on either side of the head. Of note, cervical spine collars must always be removed prior to intubation, to permit the use of the jaw-thrust maneuver if required to open the airway. While MILS is a necessity in the patient at risk for cervical spine injury, it must be remembered that any manipulation of the airway with direct laryngoscopy will result in some movement of the cervical spine.

Loss of the Neurological Exam

The inability to monitor the clinical neurological examination is an important safety hazard following intubation. A period of several minutes (with agents such as propofol and succinylcholine) to an hour or more (with most other agents) in which the neurological exam will be obscured should be anticipated following RSI. It is therefore very important to ensure several specific steps are taken to optimize patient safety.

(a) The neurological examination, including the pupillary examination, immediately prior to intubation should be clearly documented, as appropriate to the specific patient (GCS for the trauma patient, NIH stroke scale for the ischemic stroke patient, a precise description of any involuntary movements in the patient with suspected seizures) to permit appropriate decisions to be made regarding subsequent emergent therapeutic intervention or diagnostic testing.
(b) The pupillary examination should be closely followed following intubation to quickly detect and treat cerebral herniation should it occur.
(c) Patients intubated following overt clinical seizures or clinically evident status epilepticus are at particularly high risk for subsequent non-convulsive seizures, with an incidence up to 48 % [23]. These patients should therefore be monitored with continuous electroencephalography (cEEG) following intubation. Empiric treatment with a benzodiazepine or other agent (such as propofol) is often used until cEEG can be initiated.
(d) Other appropriate neurological monitoring or diagnostic testing should be performed in lieu of the neurological examination. This includes repeat CT imaging and/or placement of an ICP monitor when a prolonged period of sedation is anticipated.

General Complications Related to Intubation

Complications of intubation include esophageal intubation, right mainstem intubation, airway injury, bleeding, pneumomediastinum, pneumothorax, and aspiration of gastric content. In addition to the precautions specific to neuroICU patients listed above, several fundamental precautions are essential to ensure safe intubation.

(a) Ensure immediate availability of a suction catheter, a bag mask, and an oxygen source. Ensure the oxygen source is connected to the bag source and that oxygen is flowing. Severe desaturation and cardiac arrest can result from inadvertent and undetected disconnection of the oxygen source.

(b) Never perform "blind" introduction of the endotracheal tube. Direct visualization of passage through the cords is essential in avoiding esophageal intubation, unless an experienced airway provider is using an endotracheal tube introducer (bougie).

(c) Bag-mask ventilation should ideally be avoided following administration of paralytic, to minimize gastric distension and the risk of aspiration, unless the patient is hypoxic or has severe ICP elevation.

(d) Once the endotracheal tube tip is seen to pass the vocal cords, the stylet should be withdrawn before the tube is advanced further, to minimize the risk of tracheal perforation, pneumomediastinum, and pneumothorax.

(e) Clinical confirmation of tracheal intubation is imperfect [24]. Additional confirmation with a CO_2 detector is essential. While CO_2 detectors that change color are useful, it must be remembered that gastric air can also sometimes produce color change following esophageal intubation and color change might be absent following tracheal intubation in the setting of cardiac arrest because of absent pulmonary perfusion. Waveform capnography is therefore the ideal tool for confirmation of tracheal placement of the tube.

(f) A rapid assessment must be made for mainstem intubation. This can be done with auscultation for equal bilateral breath sounds or with ultrasound to confirm bilateral "lung sliding"–visualization of movement of the parietal against the visceral pleura.

(g) The endotracheal tube should be secured well with a tube holder or tape and the level of insertion immediately documented.

Managing the Airway Safely: The Role of Algorithms and Airway Teams

Airway Teams

The ready availability of skilled personnel is key to the management of airway emergencies in the ICU. Several institutions have constituted airway teams with the ability to respond immediately to such emergencies. Often, the airway team will respond to all cardiac arrests as part of the designated cardiac arrest team and will also be available on a 24-h basis for the management of any airway-related issues. An airway team is composed of personnel with formal training and experience in the management of difficult airways. Typical members will be junior and senior anesthesia housestaff, a senior anesthesia faculty/staff member, and an individual with expertise in emergent surgical airways. The precise composition of the team may vary based on the availability of personnel with airway expertise at the institution–for example, emergency medicine or critical care physicians may serve on the airway team where 24-h anesthesia expertise is unavailable. The availability of skilled airway teams may increase survival to hospital discharge, decrease the need for surgical airways and the time taken to intubate [25, 26].

Airway Carts and Equipment

Personnel skilled in airway management must have ready access to the appropriate equipment in the ICU. This is often accomplished with airway carts, which contain all the equipment necessary for the management of routine as well as difficult and failed airways. The airway cart must be standardized, so that the cart in the neuroICU has the all of the equipment available in the cart in the operating room or the surgical intensive care unit, in the same location in each cart for ease of access by the airway team serving the entire institution. The cart should typically contain a sealed pharmacy box with all of the typically used RSI drugs, oral and nasal airways, multiple sizes and types of laryngoscope blades, laryngoscope handles, a variety of endotracheal tube sizes, supraglottic airways of different sizes, bougies, CO_2 detectors, syringes, endotracheal tube exchange catheters, and all other equipment required to handle the difficult airway. In addition, many ICUs will have at least one video laryngoscope available on the unit at all times and a fiberoptic bronchoscope either on the unit or available at a few minutes' notice.

The Difficult Airway and Failed Airway Algorithms

Since difficult airways are infrequent but extremely high-risk events, the importance of the difficult airway algorithm cannot be overemphasized. The American Society of Anesthesiologists publishes guidelines and an algorithm for the management of the difficult airway (Fig. 2.2) [27]. While an in-depth discussion of the difficult airway algorithm is beyond the scope of this chapter, all neurocritical care providers must be familiar with the basic approach to the difficult airway. The approach to the difficult airway, which may be identified using the criteria mentioned earlier, is based on a few fundamental questions.

Is This a Failed Airway?

A failed airway is present when there is a failure to effect gas exchange *in a patient who cannot do so on his or her own*. This is the "cannot intubate, cannot ventilate situation" when there is an inability to perform tracheal intubation (with even a single attempt) AND an inability to ventilate the patient adequately with a bag and mask to maintain oxyhemoglobin saturations above 90 %. A second form of failed

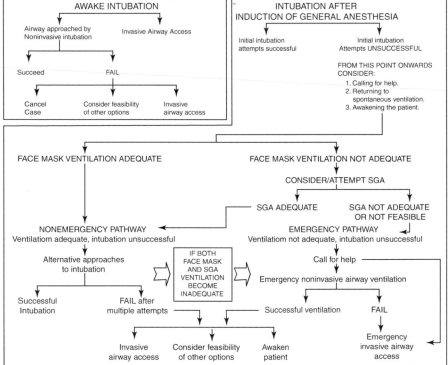

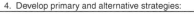

Fig. 2.2 Difficult airway algorithm. American Society of Anesthesiologists Practice Guidelines 2013 for the management of the difficult airway (From Osborn et al. [48]: Springer, with permission)

airway is the "cannot intubate, CAN ventilate" scenario, where there have been three failed attempts to intubate by an experienced operator, and bag-mask ventilation is capable of maintaining adequate oxyhemoglobin saturation [28]. For the purposes of this chapter, the "cannot intubate" scenario is assumed to be present when the best available laryngoscopic equipment (i.e., video vs direct laryngoscopy) and expertise has been used and is unsuccessful. When the "cannot intubate, cannot ventilate" scenario is present, a surgical airway must be established immediately. It is reasonable to make one attempt at placement of an extraglottic airway while preparations for the surgical airway are underway. The surgical airway of choice in this situation is the cricothyroidotomy, which can be performed using either a surgical or percutaneous needle-and-guidewire approach. The surgical airway must never be delayed in this scenario, while several futile attempts are made to intubate or use alternative techniques. In the "cannot intubate, CAN ventilate scenario," there is time to attempt alternative approaches. It is best to have one "go to" alternative that the operator is familiar with rather than attempt a new and unfamiliar alternative in this situation. Extraglottic airways, such as the KingLT©, Combitube™ and Laryngeal Mask Airways (LMA)© are commonly used as alternatives. The LMA© is introduced along the palate until resistance is encountered and creates a mask seal over the laryngeal inlet to ventilate and oxygenate patients for limited periods of time. The LMA© may or not have an inflatable rim to create the seal to permit ventilation. The Intubating LMA (ILMA)© can be used to facilitate blind or fiberoptically guided passage of an endotracheal tube through the LMA© into the trachea. The Combitube™ is a dual-lumen, dual-cuff airway that is blindly introduced and can be placed with either the trachea or the esophagus, although esophageal placement is the rule. One cuff typically lies above the glottis and the other below the glottis in the esophagus, thereby isolating the laryngeal inlet and allowing for side-stream ventilation into the trachea. The King LT© is similar to the Combitube™, but has only a single large lumen with two cuffs inflated through a single valve and is always inserted with the tip in the esophagus. This results in a pharyngeal cuff and an esophageal cuff, with a port between the cuffs at the level of the laryngeal inlet to allow side-stream gas exchange.

Is RSI Reasonable?

In the absence of a failed airway, a decision must be made if in the presence of the difficult airway, an attempt at RSI is reasonable. An attempt at RSI is reasonable if the operator believes that, given his/her specific expertise, the specific equipment available (i.e., direct vs video laryngoscopy), and the specific situation at hand RSI is likely to be successful AND bag-mask ventilation can be performed easily. Of note, video laryngoscopy results in a much superior view of the laryngeal inlet compared to direct laryngoscopy and is associated with a higher rate of intubation success [29, 30]. When video laryngoscopy is readily available, this may therefore be the preferred tool for RSI in the patient with the difficult airway. Several specific maneuvers may be useful in improving the laryngoscopic grade in the patient with the difficult airway. These include Sellick's maneuver (downward pressure on the cricoid cartilage), the BURP maneuver (Backward Upward Rightward and Posterior displacement of the thyroid cartilage using the right hand) and RAMP positioning (stacking linens under the shoulder blades and neck so the external auditory meatus and the sternal notch are in a straight line).

The use of an *endotracheal tube introducer (bougie)* may also facilitate intubation in patients with a visible epiglottis to laryngoscopy but minimal or no visibility of the glottis inlet (Cormack–Lehane grades 2 and 3). Once the epiglottis is visualized, the tip of the bougie is introduced in the midline with the angled tip pointing anteriorly. The tactile sensation of the tracheal rings must be appreciated as the bougie is advanced. Tracheal insertion is also confirmed by the resistance encountered as the bougie reaches the carina or the more distal bronchial passages. With the laryngoscopic blade still in place the endotracheal tube is then railroaded over the bougie.

If RSI is not a reasonable option, then the patient should be assessed for awake intubation vs an alternative technique, such as an extraglottic airway.

Is Awake Intubation Reasonable?

When RSI is not considered reasonable or optimal, an awake intubation can be considered. Awake intubation is the visualization of and intubation through the laryngeal inlet using light to moderate sedation and topical anesthesia only, with a direct laryngoscope, video laryngoscope, or flexible endoscope. Often, a "look" with a video or direct laryngoscope is performed under moderate sedation to assess the feasibility of RSI. When RSI is not considered reasonable, *AND the patient is able to spontaneously sustain sufficient oxygenation with supplemental oxygen delivery alone*, fiberoptic intubation is often attempted in the patient with the difficult airway. A fiberoptic bronchoscope is introduced through the nose or mouth following administration of topical anesthetic and guided into the laryngeal inlet. Once tracheal rings and the carina are visualized, the endotracheal tube is railroaded in over the bronchoscope. Where an "awake" intubation is not considered reasonable, typically because of patient instability, an alternative approach, such as an extraglottic airway, may be attempted. *If at any time criteria for a failed airway are met, the failed airway algorithm (Section "a" above) should be used.*

Extubation Safety

Case 3

A 64-year-old woman with severe rheumatoid arthritis and morbid obesity undergoes cervical spine surgery in the prone position. She is brought to the ICU intubated late in the evening after the surgery. She is awake and alert and the rapid shallow breathing index is 40. Assessment for a cuff leak is performed with the patient still connected to the ventilator and deflation of the cuff, an audible leak is reported. She is extubated. Immediately following extubation she is seen to be in severe distress with ineffective respiratory effort and paradoxical abdominal movement. No air entry is present to auscultation. She desaturates within a few minutes. Bag-mask ventilation is ineffective and the patient suffers a cardiac arrest during attempts to establish a surgical airway. A surgical airway is eventually obtained and gas exchange reestablished, however, the patient suffers severe anoxic injury and care is withdrawn several days later.

Risks to Patient Safety

Extubation failure is typically defined as the need to reintubate within 72 h of extubation. In one series of neurocritical care patients, the rate of extubation failure was 6 %, with "altered mental status" being the most common reason [31]. The following section will focus on risks to patient safety specifically associated with the airway during extubation of the neurocritical care patient. Predictors of weaning success, methods of weaning from mechanical ventilation, and management of extubation failure unrelated to the airway will not be reviewed in this chapter.

Post-extubation Stridor (PES)

The overall incidence of post-extubation stridor (PES) is about 3–30 % across varied populations of patients, with the rate of reintubation for PES being about 1–4 % [32]. While mortality specifically attributable to PES is uncertain, several patients in the neuroICU are at risk for the development of acute upper airway compromise and stridor following extubation. Compromise of the upper airway mostly occurs because of upper airway edema or laxity of musculature and loss of tone, although other less common causes, such as laryngospasm and vocal cord paralysis, must also be kept in mind. The clinical presentation can range from a relatively mild, mostly inspiratory, audible stridor to respiratory distress and complete occlusion of the airway, as occurred in the case described above. The best recognized risk factor for post-extubation stridor is probably female gender [32]. Most, but not all studies, also identify duration of intubation, traumatic or difficult intubation, and high cuff pressures as risk factors for post-extubation stridor [32]. Certain neurosurgical patients may in specific be at increased risk for PES. Patients who undergo major posterior spine surgery often remain in the prone position for several hours, resulting in dependent edema in the pharynx and larynx. The risk may be increased particularly when the surgery is of long duration and large volumes of fluid are used. Patients undergoing posterior fossa surgery may also be at increased risk, again because of the need for prone positioning but also because of brainstem dysfunction from direct injury or edema. Pathology in the brainstem, such as a stroke, hemorrhage, trauma, or postoperative edema can result in diminished bulbar function and consequent loss of tone in the pharyngeal muscles resulting in compromise of the upper airway. Injury to the lower cranial nerves may occur with subarachnoid hemorrhage and result in loss of pharyngeal tone as well as vocal cord paralysis. A variety of neuromuscular diseases such as myasthenia gravis, acute inflammatory demyelinating polyneuropathy, and amyotrophic lateral sclerosis may result in bulbar dysfunction.

Predicting PES

The prevention of PES is dependent on the ability to predict its occurrence. This is primarily done through assessment for a cuff leak. The endotracheal tube cuff is deflated. Ideally, this should elicit a cough as well as audible movement of air around the cuff. The cuff leak can be quantified by measuring the difference between the delivered and exhaled tidal volume. Unfortunately there is much variation in how the cuff leak is assessed and much variability in its predictive value—sensitivities of 15–85 % and specificities of 72–99 % have been reported [32]. One study describes assessment of both post-deflation cough as well as audible cuff leak following disconnection from the ventilator and occlusion of the endotracheal tube with a finger. No patient with both cough and audible leak developed stridor while patients with both absent were ten times more likely to develop PES [33]. Some studies suggest that the quantitative cuff leak may also be useful—almost no patients with cuff leak volume >110 mL developed PES, although when a leak <110 mL was present, only two-thirds of patients developed PES [34]. Assessment of a cuff leak should therefore be made either along with assessment for a cough and occlusion of the tube with a finger following disconnection from the ventilator, or by measuring a quantitative leak, rather than simply by listening for a leak following cuff deflation with the patient still connected to the ventilator.

Prevention of PES

Two randomized controlled trials have demonstrated that the use of glucocorticoids at least 4 h prior to extubation in high-risk patients (selected using a quantitative cuff leak) decreases both the incidence of PES as well as the need for reintubation [35, 36]. The use of methylprednisolone 20 mg IV every 4 h starting 12 h prior to extubation in patients with a quantitative leak <24 % or absent audible leak following tube occlusion is a reasonable approach.

Risk–Benefit Analysis and the Decision to Extubate

Patients with both a post-deflation cough and an audible leak OR a quantitative leak >110 mL (or >12–24 % of tidal volume) should likely be extubated. When a cuff leak is absent or the quantitative leak is low, a significant number of patients will nevertheless tolerate extubation and judgment should be used and a risk–benefit assessment performed. If the patient has no risk factors for either PES or difficult intubation, it is reasonable to extubate while preparing for management of PES and reintubation should it become necessary. When risk factors for either PES or difficult airway are present, it is reasonable to delay extubation for 12–24 h and treat with glucocorticoids as described above. Most patients should likely be extubated following at least 12 h of glucocorticoid treatment. In patients with risk factors for difficult airway, an airway exchange catheter should likely be inserted prior to removal of the endotracheal tube, with careful attention to the depth of insertion of the exchange catheter being similar to the depth of endotracheal tube placement while intubated. Should extubation failure occur, the endotracheal tube can be rapidly inserted back into the trachea over the exchange catheter. The exchange catheter is typically very uncomfortable, however, and can provoke unremitting coughing and gagging, potentially increasing the risk of raised intracranial pressure, postoperative hemorrhage and aspiration. It should therefore likely be removed within a reasonable time frame (10–30 min) if the patient is doing well.

Management of PES

The patient with PES unable to maintain adequate gas exchange or in severe respiratory distress at any time should be emergently reintubated, over an airway exchange catheter, if one was used. Reintubation through a narrow airway can be facilitated by use of a smaller sized endotracheal tube than previously used and, when an airway exchange catheter was not used, with the use of an endotracheal tube introducer (bougie). In the patient with only audible stridor and perhaps some use of accessory muscles of respiration, it is reasonable to first treat with nebulized racemic epinephrine 0.05 ml /kg of a 2.25 % solution diluted to 3 mL total volume with normal saline via nebulizer over 15 min [37]. Rebound PES can occur following initial treatment with nebulized epinephrine [38]. Glucocorticoids are also typically administered (IV methylprednisolone 20–60 mg) although no clinical benefit from steroids can be expected for several hours. Other reasonable options include a 30–60 min trial of noninvasive ventilation and the use of heliox. It should be noted that none of the above measures have had efficacy demonstrated in randomized controlled trials.

Inability to Protect the Airway

A more common cause of extubation failure in the neurocritical care patient than PES is the inability to protect the airway [31]. Occasionally, the inability to protect the airway occurs as a result of poor mental status and the loss of muscle tone in the upper airway as described above in the section on PES. Patients with GCS < 8 at the time of extubation are more likely to suffer extubation failure [3]. A more important cause of extubation failure in neurocritical care patients, however, may be the inability to protect the airway related to a poor cough and the inability to handle secretions [4]. Adequacy of coughing can be assessed objectively, with the ability to achieve peak expiratory flow (PEF) >60 L/mt [5], or the ability to moisten an index card held 1–2 cm from the endotracheal tube while the patient is coughing [39]. Patients with more than 2.5 mL/h of secretions are also more likely to fail extubation [5].

Risk–Benefit Assessment and the Decision to Extubate

Patients meeting other parameters for extubation with a GCS ≥ 8 and a cough reflex adequate to handle secretions should be extubated. When the GCS is <8 or the patient's cough is judged to be poor or inadequate for the volume of secretions, the decision to extubate should be made on a case-by-case basis. Of note, when the inability to protect the airway is the primary reason to defer extubation, early tracheostomy may have a role in hastening liberation from mechanical ventilation [40].

Difficult Airway

Patients known to have been difficult to intubate or those with risk factors for difficult airway described in the section above, may be at significant risk for difficult or failed reintubation. The use of an airway exchange catheter, as described in the section on PES, should be considered in these patients. The patient with risk factors for difficult airway or PES should ideally be extubated early in the day when most skilled and ancillary personnel can be expected to be immediately available.

Airway Emergencies in the Intubated Patient

Case 4
A 26-year-old man is admitted following traumatic brain injury with multiple facial fractures. Copious blood stained secretions are suctioned from the endotracheal tube every hour. Six hours following admission the patient abruptly develops very high peak airway pressures and very low delivered tidal volumes with rapid desaturation and cardiac arrest. Severe resistance is encountered when manual bag ventilation is attempted and a suction catheter cannot be passed through the endotracheal tube. The endotracheal tube is removed under direct laryngoscopic vision and the patient is emergently reintubated with immediate restoration of oxygenation and spontaneous circulation. The endotracheal tube is found to be occluded with blood and inspissated mucus. The patient eventually makes a good recovery and is extubated.

Risks to Patient Safety

Among the important preventable adverse events related to the airway in the intubated patient are occlusion of the airway and unplanned extubations.

Airway Occlusion

This is a potentially catastrophic event, as described in the illustrative case above. The primary causes of occlusion of the endotracheal tube are blood in the airway and inspissated mucus. Airway occlusion typically presented with high peak airway pressures (but unchanged plateau pressures) that can eventually limit breath delivery and potentially cause failure of gas exchange and cardiac arrest. *The immediate response to suspected airway occlusion should be disconnection of the tube from the ventilator and manual bag ventilation.* Tube occlusion can be confirmed by the inability to pass a suction catheter or by direct bronschoscopic visualization, if the patient's condition permits. Bag ventilation will exclude all potential problems with the ventilator circuit, such as occluded filters or water logging and permit assessment of resistance to manual ventilation. Airway occlusion is, however, a potentially entirely preventable event [41]. Vital to prevention are the following.

(a) *Adequate humidification of the airway:* This is typically achieved with heated humidifiers attached to the ventilator circuit. While humidification can sometimes be achieved with heat–moisture exchangers alone, heated humidifiers appear to be more effective in preventing airway occlusion [41].
(b) Adequate patient hydration.
(c) Diligent suctioning, as required to prevent inspissation of secretions within the tube.

Unplanned Extubation

Unplanned extubation occurs in 3–12 % of intubated patients [42, 43]. It is more common in patients who are agitated, are only lightly sedated, or are physically restrained [44, 45]. While most unplanned extubations are obvious, in other cases the tube may be pulled to a position immediately above the glottis inlet, resulting in an audible cuff leak, high airway pressures, and low delivered volumes with eventual desaturation depending on the patient's condition. While failed extubations in general are associated with increased mortality [46], it is important to note that about 40 % of patients who suffer unplanned extubation will not require reintubation within the next 12 h [47], suggesting that an undue delay in extubation may be the underlying problem in many of these patients. Important precautions to avoid unplanned extubations include the following.

(a) *Do not delay extubation* in patients meeting criteria for respiratory function, airway protection, and airway patency.

(b) Perform regular assessment of pain and depth of sedation using widely used sedation scales (such as the Richmond Agitation Sedation Scale) and ensure sedation and pain control goals are met with appropriate use of analgesia and sedatives.
(c) Periodically reassess the need for and adequacy of physical restraints.
(d) Document depth of insertion of the endotracheal tube every few hours.
(e) Obtain daily chest x-ray to assess the position of the endotracheal tube.

Dislodgement of Tracheostomy Tube

This is a specific type of unplanned extubation. Reinsertion of the tube is typically straightforward 5 or more days following tracheostomy, once a track is established. The head must be extended, and the stoma clearly visible. The tracheostomy tube, with an obturator in place is then initially inserted at a 90° angle to the neck then rotated in parallel to the neck as it is advanced into the track. An appropriately sized obturator, spare tracheostomy tubes of equal and smaller size, and a document describing the dimensions and specifics of the tracheostomy tube should be immediately available at all times within the patient's room. When the track is less than 5 days old, however, reinsertion of the tube through the stoma often results in false passage into pretracheal tissue. Orotracheal intubation is often required in these patients, although a single attempt at reinsertion through the stoma by an experienced provider, often through initial introduction of a bougie into the stoma, is reasonable while preparations for reintubation are underway.

Dos and Don'ts

Dos

- Anticipate the need for airway protection in a patient likely to suffer neurological decline.
- Perform bedside wound opening prior to intubation in the patient with the neck hematoma and airway compromise.
- Perform an assessment for difficult airway using the LEMON criteria and for difficult bag-mask ventilation using the MOANS criteria in all admissions to the neuroICU.
- Perform rapid sequence intubation in the patient with raised intracranial pressure.
- Utilize waveform capnography to confirm endotracheal tube placement and avoid hypo- and hyper- ventilation following intubation.
- Document clearly the focused clinical neurological examination prior to intubation.
- Perform frequent pupillary assessment in the patient with raised intracranial pressure immediately following rapid sequence intubation.

- Obtain appropriate monitoring (ICP, EEG) and repeat imaging following intubation in lieu of the clinical neurological exam.
- Maintain cerebral perfusion pressure >50–60 mmHg following intubation.
- Remove the cervical collar and use manual in-line stabilization during intubation.
- Call for help early, when dealing with the difficult airway.
- Use glucocorticoids in patients with an inadequate cuff leak to decrease the risk of post-extubation stridor.
- Consider use of an airway exchange catheter in high-risk extubations, including patients with risk factors for difficult airway or post-extubation stridor
- Ensure adequate humidification and appropriate suctioning to decrease the risk of airway occlusion.
- Perform regular assessment of pain and discomfort using standardized sedation and pain scores and treat appropriately to decrease the risk of unplanned extubation.

Don'ts

- Delay intubation in a patient with poor mental status, inadequate cough, or inability to clear secretions.
- Use the gag reflex to make decisions on intubation.
- Use succinylcholine to intubate a patient with significant paralysis for more than 48–72 h.
- Hypoventilate the patient with raised intracranial pressure during intubation.
- Hyperventilate the patient following intubation unless treating cerebral herniation.
- Delay a surgical airway in the patient with a failed airway.
- Attempt rapid sequence intubation in the patient with difficult airway when you are uncertain of success—consider awake fiberoptic intubation.
- Assess a cuff leak with the patient connected to the ventilator—disconnect and occlude the tube with a finger, then check for both cough and cuff leak on deflation. Alternatively, measure the volume of leak.
- Delay extubation in patients meeting criteria for respiratory function, airway protection, and airway patency
- Delay reintubation following extubation failure.

References

1. Office of Health Care Quality. Maryland Hospital Patient Safety Program annual report fiscal year 2006. Annapolis: Office of Health Care Quality; 2007.
2. Chan B, Gaudry P, Grattan-Smith TM, McNeil R. The use of Glasgow Coma Scale in poisoning. J Emerg Med. 1993;11(5):579.
3. Namen AM, Ely EW, Tatter SB, Case LD, Lucia MA, Smith A, Landry S, Wilson JA, Glazier SS, Branch CL, Kelly DL, Bowton DL, Haponik EF. Predictors of successful extubation in neurosurgical patients. Am J Respir Crit Care Med. 2001;163(3 Pt 1):658.

4. Coplin WM, Pierson DJ, Cooley KD, Newell DW, Rubenfeld GD. Implications of extubation delay in brain-injured patients meeting standard weaning criteria. Am J Respir Crit Care Med. 2000;161(5):1530.
5. Salam A, Tilluckdharry L, Amoateng-Adjepong Y, Manthous CA. Neurologic status, cough, secretions and extubation outcomes. Intensive Care Med. 2004;30(7):1334.
6. Christ A, Arranto CA, Schindler C, Klima T, Hunziker PR, Siegemund M, Marsch SC, Eriksson U, Mueller C. Incidence, risk factors, and outcome of aspiration pneumonitis in ICU overdose patients. Intensive Care Med. 2006;32(9):1423.
7. Murphy M, Walls RM. Identification of the difficult and failed airway. In: Walls RM, Murphy MF, Luten RC, editors. Manual of emergency airway management. Philadelphia: Lippincott Williams & Wilkins; 2004. p. 70.
8. Reed MJ, Dunn MJ, McKeown DW. Can an airway assessment score predict difficulty at intubation in the emergency department? Emerg Med J. 2005;22(2):99.
9. Mallampati SR, Gatt SP, Gugino LD, Desai SP, Waraksa B, Freiberger D, Liu PL. A clinical sign to predict difficult tracheal intubation: a prospective study. Can Anaesth Soc J. 1985;32(4):429.
10. Cormack RS, Lehane J. Difficult tracheal intubation in obstetrics. Anaesthesia. 1984;39(11):1105.
11. Walls RM, Murphy MF. Manual of emergency airway management. 3rd ed. Philadelphia: Lippincott Williams & Wilkins; 2008.
12. Moorthy SS, Greenspan CD, Dierdorf SF, Hillier SC. Increased cerebral and decreased femoral artery blood flow velocities during direct laryngoscopy and tracheal intubation. Anesth Analg. 1994;78(6):1144.
13. Bilotta F, Branca G, Lam A, Cuzzone V, Doronzio A, Rosa G. Endotracheal lidocaine in preventing endotracheal suctioning-induced changes in cerebral hemodynamics in patients with severe head trauma. Neurocrit Care. 2008;8(2):241.
14. Samaha T, Ravussin P, Claquin C, Ecoffey C. Prevention of increase of blood pressure and intracranial pressure during endotracheal intubation in neurosurgery: esmolol versus lidocaine. Ann Fr Anesth Reanim. 1996;15(1):36.
15. Splinter WM, Cervenko F. Haemodynamic responses to laryngoscopy and tracheal intubation in geriatric patients: effects of fentanyl, lidocaine and thiopentone. Can J Anaesth. 1989;36(4):370.
16. Wyte SR, Shapiro HM, Turner P, Harris AB. Ketamine-induced intracranial hypertension. Anesthesiology. 1972;36(2):174–6.
17. Bourgoin A, Albanèse J, Léone M, Sampol-Manos E, Viviand X, Martin C. Effects of sufentanil or ketamine administered in target-controlled infusion on the cerebral hemodynamics of severely brain-injured patients. Crit Care Med. 2005;33(5):1109.
18. Qureshi AI, Geocadin RG, Suarez JI, Ulatowski JA. Long-term outcome after medical reversal of transtentorial herniation in patients with supratentorial mass lesions. Crit Care Med. 2000;28(5):1556–64.
19. Koenig MA, Bryan M, Lewin 3rd JL, Mirski MA, Geocadin RG, Stevens RD. Reversal of transtentorial herniation with hypertonic saline. Neurology. 2008;70(13):1023–9.
20. Seder DB, Mayer SA. Critical care management of subarachnoid hemorrhage and ischemic stroke. Clin Chest Med. 2009;30:103–22.
21. Muizelaar JP, Marmarou A, Ward JD, Kontos HA, Choi SC, Becker DP, Gruemer H, Young HF. Adverse effects of prolonged hyperventilation in patients with severe head injury: a randomized clinical trial. J Neurosurg. 1991;75(5):731.
22. Davis DP, Dunford JV, Ochs M, Park K, Hoyt DB. The use of quantitative end-tidal capnometry to avoid inadvertent severe hyperventilation in patients with head injury after paramedic rapid sequence intubation. J Trauma. 2004;56(4):808.
23. DeLorenzo RJ, Waterhouse EJ, Towne AR, Boggs JG, Ko D, DeLorenzo GA, Brown A, Garnett L. Persistent nonconvulsive status epilepticus after the control of convulsive status epilepticus. Epilepsia. 1998;39(8):833–40.

24. Grmec S. Comparison of three different methods to confirm tracheal tube placement in emergency intubation. Intensive Care Med. 2002;28(6):701.
25. Sample G, McCabe P, Vandruff T. Code critical airway teams improves patient safety. Crit Care. 2010;14 Suppl 1:231.
26. Rochlen L. Proceedings from the Annual Meeting of the American Society Anesthesiologists. Designated airway emergency team may improve survival rates at hospital discharge; 17–21 Oct 2009; New Orleans.
27. Apfelbaum JL, Hagberg CA, Caplan RA, Blitt CD, Connis RT, Nickinovich DG, Hagberg CA, Caplan RA, Benumof JL, Berry FA, Blitt CD, Bode RH, Cheney FW, Connis RT, Guidry OF, Nickinovich DG, Ovassapian A, American Society of Anesthesiologists Task Force on Management of the Difficult Airway. Practice guidelines for management of the difficult airway: an updated report by the American Society of Anesthesiologists Task Force on Management of the Difficult Airway. Anesthesiology. 2013;118(2):251–70.
28. Walls RM. The emergency airway algorithms. In: Walls RM, Murphy MF, editors. Manual of emergency airway management. 4th ed. Philadelphia: Lippincott Williams & Wilkins; 2012. p. 22.
29. Nouruzi-Sedeh P, Schumann M, Groeben H. Laryngoscopy via Macintosh blade versus GlideScope: success rate and time for endotracheal intubation in untrained medical personnel. Anesthesiology. 2009;110(1):32.
30. Griesdale DE, Liu D, McKinney J, Choi PT. Glidescope®video-laryngoscopy versus direct laryngoscopy for endotracheal intubation: a systematic review and meta-analysis. Can J Anaesth. 2012;59(1):41–52. Epub 2011 Nov 1.
31. Karanjia N, Nordquist D, Stevens R, Nyquist P. A clinical description of extubation failure in patients with primary brain injury. Neurocrit Care. 2011;15(1):4–12.
32. Wittekamp BH, van Mook WN, Tjan DH, Zwaveling JH, Bergmans DC. Clinical review: post-extubation laryngeal edema and extubation failure in critically ill adult patients. Crit Care. 2009;13(6):233.
33. Maury E, Guglielminotti J, Alzieu M, Qureshi T, Guidet B, Offenstadt G. How to identify patients with no risk for postextubation stridor? J Crit Care. 2004;19(1):23.
34. Miller RL, Cole RP. Association between reduced cuff leak volume and postextubation stridor. Chest. 1996;110:1035–40.
35. Cheng KC, Hou CC, Huang HC, Lin SC, Zhang H. Intravenous injection of methylprednisolone reduces the incidence of postextubation stridor in intensive care unit patients. Crit Care Med. 2006;34(5):1345.
36. François B, Bellissant E, Gissot V, Desachy A, Normand S, Boulain T, Brenet O, Preux PM, Vignon P, Association des Réanimateurs du Centre-Ouest (ARCO). 12-h pretreatment with methylprednisolone versus placebo for prevention of postextubation laryngeal oedema: a randomised double-blind trial. Lancet. 2007;369(9567):1083.
37. MacDonnell SP, Timmins AC, Watson JD. Adrenaline administered via a nebulizer in adult patients with upper airway obstruction. Anaesthesia. 1995;50:35–6.
38. Irwin RS, Rippe JM. Irwin and Rippe's intensive care medicine. 6th ed. Philadelphia: Lippincott Williams & Wilkins; 2007.
39. Khamiees M, Raju P, DeGirolamo A, Amoateng-Adjepong Y, Manthous CA. Predictors of extubation outcome in patients who have successfully completed a spontaneous breathing trial. Chest. 2001;120(4):1262.
40. Alali AS, Scales DC, Fowler RA, Mainprize TG, Ray JG, Kiss A, de Mestral C, Nathens AB. Tracheostomy timing in traumatic brain injury: a propensity-matched cohort study. J Trauma Acute Care Surg. 2014;76(1):70–6; discussion 76–8.
41. Doyle A, Joshi M, Frank P, Craven T, Moondi P, Young P. A change in humidification system can eliminate endotracheal tube occlusion. J Crit Care. 2011;26(6):637.e1–4.
42. Vassal T, Anh NG, Gabillet JM, Guidet B, Staikowsky F, Offenstadt G. Prospective evaluation of self-extubations in a medical intensive care unit. Intensive Care Med. 1993;19(6):340.
43. Tindol Jr GA, DiBenedetto RJ, Kosciuk L. Unplanned extubations. Chest. 1994;105(6):1804.

44. Chevron V, Ménard JF, Richard JC, Girault C, Leroy J, Bonmarchand G. Unplanned extubation: risk factors of development and predictive criteria for reintubation. Crit Care Med. 1998;26(6):1049.
45. Curry K, Cobb S, Kutash M, Diggs C. Characteristics associated with unplanned extubations in a surgical intensive care unit. Am J Crit Care. 2008;17(1):45.
46. Epstein SK, Ciubotaru RL. Independent effects of etiology of failure and time to reintubation on outcome for patients failing extubation. Am J Respir Crit Care Med. 1998;158(2):489.
47. Boulain T. Unplanned extubations in the adult intensive care unit: a prospective multicenter study. Association des Réanimateurs du Centre-Ouest. Am J Respir Crit Care Med. 1998; 157(4 Pt 1):1131.
48. Osborn IP, Kleinberger AJ, Gurudutt VV. Airway emergencies and the difficult airway. In: Levine AI, Govindaraj S, DeMaria Jr S, editors. Anesthesiology and otolaryngology. New York: Springer; 2013.

Chapter 3
Mechanical Ventilation in the Neuro-ICU

Sang-Beom Jeon and Younsuck Koh

Introduction

In a modern Neuro-ICU, patients are treated for their acute brain injury, such as aneurysmal subarachnoid hemorrhage, intracerebral hemorrhage, malignant ischemic stroke, status epilepticus and traumatic brain injury. Not only do the patients have primary injury on their brains at the time of the insults, but they are also frequently followed by secondary brain injury during admission to the Neuro-ICU. The complications are not limited to the brain with frequent impairments of other organs, especially the lungs. There is a complex interaction between the brain and lungs. Brain injury is often complicated by pulmonary edema and pneumonia possibly due to impairments of the autonomic and immune system as well as aspiration [1]. Alternatively, hypoxemia and inflammation induced by lung injury can accelerate the secondary brain injury including ischemia and brain swelling [1].

Thus, it is often very challenging to manage patients with both brain and lung injury. The appropriate treatment of one may be contradictory to the management of the other, as described below.

S.-B. Jeon, MD, PhD
Department of Neurology, Asan Medical Center, Seoul, Republic of Korea

Y. Koh, MD, PhD, FCCM (✉)
Department of Pulmonary and Critical Care Medicine, Asan Medical Center,
Seoul, Republic of Korea
e-mail: yskoh@amc.seoul.kr

© Springer International Publishing Switzerland 2015
K.E. Wartenberg et al. (eds.), *Neurointensive Care: A Clinical Guide
to Patient Safety*, DOI 10.1007/978-3-319-17293-4_3

Case

A 56-year-old woman with a history of hypertension presented to the Neuro-ICU with a sudden onset of severe headache followed by stuporous mental status. On neurological examination, her arms and legs withdrew to noxious stimuli and brain stem reflexes were intact. Her brain CT revealed thick hemorrhage in the basal cistern, bilateral sylvian fissures and ventricles along with evidence for global cerebral edema and hydrocephalus, compatible with acute subarachnoid hemorrhage (Fig. 3.1a). She was intubated for airway protection and mechanical ventilation, with sedation and analgesia for the control of intracranial hypertension. External ventricular drain was placed, and ruptured right middle cerebral artery aneurysm was clipped. Six days after the bleeding, she developed flexor posturing of her left arms and legs. CT angiography revealed severe narrowing of the right middle cerebral artery M1 and anterior cerebral artery A1. Rapid infusion of normal saline and induced hypertension with continuous infusion of phenylephrine was attempted. Balloon angioplasty and intra-arterial injection of verapamil were also performed for the therapy of vasospasm.

Three days after the commencement of hypervolemia and induced hypertension, she developed fever, increased amount of sputum and leukocytosis. Her chest radiograph showed bilateral lung infiltrates (Fig. 3.1b). Under mechanical ventilation support of pressure control mode with positive end-expiratory pressure (PEEP) of 18 cm H_2O, her airway pressure was 35 cm H_2O and the oxygen saturation is 88 % on FiO_2 of 1.0. The arterial blood gas shows pH of 7.28, $PaCO_2$ of 48 mmHg, and PaO_2 of 55 mmHg with normal cardiac function, suggesting that she has acute respiratory distress syndrome (ARDS). In addition to antibiotics, low tidal volume with

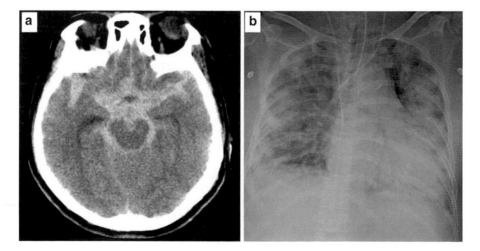

Fig. 3.1 (a) An axial CT image of the brain shows acute subarachnoid hemorrhage. (b) A chest radiograph reveals bilateral infiltrations of the lungs suggesting acute respiratory distress syndrome

higher PEEP and/or prone positioning seems to be required to improve her oxygenation. However, because of her intracranial pressure (ICP) of 25 mmHg, there are concerns about her reduced brain compliance. Can such lung-protective ventilation strategy for ARDS be safely applied to her without inducing additional brain injury?

Risks of Patient Safety

The skull is a rigid container filled with the brain, blood and cerebrospinal fluid. Expansion of one component occurs at the expense of the others, with the elevation of ICP (the Monro-Kellie doctrine). The consequences of elevated ICP, i.e., intracranial hypertension, have been generally attributed to secondary cerebral ischemia. ICP surge can compromise cerebral perfusion and lead to secondary cerebral ischemia/infarction. Such circumstances faced in the Neuro-ICU include subarachnoid hemorrhage, traumatic brain injury, intracerebral hemorrhage, cerebral infarction, meningo-encephalitis, status epilepticus, etc.

In the above case of subarachnoid hemorrhage, global cerebral edema and hydrocephalus along with subarachnoid blood would contribute to the elevation of ICP. To avert delayed cerebral ischemia and ongoing process of secondary cerebral infarction, cerebral perfusion should be maintained. For this purpose, hemodynamic augmentation has been a mainstay in the management of patients with subarachnoid hemorrhage during vasospasm period, usually from post-bleed day 3 to day 14. The traditional components of hemodynamic augmentation are volume expansion, induced hypertension and hemodilution. However, this therapy is not based on strong scientific evidences and increases the risk of pulmonary edema. Recently, the consensus statement from the Neurocritical Care Society for the management of subarachnoid hemorrhage supported (1) maintaining euvolemia and considering a saline bolus to increase cerebral blood flow in areas of ischemia as a prelude to other interventions, (2) induced hypertension with/without inotropic agents, and (3) no hemodilution in an attempt to improve rheology except in cases of erythrocythemia [2].

The other body organs also become vulnerable to medical complications after acute severe brain injury. Among variable complications, pulmonary dysfunction is one of the most commonly encountered detrimental impairments. Decreased mental status, oropharyngeal weakness, decrease or absence of gag reflexes and cough reflexes and impaired immune functions increase the risk of aspiration pneumonia. Pulmonary edema may also be triggered by excessive fluid therapy and induced hypertension for improving cerebral perfusion as seen in the above subarachnoid hemorrhage case. Otherwise, neurogenic pulmonary edema (NPE) is as common as up to 40 % after subarachnoid hemorrhage and 20 % after traumatic brain injury [3, 4]. Some authors, however, argue that true frequency of this is very low [5–7]. NPE is caused by the extravasation of a proteinaceous fluid across the alveolar membrane of the lungs by Starling's force, presumably acting via the catecholamine storm associated with severe brain injury and/or intracranial hypertension [8]. In a subset of patients, depressed cardiac contractility after brain injury results in NPE (neuro-cardiac NPE) [9]. Patients with NPE have a higher mortality rate, but many cases are well tolerated and require nothing more than supplemental oxygen, and resolution typically occurs within 3 days [3].

ARDS is a severe form of pulmonary edema induced by the increase in the permeability of pulmonary capillary endothelial cells and alveolar epithelial cells [10, 11]. The Berlin definition of ARDS is (1) within 1 week of a known clinical insult such as acute brain injury or new or worsening respiratory syndrome, (2) bilateral opacities on chest imaging, which are not fully explained by effusions, lobar/lung collapse, or nodules, (3) respiratory failure not fully explained by cardiac failure or fluid overload, which needs objective assessment (e.g., echocardiography) to exclude hydrostatic edema if no risk factor present, and (4) impaired oxygenation (mild, 200 mmHg $< PaO_2/FiO_2 \leq 300$ mmHg with PEEP or CPAP ≥ 5 cm H_2O; moderate, 100 mmHg $< PaO_2/FiO_2 \leq 200$ mmHg with PEEP ≥ 5 cm H_2O; severe, $PaO_2/FiO_2 \leq 100$ mmHg with PEEP ≥ 5 cm H_2O) [12]. This syndrome is found in 10–50 % of patients who have severe brain injury, especially in patients with traumatic brain injury or aneurysmal subarachnoid hemorrhage, and is a predictor of poor outcome in this setting [4, 13–18].

Safety Barriers

In patients with brain injury, inappropriate managements can produce damage of the lungs as well as the brain. Catecholamine-driven pulmonary dysfunction may occur after acute brain injury, as described above. Moreover, attempts to improve cerebral perfusion with volume infusion and induced hypertension can further aggravate volume overload in pulmonary circulation. This is driven by pulmonary vascular hydrostatic pressure in the setting of increased vascular endothelial and alveolar epithelial permeability [19].

In addition, mechanical ventilation per se can cause injury of the lungs [16]. Such complication is mostly attributed to end-inspiratory over-distension and a low end-expiratory lung volume allowing repeated collapse and re-expansion in each respiratory cycle. The result of this tidal recruitment is high shear force on alveolar walls and small airways during inflation, especially at the interfaces between collapsed and aerated alveoli [16]. In order to prevent ventilator-induced lung injury, a strategy to limit the tidal volume to 6–8 mL/kg of predicted body weight and to apply PEEP, permissive hypercapnia, is recommended [20]. However, provision of limited tidal volume may induce hypercapnia, which potentially increases intracranial blood volume via acidosis-induced vasodilatation of cerebral vessels. This may put patients at risk for intracranial hypertension. Therefore, patients with elevated ICP have notably been excluded from studies on permissive hypercapnia [20]. Ventilator support under prone position has been highly recommended to improve oxygenation and survival of patients with severe ARDS [21]. However, this procedure could not be applied to patients with intracranial hypertension due to the concern of elevating ICP [21]. The mechanism of increased ICP after prone positioning has been attributed to the increase in cerebral venous pressure [22].

Discussion

The current standard treatment of patients with ARDS consists of correcting the predisposing condition, appropriate organ support and lung-protective ventilation. The "lung-protective" ventilation is, as shown in Table 3.1, composed of application of low tidal volume, optimal setting of PEEP and limiting plateau pressure less than 28 cm H_2O. It has been recommended to tolerate hypercapnia (permissive hypercapnia) resulting from low tidal volume ventilation strategy for improving oxygenation.

No large studies, however, have systematically examined the role of different mechanical ventilation strategies on brain oxygenation as well as lung oxygenation. Thus, it is not clear that lung-protective ventilation can be also "brain-protective," as described previously. It has been reported that interventions known to increase arterial oxygen level, such as increasing fraction of inspired oxygen (FiO_2), increasing PEEP, increasing minute ventilation, paralysis with neuromuscular blockade, augmenting blood pressure, sedation and transfusion, also increase brain tissue oxygen level [23, 24]. Alternatively, hypoxemia not only decreases cerebral oxygen delivery but also results in cerebral vasodilation, therefore further increasing ICP.

Here, we discuss about the contradictory aspects of the mechanical ventilation in the management of patients with both acute brain injury and ARDS.

Positive End-Expiratory Pressure

PEEP is a pressure for the prevention of alveolar derecruitment during expiration. The level of PEEP has been determined by the level of required FiO_2 (Table 3.1). The way to select optimal PEEP to prevent repetitive opening and collapse during tidal cycling along with the minimization of alveolar over-distension has not been determined. In severe ARDS, alveolar recruitment maneuver followed by a decremental PEEP trial has been tried. Alveolar recruitment maneuver helps the heterogeneous tidal compliance of injured alveoli be more homogeneous, and a decremental PEEP trial leads the lungs to remain more open at the end-expiration. It has not been well addressed whether a short period of high airway pressure during alveolar recruitment maneuver is safe in patients with acute brain injury. Moreover, there have been controversies about the effect of PEEP on cerebral physiology. Increase

Table 3.1 Protocol for mechanical ventilation in ARDS

Variable	Goal and adjustment
Oxygenation goal	PaO_2 55–80 mmHg or SpO_2 88–95 %
Tidal volume	
Initial V_T	8 mL/kg
Final V_T	6 mL/kg (reduce V_T by 1 mL/kg at interval $\leq$2 h)
Plateau pressure goal	$\leq$30 cm H_2O
If P_{plat} >30 cm H_2O	Decrease V_T by 1 mL/kg steps to 4 mL/kg
If P_{plat} <25 cm H_2O and V_T <6 mL/kg	Increase V_T by 1 mL/kg until P_{plat} >25 cm H_2O or V_T=6 mL/kg
If P_{plat} <30 cm H_2O and Breath stacking or dyssynchrony occurs	Increase V_T by 1 mL/kg to 7–8 mL/kg if P_{plat} $\leq$30 cm H_2O
pH goal	7.30–7.45
If pH 7.15–7.30	Increase RR (max=35) until pH >7.30 or $PaCO_2$<25
If pH <7.15	Increase RR up to 35/min. Increase V_T in 1 mL/kg steps until pH >7.15. Give $NaHCO_3$
pH >7.45	Decrease RR
Combinations of FiO_2 and PEEP (cm H_2O)	
	0.3 and 5
	0.4 and 5
	0.4 and 8
	0.5 and 8
	0.5 and 10
	0.6 and 10
	0.7 and 10
	0.7 and 12
	0.7 and 14
	0.8 and 14
	0.9 and 14
	0.9 and 16
	0.9 and 18
	1.0 and 18–24

Modified protocol from NIH NHLBI ARDS Clinical Network (www.ardsnet.org) with permission
VT tidal volume, *kg* predicted body weight (kilogram), *Pplat* plateau pressure, *RR* respiratory rate

in PEEP can mediate a change in ICP [25]. Increased thoracic pressure caused by PEEP increment is directly transmitted through the neck vein to the cranium [26, 27]. Increased peak inspiratory and mean airway pressure caused by the increase of PEEP decrease mean arterial pressure as well as venous return and cardiac output [28]. Additionally, reduced jugular venous return due to elevated intrathoracic pressure can increase the volume of blood and cerebrospinal fluid in a rigid cranial vault, which leads to intracranial hypertension. In patients with severe lung injury, the effects of PEEP on the increase in intrathoracic pressure are often amplified. Therefore, PEEP could affect cerebral perfusion pressure (CPP) as well as ICP, because CPP is determined by the difference between mean arterial pressure and

ICP [28–30]. Reduced plateau pressures by lower tidal volume may offset the harmful effects of PEEP on ICP [31].

However, the safe level of PEEP in acute brain injury has not been well addressed. Recent studies have shown that the application of PEEP may not have deleterious effects on ICP. In patients with acute ischemic stroke, a study increased PEEP up to 12 cm H_2O, but ICP remained unchanged or demonstrated a slight decline [32]. Marked changes in CPP were observed, but these were mediated through the decrease in mean arterial pressure. In another study of patients with traumatic brain injury, escalating PEEP levels up to 11–15 cm H_2O decreased ICP and increased CPP slightly. PEEP did not worsen intracranial hypertension [25]. In patients with high-grade SAH, with increase in PEEP up to 20 cm H_2O, stepwise elevation of PEEP resulted in a significant decrease of mean arterial pressure and regional cerebral blood flow [33]. Normalization of mean arterial pressure restored regional cerebral blood flow to baseline values, despite the persisting increase in PEEP. Application of PEEP did not impair ICP or regional cerebral blood flow per se but indirectly affected cerebral perfusion via its negative effects on mean arterial pressure in the setting of disturbed cerebrovascular autoregulation.

Therefore, increasing PEEP up to 20 cm H_2O may not have deleterious effects on ICP, as long as the baseline ICP is not high (<20 mmHg). To preserve cerebral perfusion and cerebral blood flow, maneuvers to keep mean arterial pressure should always be pursued. The benefit of PEEP could outweigh the risks after acute brain injury through the correction of hypoxemia. In the setting of intracranial hypertension, therefore, PEEP settings should be individualized according to oxygenation, hemodynamics and cerebral physiological conditions. Neurological examination and neuro-monitoring variables, such as ICP, CPP, cerebral oxygen partial pressure, cerebral blood flow, arterial oxygenation and hemodynamic indexes, are the determining factors to set an appropriate level of PEEP.

Permissive Hypercapnia

As a consequence of low tidal volume, carbon dioxide (CO_2) elimination via the lungs is reduced, and hypercapnia and respiratory acidosis could be ensued. Hypercapnia can cause stimulation of brain stem respiratory center with subsequent hyperventilation, which may produce ventilator dyssynchrony and require oversedation or neuromuscular blockades. Cerebral blood flow is sensitive to a change in $PaCO_2$. Lowering $PaCO_2$ from 40 to 20 mmHg reduces cerebral blood flow by 40 %, whereas raising $PaCO_2$ up to 80 mmHg nearly doubles cerebral blood flow, causing increase in ICP [34]. Hypercapnia can also cause increase in ICP and decrease in CPP and cerebral blood flow. In normal brain, persistent hypercapnia causes an elevation in ICP and cerebral blood flow lasting less than 12 h [35]. In patients with poor intracerebral compliance, the limit of tolerance to hypercapnia and respiratory acidosis is unclear, but marked elevation of ICP could be induced by even modest hypercapnia [36, 37].

This potential side effect of hypercapnia makes physicians become reluctant to apply lung-protective ventilation to patients who are vulnerable to secondary brain injury. However, lung-protective ventilation does not necessarily imply hypercapnia, respiratory acidosis and increased ICP. Moreover, the risk of elevated ICP as a consequence of mild permissive hypercapnia has not been proven, and an effect on outcomes after brain injury has not been demonstrated [36]. In fact, a study of patients with subarachnoid hemorrhage and ARDS did not show increase of ICP due to hypercapnia (PCO_2 50–60 mmHg). Given that the mortality benefit of lung-protective ventilation was demonstrated in a large clinical trial, mild hypercapnia as a result of this strategy may be allowed with individualizing a patient depending on cerebral physiological conditions.

Prone Positioning

Prone positioning can effectively improve oxygenation in ARDS. Prone ventilation leads to decreased mortality when applied early (<36 h after intubation and mechanical ventilation) in the course of severe ARDS (PaO_2:FiO_2 ratio <150 mmHg with an $FiO_2 \geq 0.6$ and a PEEP ≥ 5 cm H_2O) [21]. The mechanism of beneficial effects of prone positioning seems to be shifting atelectatic lung from dependent to nondependent areas, decreasing shunt fraction by improving ventilation/perfusion matching, facilitating secretion drainage, relieving cardiac compression of the lungs and increasing the functional residual capacity of the lungs. However, patients with reduced intracranial compliance have been excluded in clinical trials. In such patients, prone positioning itself may have potential to exacerbate intracranial hypertension with the risk of additional cerebral ischemia, as described previously.

Although implementing prone positioning is controversial for patients with intracranial lesions and is not advocated by some authors, it should still be considered for the treatment of acutely brain-injured patients with severe ARDS while adjusting head position to the lowest ICP. In high-grade subarachnoid hemorrhage, prone positioning showed a significantly increased arterial oxygen level joined by an improved brain tissue oxygenation [38]. In this study, patients were positioned with the head midline or turned slightly laterally and elevated 15–20°. They were returned to the supine position earlier if ICP continuously exceed 25 mmHg and if the intensity of intracranial hypertension treatment had to be continuously increased. Despite a small increase in ICP and decrease in CPP, arterial and brain tissue oxygen levels improved. In a study of patients with neurogenic pulmonary edema, prone positioning was also effective in improving oxygenation [39].

One pitfall of prone ventilation is that such position is not easy to be applied to patients who have invasive neuro-monitoring devices, such as intraparenchymal ICP or oxygen tension monitoring probes. However, it should be considered in the event of severe ARDS. Neuro-monitoring devices can give physicians a useful guide to the prevention of secondary ischemic insults after severe acute brain injury.

Adjunctive Therapy

Interventional Lung Assist

Advanced management to eliminate CO_2 may be considered for patients with high ICP and marked hypercapnia. Pumpless extracorporeal lung assist combined with lung-protective ventilation has been applied for this purpose in patients with ARDS and severe traumatic brain injury [40]. With this device, hypercapnia was successfully eliminated, and the minute volume of artificial ventilation could be reduced enough to avoid lung damage. As a result, ICP was reduced, and systemic hemodynamic variables and CPP remained stable. Whether this combination could improve survival in acutely brain-injured patients with ARDS remains to be substantiated.

Nitric Oxide Inhalation

A paucity of evidence exists regarding the safety of inhaled nitric oxide in acutely brain-injured patients. Anecdotal reports have suggested beneficial effects of nitric oxide on the cerebral hemodynamics including decrease in ICP [41, 42]. Increased oxygenation or anti-inflammatory effects of inhalation of NO may decreased ICP [43].

Neuromuscular Blocking Agents

Paralysis with neuromuscular blocking agents can improve oxygenation through increasing chest wall compliance, eliminating patient-ventilator dyssynchrony, facilitating lung recruitment and reducing oxygen consumption [44]. A recent randomized clinical trial has shown that early administration of cisatracurium for 48 h improved survival as well as oxygenation in patients with severe ARDS defined as a PaO_2:FiO_2 ratio < 150, a PEEP ≥5 cm H_2O and a tidal volume of 6–8 mL/kg of predicted body weight [45]. In this study, cisatracurium did not increase the risk of ICU-acquired weakness.

However, there are controversies about the effect of neuromuscular blocking agents on ICP. In neurosurgical patients, a study showed that the atracurium bolus resulted in transient decrease in ICP, CPP and mean arterial pressure, whereas the cisatracurium bolus did not [46]. Other studies failed to show the relationship of neuromuscular blocking agents (cisatracurium and doxacurium) to ICP, CPP and mean arterial pressure [47, 48]. However, neuromuscular blocking agents may be beneficial in reducing ICP at least in patients with both intracranial and intraabdominal hypertension [49]. Relaxation of abdominal muscle tone with these drugs results in reduction of intraabdominal pressure which is one of the contributing factors of ICP elevation [49]. Thus, neuromuscular blocking agents should be considered in patients with severe ARDS and intractable ICP crisis.

Neuro-Monitoring

After acute injury, the brain often becomes less compliant and more vulnerable to secondary ischemia. As intracranial volume expands, only a small addition of extra-volume may result in a surge in ICP followed by plummeting in CPP, cerebral blood flow and brain tissue oxygen tension. Thus, reviewing neuro-imaging, such as brain CT and MRI, is insufficient and direct measurements of brain physiologic variables are needed at least for comatose patients with ICP crisis. In patients with external ventricular drain, ICP can be measured without other devices. Fiberoptic ICP probes may also be inserted into the brain parenchyma. Direct measurement of ICP allows calculation of CPP. In case of constant cerebrovascular resistance, CPP will reflect cerebral blood flow. However, cerebral physiology is dynamic and cerebrovascular resistance is not constant in many cases and cerebral blood flow cannot be measured only with CPP. Fortunately, real-time measurements of quantitative cerebral blood flow are available with thermal diffusion flowmetry technique [50]. Brain tissue oxygen tension or jugular venous oxygen saturation can also be measured, through which cerebral oxygenation can be assessed. Metabolic components at brain mito-chondrial level, such as glucose, pyruvate and lactate, may be evaluated through microdialysis. All of these modalities can be measured at bedside continuously [50].

It is imperative to detect secondary brain injury while permanent damage can be prevented. Neurological examination remains the gold standard for the assessment of brain-injured patients. However, most patients with acute brain injury and ARDS are unconscious due to brain dysfunction and/or sedatives or analgesics for mechanical ventilation, and clinical examination of such patients are usually very limited. For the proactive treatment to prevent secondary neuronal injury, it would be worthwhile to employ aforementioned multimodal neuro-monitoring.

Summary

Implementing lower tidal volume and optimal PEEP is crucial to improve survivals in patients with severe pulmonary dysfunction, such as ARDS. During this therapy, hypercapnia may ensue, and prone positioning may be needed in severe ARDS. As long as these managements improve oxygenation of the lungs and arterial blood, they will improve brain oxygenation and decrease the risk of cerebral ischemia. Clinicians should be balanced between the benefit and the risks. To perform neuro-monitoring as well as careful neurological examination for comatose patients with ICP crisis and severe ARDS is mandatory. In neuro-critically injured patients, careful approach with seemingly conflicting therapeutic strategies requires individualization until convincing data from large clinical trials are available.

Dos and Don'ts

Dos

- Low tidal volume (6–8 mL/kg predicted body weight)
- Set a PEEP to $\geq$5 cm H_2O
- Keep a plateau pressure $\leq$30 cm H_2O
- Avoid hypercapnia if possible
- Moderate permissive hypercapnia for better oxygenation
- Early (<36 h) prone positioning if other measures fail to avoid desaturation (PaO_2:FiO_2 < 150 mmHg)
- Consider neuro-monitoring in patients with ICP crisis and severe ARDS

Don'ts

- Hypervolemic therapy in patients with ARDS
- High tidal volume (>8 mL/kg predicted body weight)
- No implementation of PEEP due to concerns for ICP
- High PEEP (>20 cm H_2O) without neurological examination and neuro-monitoring during ICP crisis
- Excessive hypercapnia without neurological examination and neuro-monitoring during ICP crisis

References

1. Gonzalvo R, Marti-Sistac O, Blanch L, Lopez-Aguilar J. Bench-to-bedside review: brain-lung interaction in the critically ill–a pending issue revisited. Crit Care. 2007;11(3):216.
2. Diringer MN, Bleck TP, Claude Hemphill 3rd J, et al. Critical care management of patients following aneurysmal subarachnoid hemorrhage: recommendations from the Neurocritical Care Society's Multidisciplinary Consensus Conference. Neurocrit Care. 2011;15(2):211–40.
3. Fontes RB, Aguiar PH, Zanetti MV, Andrade F, Mandel M, Teixeira MJ. Acute neurogenic pulmonary edema: case reports and literature review. J Neurosurg Anesthesiol. 2003;15(2): 144–50.
4. Bratton SL, Davis RL. Acute lung injury in isolated traumatic brain injury. Neurosurgery. 1997;40(4):707–12; discussion 712.
5. Baumann A, Audibert G, McDonnell J, Mertes PM. Neurogenic pulmonary edema. Acta Anaesthesiol Scand. 2007;51(4):447–55.
6. Colice GL. Neurogenic pulmonary edema. Clin Chest Med. 1985;6(3):473–89.
7. Fein IA, Rackow EC. Neurogenic pulmonary edema. Chest. 1982;81(3):318–20.
8. Berthiaume Y, Broaddus VC, Gropper MA, Tanita T, Matthay MA. Alveolar liquid and protein clearance from normal dog lungs. J Appl Physiol. 1988;65(2):585–93.
9. Davison DL, Terek M, Chawla LS. Neurogenic pulmonary edema. Crit Care. 2012;16(2):212.

10. Darragh TM, Simon RP. Nucleus tractus solitarius lesions elevate pulmonary arterial pressure and lymph flow. Ann Neurol. 1985;17(6):565–9.
11. Greenhoot JH, Reichenbach DD. Cardiac injury and subarachnoid hemorrhage. A clinical, pathological, and physiological correlation. J Neurosurg. 1969;30(5):521–31.
12. Force ADT, Ranieri VM, Rubenfeld GD, et al. Acute respiratory distress syndrome: the Berlin Definition. JAMA. 2012;307(23):2526–33.
13. Holland MC, Mackersie RC, Morabito D, et al. The development of acute lung injury is associated with worse neurologic outcome in patients with severe traumatic brain injury. J Trauma. 2003;55(1):106–11.
14. Gruber A, Reinprecht A, Gorzer H, et al. Pulmonary function and radiographic abnormalities related to neurological outcome after aneurysmal subarachnoid hemorrhage. J Neurosurg. 1998;88(1):28–37.
15. Kahn JM, Caldwell EC, Deem S, Newell DW, Heckbert SR, Rubenfeld GD. Acute lung injury in patients with subarachnoid hemorrhage: incidence, risk factors, and outcome. Crit Care Med. 2006;34(1):196–202.
16. Mascia L, Mastromauro I, Viberti S. High tidal volume as a predictor of acute lung injury in neurotrauma patients. Minerva Anestesiol. 2008;74(6):325–7.
17. Robertson CS, Valadka AB, Hannay HJ, et al. Prevention of secondary ischemic insults after severe head injury. Crit Care Med. 1999;27(10):2086–95.
18. Schirmer-Mikalsen K, Vik A, Gisvold SE, Skandsen T, Hynne H, Klepstad P. Severe head injury: control of physiological variables, organ failure and complications in the intensive care unit. Acta Anaesthesiol Scand. 2007;51(9):1194–201.
19. Contant CF, Valadka AB, Gopinath SP, Hannay HJ, Robertson CS. Adult respiratory distress syndrome: a complication of induced hypertension after severe head injury. J Neurosurg. 2001;95(4):560–8.
20. Network TARDS. Ventilation with lower tidal volumes as compared with traditional tidal volumes for acute lung injury and the acute respiratory distress syndrome. The Acute Respiratory Distress Syndrome Network. N Engl J Med. 2000;342(18):1301–8.
21. Guerin C, Reignier J, Richard JC, et al. Prone positioning in severe acute respiratory distress syndrome. N Engl J Med. 2013;368(23):2159–68.
22. Beuret P, Ghesquieres H, Fol S, Pirel M, Nourdine K, Ducreux JC. [Prone position and severe pneumopathy in a patient with head injuries and intracranial hypertension]. Ann Fr Anesth Reanim. 2000;19(8):617–9.
23. Maloney-Wilensky E, Gracias V, Itkin A, et al. Brain tissue oxygen and outcome after severe traumatic brain injury: a systematic review. Crit Care Med. 2009;37(6):2057–63.
24. Pascual JL, Georgoff P, Maloney-Wilensky E, et al. Reduced brain tissue oxygen in traumatic brain injury: are most commonly used interventions successful? J Trauma. 2011;70(3): 535–46.
25. Huynh T, Messer M, Sing RF, Miles W, Jacobs DG, Thomason MH. Positive end-expiratory pressure alters intracranial and cerebral perfusion pressure in severe traumatic brain injury. J Trauma. 2002;53(3):488–92; discussion 492–3.
26. Abbushi W, Herkt G, Speckner E, Birk M. [Intracranial pressure – variations in brain-injured patients caused by PEEP-ventilation and lifted position of the upper part of the body (author's transl)]. Anaesthesist. 1980;29(10):521–4.
27. Lodrini S, Montolivo M, Pluchino F, Borroni V. Positive end-expiratory pressure in supine and sitting positions: its effects on intrathoracic and intracranial pressures. Neurosurgery. 1989;24(6):873–7.
28. Nyquist P, Stevens RD, Mirski MA. Neurologic injury and mechanical ventilation. Neurocrit Care. 2008;9(3):400–8.
29. Apuzzo JL, Wiess MH, Petersons V, Small RB, Kurze T, Heiden JS. Effect of positive end expiratory pressure ventilation on intracranial pressure in man. J Neurosurg. 1977;46(2): 227–32.
30. Burchiel KJ, Steege TD, Wyler AR. Intracranial pressure changes in brain-injured patients requiring positive end-expiratory pressure ventilation. Neurosurgery. 1981;8(4):443–9.

31. Chang WT, Nyquist PA. Strategies for the use of mechanical ventilation in the neurologic intensive care unit. Neurosurg Clin N Am. 2013;24(3):407–16.
32. Georgiadis D, Schwarz S, Baumgartner RW, Veltkamp R, Schwab S. Influence of positive end-expiratory pressure on intracranial pressure and cerebral perfusion pressure in patients with acute stroke. Stroke. 2001;32(9):2088–92.
33. Muench E, Bauhuf C, Roth H, et al. Effects of positive end-expiratory pressure on regional cerebral blood flow, intracranial pressure, and brain tissue oxygenation. Crit Care Med. 2005;33(10):2367–72.
34. Harper AM, Glass HI. Effect of alterations in the arterial carbon dioxide tension on the blood flow through the cerebral cortex at normal and low arterial blood pressures. J Neurol Neurosurg Psychiatry. 1965;28(5):449–52.
35. Christensen MS, Brodersen P, Olesen J, Paulson OB. Cerebral apoplexy (stroke) treated with or without prolonged artificial hyperventilation. 2. Cerebrospinal fluid acid-base balance and intracranial pressure. Stroke. 1973;4(4):620–31.
36. Lowe GJ, Ferguson ND. Lung-protective ventilation in neurosurgical patients. Curr Opin Crit Care. 2006;12(1):3–7.
37. Leech P, Miller JD. Intracranial volume–pressure relationships during experimental brain compression in primates. 3. Effect of mannitol and hyperventilation. J Neurol Neurosurg Psychiatry. 1974;37(10):1105–11.
38. Reinprecht A, Greher M, Wolfsberger S, Dietrich W, Illievich UM, Gruber A. Prone position in subarachnoid hemorrhage patients with acute respiratory distress syndrome: effects on cerebral tissue oxygenation and intracranial pressure. Crit Care Med. 2003;31(6):1831–8.
39. Fletcher SJ, Atkinson JD. Use of prone ventilation in neurogenic pulmonary oedema. Br J Anaesth. 2003;90(2):238–40.
40. Bein T, Kuhr LP, Metz C, Woertgen C, Philipp A, Taeger K. ARDS and severe brain injury. Therapeutic strategies in conflict. Anaesthesist. 2002;51(7):552–6.
41. Papadimos TJ, Medhkour A, Yermal S. Successful use of inhaled nitric oxide to decrease intracranial pressure in a patient with severe traumatic brain injury complicated by acute respiratory distress syndrome: a role for an anti inflammatory mechanism? Scand J Trauma Resusc Emerg Med. 2009;17:5.
42. Vavilala MS, Roberts JS, Moore AE, Newell DW, Lam AM. The influence of inhaled nitric oxide on cerebral blood flow and metabolism in a child with traumatic brain injury. Anesth Analg. 2001;93(2):351–3, 353rd contents page.
43. Papadimos TJ. The beneficial effects of inhaled nitric oxide in patients with severe traumatic brain injury complicated by acute respiratory distress syndrome: a hypothesis. J Trauma Manag Outcomes. 2008;2(1):1.
44. Greenberg SB, Vender J. The use of neuromuscular blocking agents in the ICU: where are we now? Crit Care Med. 2013;41(5):1332–44.
45. Papazian L, Forel JM, Gacouin A, et al. Neuromuscular blockers in early acute respiratory distress syndrome. N Engl J Med. 2010;363(12):1107–16.
46. Schramm WM, Papousek A, Michalek-Sauberer A, Czech T, Illievich U. The cerebral and cardiovascular effects of cisatracurium and atracurium in neurosurgical patients. Anesth Analg. 1998;86(1):123–7.
47. Schramm WM, Jesenko R, Bartunek A, Gilly H. Effects of cisatracurium on cerebral and cardiovascular hemodynamics in patients with severe brain injury. Acta Anaesthesiol Scand. 1997;41(10):1319–23.
48. Prielipp RC, Robinson JC, Wilson JA, MacGregor DA, Scuderi PE. Dose response, recovery, and cost of doxacurium as a continuous infusion in neurosurgical intensive care unit patients. Crit Care Med. 1997;25(7):1236–41.
49. An G, West MA. Abdominal compartment syndrome: a concise clinical review. Crit Care Med. 2008;36(4):1304–10.
50. Wartenberg KE, Schmidt JM, Mayer SA. Multimodality monitoring in neurocritical care. Crit Care Clin. 2007;23(3):507–38.

Chapter 4
Nutrition in Neuro-ICU

Sandeep Kantor, Maher J. Albahrani, and Sadanandan Prakash

Introduction

There are many challenges in providing adequate enteral nutrition (EN) to neurologically injured patients. These include alterations in gastrointestinal motility, elevated intracranial pressure, altered levels of consciousness and overall neurologic dysfunction. Patients with acute neurological insults, such as brain trauma or stroke, may have been previously well-nourished or malnourished. When severe neurological injury occurs along with a phase of starvation, a hypermetabolic state ensues. The associated increase in oxygen consumption and caloric demands may persist for some time into recovery and can affect patient's ability to survive [1]. The increase in metabolism and protein loss is due to persistent inflammatory response and prolonged immobility due to injury. Increased levels of catecholamines, glucocorticoid, glucagon and growth hormone along with increased insulin resistance lead to hyperglycemia, even in nondiabetic patients. Muscle tone abnormalities such as spasticity, decorticate or decerebrate posturing, and periodic sympathetic discharges ("storming") are all associated with increased caloric needs [2]. Brain injury leads to delayed gastric emptying evidenced as increased gastric residue volume (GRV) in patients receiving EN [3]. Inadequate nutrition support in neurocritically ill patients, even well past the initial injury, may result in malnutrition and muscle wasting. This increases the difficulty in mobility and functional rehabilitation, and promotes the development of medical complications such as decubitus ulcers, pneumonia, urinary tract infections, and venous thromboembolism [4].

S. Kantor, MBBS, DA, MD, FCCP, FCCM (✉) • M.J. Albahrani, MBChB
S. Prakash, MBBS, DA, MD, FFARCS (I), EDIC
Department of Anesthesia and Critical Care, Royal Hospital, Muscat, Oman
e-mail: annsash@gmail.com

© Springer International Publishing Switzerland 2015
K.E. Wartenberg et al. (eds.), *Neurointensive Care: A Clinical Guide to Patient Safety*, DOI 10.1007/978-3-319-17293-4_4

Early enhanced EN appears to accelerate neurologic recovery and reduces both the incidence of major complications and post-injury inflammatory responses [5]. The preferred route of nutrient administration is the gastric route, but if targeted volume of more than 60 % is not achieved, alternatives are post-pyloric route or mixed enteral/parenteral nutrition. Most of these patients require prolonged mechanical ventilation related to their low neurological status. In patients with anticipated prolonged enteral feeding, such as those with major hemispheric or brain stem ischemic stroke or in prolonged coma, early placement of percutaneous endoscopic gastrostomy (PEG) tube might be useful.

Although well established guidelines for providing nutrition in the general critically ill population are available, this is not the case in patients with neurological injury. In this chapter, we shall highlight safe practices of nutrition support in neurocritical patients using the following case as an example.

Case

A 62-year-old gentleman was brought to emergency room (ER) with acute onset of impaired speech and comprehension along with left-sided weakness. The patient had a history of hypertension and hyperlipidemia. He was on two antihypertensive medications and a statin, and was not receiving any antiplatelet medication. On arrival to ER, he was found to have global aphasia, left homonymous hemianopia, left hemiplegia, and hemisensory loss. His vital signs were as follows: blood pressure 126/60 mmHg, pulse 120 beats/min, respiratory rate 36 breaths/min and oxygen saturation (SaO_2) of 85 %. He was intubated and ventilated after appropriate sedation and neuromuscular blockade. Non-contrast head CT showed dense right middle cerebral artery infarct without any evidence of intracranial bleed. ECG showed multifocal atrial ectopics, and chest X-ray revealed endotracheal tube in proper position with bilateral lower lobe infiltrates.

On arrival in neurocritical ICU, his temperature was 36.5 °C, heart rate 132/m (with multifocal ectopics), respiratory rate 14 breaths/min, blood pressure 114/52 mmHg and SaO_2 of 100 %. On physical examination he appeared pale and cachectic. The carotid pulses were equal, without any bruit. There were bilateral basal crepitations on chest auscultation, with normal heart sounds. Both upper limbs and lower limbs were adequately perfused and warm. Abdomen was soft and non-distended with diminished bowel sounds. His laboratory tests are shown in Table 4.1.

The patient was known for chronic alcohol use and smoked two packs of cigarettes/day. He had not been eating well for the last 6 months and had lost 7 kg during that period. His most recent weight was 60 kg. His height was 172 cm.

The patient was sedated with fentanyl and propofol infusion. Nasogastric (NG) tube was used for continuous drainage. Since the drainage was large in volume, the patient was started on parenteral nutrition (PN) after 72 h of admission. However, the patient developed severe electrolyte disturbance (hypokalemia, hypophosphatemia and hypomagnesemia) and hyperglycemia. Electrolyte correction was attempted

Table 4.1 Patient laboratory test results

Laboratory test	Value	Normal range
Hemoglobin	9 g/dL	11.5–15.5 g/dL
Hematocrit	35 %	41–55 %
White blood cell count	$18 \times 10^3/\mu L$	$4.5–11 \times 10^3/\mu L$
Platelets	$575 \times 10^3/\mu L$	$150–350 \times 10^3/\mu L$
C-reactive protein	35 mg/L	<5 mg/L
Sodium	149 mmol/L	136–145 mmol/L
Potassium	5.0 mmol/L	3.6–4.9 mmol/L
Chloride	114 mmol/L	101–111 mmol/L
CO_2	20 mmol/L	23–31 mmol/L
BUN	31 mg/dL	23–31 mg/dL
Creatinine	1.8 mg/dl (159 μmol/L)	0.6–1.0 mg/dL (53–84 μmol/L)
Blood glucose	240 mg/dl (13.3 mmol/L)	80–120 mg/dL (4.5–6.5 mmol/L)
Albumin	2.5 g/dL	4.0–5.5 g/dL

with difficulty. The patient was started on insulin infusion to target blood sugar between 70 and 110 mg/dL. These tight blood sugar controls lead to frequent hypoglycemic episodes. At this stage, the clinical dietician was consulted and the patient was started on isomeric feeds enterally to aim caloric/volume goal at 48–72 h. The patient's underlying pathology and concurrent use of vasopressors resulted in increase of GRV, which lead to frequent interruptions of enteral feeding. Prokinetic drugs were initiated and EN was continued.

On seventh day of admission, the patient developed localized twitching of face, and subsequent EEG revealed an epileptiform focus, for which antiepileptic drugs were started. Following this, there were further interruptions to EN related to intolerance. The patient required prolonged ventilation due to muscle weakness, low levels of consciousness and frequent episodes of pneumonia. Percutaneous tracheostomy was performed on day 16. However, liberation from ventilator was not successful. The patient was transferred to residential care facility on ventilator, with PEG tube in place for continued enteral feeding.

Safety Concerns in Our Patient

The following safety gaps were there in our patient:

(a) There was no proper nutritional assessment done in this patient before initiation of feeding. This patient was already malnourished with chronic alcoholism and was at a risk of developing refeeding syndrome (RFS).
(b) The patient was kept fasting for more than 72 h, on account of large GRV.
(c) No attempt was made to start early EN in this patient. Instead, early PN was initiated.
(d) There were frequent alterations of blood sugar in our patient, as a result of initiation of PN and tight glucose control.

(e) The patient should have been started on early prokinetic drugs, to improve EN tolerance.
(f) Since there were frequent interruptions to gastric feeding due to multiple factors, transpyloric route for administration of feeds should have been considered as an alternative.
(g) Periodic assessment of nutritional status should have been done, with careful allowance given to calories supplied by drugs like propofol infusion which deliver a significant amount of calories: 1.1 cal/mL.

Challenges in Providing Nutrition in Neuro ICU

Neurocritical patients with brain injury, ischemic or bleeding stroke, or tumor disease often differ from critically ill patients in several aspects:

1. Age distribution of neurocritically ill patients varies according to pathology. Traumatic brain injury (TBI) has a greater incidence in young people, whereas vascular bleeds like subarachnoid usually affect patients between fourth and sixth decades of life. Other vascular conditions of brain are more commonly seen in older patients with associated comorbidities such as diabetes, hypertension and hyperlipidemia, resulting in prolonged morbidity and length of ICU stay [6].
2. Neurocritical conditions leading to seizure disorders, delirium or infection cause increased metabolic demand and lead to a catabolic state with net protein breakdown. This has deleterious effects on immune function. Drug therapies during this critical phase such as sedatives, analgesics, antiepileptics and muscle relaxation also modify this metabolic status. The neurocritical patient of traumatic etiology develops hypermetabolic and hypercatabolic responses, not clearly related to severity levels as measured by the Glasgow Coma Scale (GCS) [7].
3. Brain injury leads to delayed gastric emptying, evidenced as increased GRV in patients receiving EN.
4. Neurocritically ill patients generally require long periods of mechanical ventilation related to their low neurological level.

Nutritional Requirement

Nutritional Assessment

Prior to prescribing nutritional support, the following assessment should be performed:

(a) The current and prior nutritional status
(b) Comorbid conditions,

(c) The underlying disease progression,

(d) Severity and time since injury and the associated catabolic effects.

Among all the methods used to assess the nutritional status, no single method is sufficiently accurate to be considered as the gold standard in critically ill patients. An overall subjective assessment is a simple, affordable and reproducible technique. Measures such as body weight, height, body mass index and physical constitution should be obtained. Blood values such as serum albumin, prealbumin, transferrin and a lymphocyte count may be used for nutritional status assessment.

Nitrogen balance is a practical method for assessing protein nutrition status. Nitrogen balance may be determined by collecting a 24-h urine sample from a patient with adequate renal function and calculating the dietary nitrogen from protein intake.

Caloric Requirement

Indirect calorimetry has been deemed the gold standard of measuring resting energy expenditure. When indirect calorimetry is not available, several formulae have been proposed to determine patient's predicted energy expenditure in order to set a caloric target. Activity or stress factors are added to this predictive energy expenditure to improve its accuracy. Some of these are Harris–Benedict, Scholfield or Ireton-Jones equations. These calculations are not validated in critically ill patients, especially in those with neurological insult. Regardless of the method used, no single method of estimating energy expenditure is infallible and close monitoring of each individual patient is needed to prevent over or underfeeding. The calculation of energy requirements using kilocalories per kilogram is, however, more often used and widely accepted by clinicians than the published predictive equations because of convenience and practicality. Total caloric intake ranges from 20 to 30 kcal/kg/day, depending on the period of the clinical course.

Protein Requirement

Generally in neurocritically ill patients, protein requirement is about 1.3–1.5 g/kg/day in the acute phase and 1.5 g/kg/day from the second week [8]. Since hypercatabolism often results in excessive protein breakdown, caloric intake of protein should be higher than 20 % of total calories in such cases [9]. In acute TBI, current recommendations suggest protein provision ranging between 1.5 and 2 g/kg/day to account for the excess catabolism. These requirements should be routinely reassessed and appropriately adjusted based on the observed nitrogen balance [10].

Glutamine supplementation previously thought to be beneficial has not been shown to confer mortality and length of hospital stay benefit in critically ill patients [11]. However, this therapy reduced nosocomial infections among critically ill patients, which differed according to patient populations, modes of nutrition and glutamine dosages [12].

Micronutrients and zinc supplementation outcomes in critical illness have been inconclusive and do not demonstrate any beneficial effects on neurological recovery. Brain damage from oxidative stress is also inferred from reduced plasma levels of antioxidants, suggesting their increased consumption [13]. Consequently, the discovery and development of antioxidant agents is one of the most promising approaches in the search for more effective management of TBI [14].

Initiation of Nutrition Therapy

Early Nutrition

Nutrition therapy should start early; within 24–48 h of admission to the intensive care unit, to offset the severe catabolic response of the body [15]. Once the patient becomes hemodynamically stable, EN should be attempted [16]. The feeding should be adjusted based on the patient's nutritional requirements over the next 48–72 h.

Intolerance to Feeding

Neurocritical patients show a high incidence of gastrointestinal complications, the most common being increased GRV. This is aggravated by drugs routinely used in Neuro ICU such as analgesics, sedatives and muscle relaxants. These complications may result in ineffective EN.

Various steps may be taken to improve EN tolerance. These include

1. Early EN within first 24–48 h.
2. Use of complete and isotonic formulas.
3. Post-pyloric feeding: Patients who cannot tolerate gastric feeding may benefit from a post-pyloric small bowel tube, with improved achievement of energy targets. However, when gastric feeding was compared to transpyloric feeding, there were no significant differences in mechanical ventilation-associated pneumonia or mortality benefit [17, 18].
4. Prokinetic drugs: Pre-emptive administration of prokinetic drugs such as intravenous metoclopramide and erythromycin is recommended for patients who are intolerant to EN [16, 19]. The Canadian Clinical Practice Guidelines (CCPG)

group recommends only metoclopramide, considering the problems with erythromycin-induced bacterial resistance [18]. However, in low doses the risk is more theoretical than practical [20]. Currently, a regimen combining metoclopramide and erythromycin appears to be more effective and associated with better tolerance than the use of either drug as a single agent [21].

5. Nutrition protocols: It is critical to adopt protocols with clear target energy intakes, infusion rates, early starting times, GRV measurement, and infusion frequencies. This is for detecting cases where the infusion should be discontinued or adjusted [22]. For example, the American Society of Parenteral and Enteral Nutrition (ASPEN) recommends that gastric residuals should be measured every 4 h during gastric feeding and to avoid withholding the infusion for residues of less than 500 mL in the absence of other signs of intolerance [18].

Feed Intolerance and Aspiration Pneumonia

The usefulness of measuring GRV in preventing aspiration pneumonia has been challenged, with the postulation that the absence of gastric volume monitoring was not inferior to routine residual gastric volume monitoring in terms of development of aspiration pneumonia [23]. However, blindly feeding until the patient vomits may increase the risk of harm in patients with intolerance [24], and in general, the probability of aspiration is greater when GRV is high [25].

ASPEN and CCPG strongly recommend raising the head of the bed to 30–45° if it is not medically contraindicated in critically ill patients who are receiving EN. The semi-seated position with the head elevated to 30° reduces the risk of bronchial aspiration in addition to improving brain distensibility and reducing intracranial pressure [26].

Glycemic Control

Hyperglycemia aggravates underlying brain damage and influences both morbidity and mortality in critically ill patients [27, 28] by inducing tissue acidosis, oxidative stress and cellular immunosuppression [29], which in turn promotes the development of multiorgan failure [30]. Hypoglycemia on the other hand impairs energy supply leading to metabolic perturbation [31] and cortical depolarizations [32]. Consequently, both hyperglycemia and hypoglycemia need to be avoided to prevent aggravation of underlying brain damage. Studies evaluating the effect of insulin upon the metabolism and progress variables recommend blood glucose values between 120 and 150 mg/dL as safe in neurocritical patients [33].

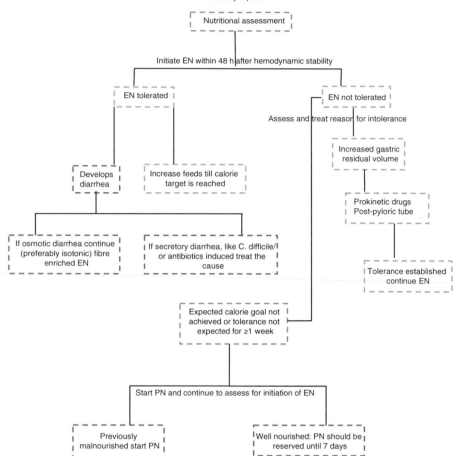

Fig. 4.1 A simple algorithm for nutrition in neurocritically ill

Parenteral Nutrition

ASPEN recommends that PN be reserved until attempts at EN for 7 days have failed in a patient who was previously healthy prior to critical illness with no evidence of protein-caloric malnutrition [16]. On the other hand, The European Society for Clinical Nutrition and Metabolism (ESPEN) guidelines for PN recommend that all critically ill patients (both previously well-nourished and malnourished) receiving less than the targeted enteral feeding after 2 days should be considered for PN [19]. In general, patients who cannot achieve early caloric goals by EN alone, adjunctive PN for short periods of time may be an option. It is our policy to start PN in previously healthy patients after 7 days, and in previously malnourished patients PN needs to be started within 2 days (Fig. 4.1).

Refeeding Syndrome

Refeeding syndrome (RFS) represents a group of clinical findings that occur in severely malnourished individuals undergoing nutritional support. Cardiac arrhythmias, multisystem organ dysfunction and death are the most severe symptoms observed. As the cachectic body attempts to reverse its adaptation to the starved state in response to the nutritional load, symptoms result from fluid and electrolyte imbalances, with hypophosphatemia playing a central role [34].

The most effective means of preventing or treating RFS are

1. Recognizing the patients at risk,
2. Providing adequate electrolyte, vitamin and micronutrient supplementation,
3. Careful fluid resuscitation,
4. Cautious and gradual energy restoration,
5. Monitoring of critical laboratory indices.

Specific Patient Groups

Traumatic Brain Injury (TBI)

The most compelling data for early nutrition after TBI comes from an analysis of a large database of 22 trauma centers in New York State [35]. The main findings from this study clearly demonstrated that any nutrition within the first 5 days after TBI is associated with a reduced mortality rate. An additional benefit was seen in the maximal level of nutrition delivered in the first week of injury where for every 10 cal/kg decrease in caloric intake there was a 30–40 % increase in mortality. There is a lack of confirmatory data to determine the proper formulation and micronutrient supplementation for patients with TBI [36].

Cerebrovascular Disease

Following stroke, dysphagia is the most important factor related to malnutrition [37]. The majority of data for nutritional status and therapy for cerebrovascular diseases is found in ischemic stroke populations. The most extensive data comes from the Feed or Ordinary Diet (FOOD) trial [38, 39]. This study demonstrated a reduction in risk of death with early tube feeding. It also showed PEG feeding to be associated with an increased risk of death or poor outcome when compared to a nasogastric route of feeding. These results led the authors to suggest the avoidance of early PEG placement in stroke patients with dysphagia. The other conclusion from the study was that neither death nor poor outcome was impacted by protein supplementation on long term follow-up.

The hypermetabolic response after subarachnoid hemorrhage is similar to that seen in severe TBI and is dependent on the clinical severity at presentation [40]. Despite early nutritional support, these patients are often in a state of negative energy balance, which has been associated with increased infectious complications.

Spinal Cord Injury (SCI)

Early nutritional support (initiated within 72 h) of spinal cord injury (SCI) patients is safe, but has not been shown to affect neurological outcome, the length of stay or the incidence of complications in patients with acute SCI [41]. The marked hypermetabolic response seen after acute TBI appears to be blunted in SCI patients due to the flaccidity of denervated musculature after spinal cord transection/injury [42].

Dysphagia is a common issue following SCI, particularly with higher-level injuries. Poor appetite, disturbances in taste and olfaction can also hinder appropriate oral caloric intake. PEG insertion may provide a safe alternative with low complication rates in patients unable to tolerate an oral diet.

Myasthenic Crisis (MC)

Adequate nutrition is important to avoid negative energy balance and worsening of muscle strength [43]. All patients should receive adequate nutritional support (25–35 cal/kg) via enteral route whenever possible. In patients with hypercarbia and a difficult weaning process, low carbohydrate feeds are the preferred solution [44]. Potassium, magnesium and phosphate depletion can exacerbate MC and these electrolytes should be replete.

Guillain–Barre Syndrome (GBS)

More than one-third of GBS patients require intensive care for mechanical ventilation or management of other medical complications related to infection or dysautonomia. These patients are at high risk for inadequate nutrition throughout the course of their illness. Gastrointestinal symptoms produce dehydration and weight loss even prior to hospital admission. Progressive bulbar dysfunction or adynamic ileus can limit or eliminate oral intake. Furthermore, GBS is a hypermetabolic and hypercatabolic state on the same order as sepsis or trauma [45]. Inadequate nutrition is associated with increased risk for fluid and electrolyte abnormalities, decubitus ulcers, as well as nosocomial infections. Early nutrition support should begin as quickly as possible by appropriate means (e.g., modified diet, nasogastric tube or PN). Close monitoring of hydration status, weight, vital proteins and nitrogen balance will help guide adjustments to this initial diet [46].

CNS Infections

These patients may develop long-term nutritional deficiencies due to ventilator dependency. Bulbar weakness is not uncommon leading to dysphagia. Nutritional therapy in this population is best guided by principles outlined for general critical care patients.

Summary

1. Global nutritional assessment should be done before starting nutrition therapy
2. It is difficult to accurately estimate caloric requirements in neurocritically ill patients. Indirect calorimetry may be helpful, if available. Consultation with a clinical dietician is strongly recommended. Suggested calorie intake ranges from 20 to 30 kcal/kg/day.
3. Early enteral nutrition is recommended to achieve calorie goal in order to accelerate neurologic recovery and reduce both the incidence of major complications and post-injury inflammatory responses. An enteral feeding protocol is advisable (Fig. 4.2).
4. Adjunctive PN for short periods of time may be an option in patients who cannot achieve early caloric goals by EN alone.
5. Head of the bed should be raised, when patients are receiving enteral nutrition.
6. GRV should be measured every 6 h during gastric feeding and withholding feeds should be avoided for residuals of less than 500 mL in the absence of other signs of intolerance.
7. Early use of prokinetic drugs is recommended in patients receiving enteral nutrition with intolerance.
8. High-protein supplementation is recommended, to provide daily intake of 1.5–2 g/kg to account for excessive catabolism, especially in patients with traumatic brain injury. These requirements should be routinely reassessed and appropriately adjusted based on the observed nitrogen balance.
9. Blood glucose control is recommended as in all other critically ill patients, to target blood glucose values between 120 and 150 mg/dL.
10. Administration of intravenous glutamine dipeptides, although not shown to confer mortality benefits, may be recommended as it has shown to reduce nosocomial infections in neurocritically ill patients.

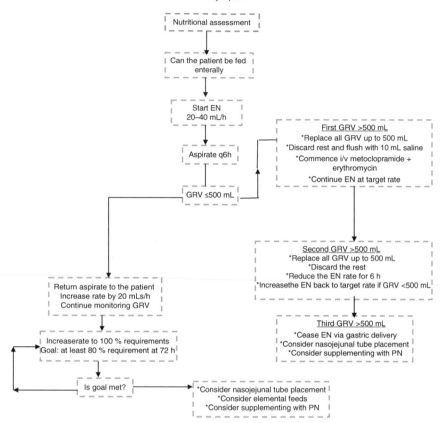

Fig. 4.2 Enteral nutrition protocol

11. Patients who cannot tolerate gastric feeding may benefit from a post-pyloric small bowel tube, to improve achievement of energy targets.
12. Recognize patients who are at risk of development refeeding syndrome. Nutrition therapy should be started slowly in these patients with careful monitoring of electrolytes.

Dos and Don'ts

Dos

- Perform initial nutrition assessment
- Establish nutrition protocols
- Early enhance enteral nutrition (EN); recommended calorie intake between 20 and 30 kcal/kg/d

- Raise head of bed to 30–45° if no contradiction
- Measure gastric residual volume (GRV)×6 h; accept ≤500 mL
- Use early prokinetic drugs to improve EN tolerance
- Keep blood glucose control between 120 and 150 mg/dL
- Perform post-pyloric tube feeding if frequent interruptions of EN
- Initiate slow and monitored feeding in malnourished patients
- Perform continuous ongoing nutrition assessment

Don'ts

- Avoid early parenteral nutrition (PN)
- Avoid extremes of blood sugar
- Avoid frequent EN interruptions
- Prevent catheter-related blood stream infection (CRBSI) when central lines are used for PN
- Don't stop feeds if there is

    - Absent bowel sound
    - Diarrhea
    - Coffee ground aspirate

References

1. Young B, Ott L, Twyman D, et al. The effect of nutritional support on outcome from severe head injury. J Neurosurg. 1987;67:668–76.
2. Cook AM, Peppard A, Magnuson B. Nutrition consideration in traumatic brain injury. Nutr Clin Pract. 2008;23:608–20.
3. Acosta Escribano JA, Carrasco Moreno R, Fernández Vivas M, Navarro Polo JN, Más Serrano P, Sánchez Payá J, et al. Gastric enteral intolerance in mechanically ventilated patients with traumatic cerebral lesion. Nutr Hosp. 2001;16:262–7.
4. Denes Z. The influence of severe malnutrition on rehabilitation in patients with severe head injury. Disabil Rehabil. 2004;26:1163–5.
5. Taylor SJ, Fettes SB, Jewkes C, Nelson RJ. Prospective, randomized, controlled trial to determine the effect of early enhanced enteral nutrition on clinical outcome in mechanically ventilated patients suffering head injury. Crit Care Med. 1999;27(11):2525–31.
6. Frontera JA, Fernández A, Claassen J, Schmidt M, Schumacher HC, Wartenberg K, Temes R, Parra A, Ostapkovich ND, Mayer SA. Hyperglycemia after SAH: predictors, associated complications, and impact on outcome. Stroke. 2006;37:199–203.
7. Foley N, Marshall S, Pikul J, Salter K, Teasell R. Hypermetabolism following moderated to severe traumatic acute brain injury: a systematic review. J Neurotrauma. 2008;25:1415–31.
8. Acosta Escribano J, Herrero Mesiguer I, Conejero Garcia-Quijada R, Metabolism and Nutrition Working Group of the Spanish Society of Intensive Care Medicine and Coronary units. Guidelines for specialized nutritional and metabolic support in the critically-ill patient: update. Consensus SEMICYUC-SENPE: neurocritical patient. Nutr Hosp. 2011;26(S2): 72–5.

9. Klein S, Kinney J, Jeejeebhoy K, Alpers D, Hellerstein M, Murray M, Twomey P. Nutrition support in clinical practice: review of published data and recommendations for future research directions. Summary of a conference sponsored by the National Institutes of Health, American Society for Parenteral and Enteral Nutrition, and American Society for Clinical Nutrition. Am J Clin Nutr. 1997;66:683–706.

10. Brain Trauma Foundation; American Association of Neurological Surgeons; Congress of Neurological Surgeons. Guidelines for the management of severe traumatic brain injury. J Neurotrauma. 2007;24 (Suppl 1):S1–106. Erratum in: J Neurotrauma. 2008;25(3):276–8.

11. Chen QH, Yang Y, He HL, Xie JF, Cai SX, Liu AR, Wang HL, Qiu HB. The effect of glutamine therapy on outcomes in critically ill patients: a meta-analysis of randomized controlled trials. Crit Care. 2014;18:R8.

12. Bollhalder L, Pfeil AM, Tomonaga Y, Schwenkglenks M. A systematic literature review and meta-analysis of randomized clinical trials of parenteral glutamine supplementation. Clin Nutr. 2013;32:213–23.

13. Huynh D, Chapman MJ, Nguyen NQ. Nutrition support in the critically ill. Curr Opin Gastroenterol. 2013;29:208–15.

14. Eghwrudjakpor PO, Allison AB. Oxidative stress following traumatic brain injury: enhancement of endogenous antioxidant defence systems and the promise of improved outcome. Niger J Med. 2010;19:14–21.

15. Doig GS, Heighes PT, Simpson F, Sweetman EA, Davies AR. Early enteral nutrition, provided within 24 h of injury or intensive care admission, significantly reduces mortality in critically ill patients: a meta-analysis of randomized controlled trials. Intensive Care Med. 2009;35:2018–27.

16. McClave SA, Martindale RG, Vanek VW, McCarthy M, Roberts P, Taylor B, Ochoa JB, Napolitano L, Cresci G, A.S.P.E.N. Board of Directors; American College of Critical Care Medicine; Society of Critical Care Medicine. Guidelines for the provision and assessment of nutrition support therapy in the adult critically Ill patient: Society of Critical Care Medicine (SCCM) and American Society for Parenteral and Enteral Nutrition (A.S.P.E.N.). JPEN J Parenter Enteral Nutr. 2009;33(3):277–316.

17. Tan M, Zhu JC, Yin HH. Enteral nutrition in patients with severe traumatic brain injury: reasons for intolerance and medical management. Br J Neurosurg. 2011;25(1):2–8.

18. Heyland DK, Dhaliwal R, Drover JW, Gramlich L, Dodek P, Canadian Critical Care Clinical Practice Guidelines Committee. Canadian clinical practice guidelines for nutrition support in mechanically ventilated, critically ill adult patients. JPEN J Parenter Enteral Nutr. 2003;27(5):355–73.

19. Singer P, Berger MM, Van den Berghe G, Biolo G, Calder P, Forbes A, Griffiths R, Kreyman G, Leverve X, Pichard C, ESPEN. ESPEN guidelines on parenteral nutrition: intensive care. Clin Nutr. 2009;28:387–400.

20. Deane AM, Fraser RJ, Chapman MJ. Prokinetic drugs for feed intolerance in critical illness: current and potential therapies. Crit Care Resusc. 2009;11:132–43.

21. MacLaren R, Kiser TH, Fish DN, Wischmeyer PE. Erythromycin vs metoclopramide for facilitating gastric emptying and tolerance to intragastric nutrition in critically ill patients. JPEN J Parenter Enteral Nutr. 2008;32:412–9.

22. Campos BB, Machado FS. Nutrition therapy in severe head trauma patients. Rev Bras Ter Intensiva. 2012;24(1):97–105.

23. Reignier J, Mercier E, Le Gouge A, Boulain T, Desachy A, Bellec F, Clavel M, Frat JP, Plantefeve G, Quenot JP, Lascarrou JB, Clinical Research in Intensive Care and Sepsis (CRICS) Group. Effect of not monitoring residual gastric volume on risk of ventilator-associated pneumonia n adults receiving mechanical ventilation and early enteral feeding: a randomized controlled trial. JAMA. 2013;309:249.

24. Heyland DK, Dhaliwal R. Measuring gastric residual volumes in enterally tube fed critically ill patients. The end of an era? In Nibble: nutrition information byte. Issue 9. http://www.criticalcarenutrition.com/docs/qi_tools/Nibble%209%20-%20GRVs.pdf.

25. Metheny NA, Schallom L, Oliver DA, Clouse RE. Gastric residual volume and aspiration in critically ill patients receiving gastric feedings. Am J Crit Care. 2008;17:512–20.
26. Ng I, Lim J, Wong HB. Effect of head posture on cerebral hemodynamics: its influence on intracranial pressure, cerebral perfusion pressure and cerebral oxygenation. Neurosurgery. 2004;54:593–7.
27. Zygun DA, Steiner LA, Johnston AJ, Hutchinson PJ, Al-Rawi PG, Chatfield D, Kirkpatrick PJ, Menon DK, Gupta AK. Hyperglycemia and brain tissue pH after traumatic brain injury. Neurosurgery. 2004;55:877–81.
28. Diaz-Parejo P, Ståhl N, Xu W, Reinstrup P, Ungerstedt U, Nordström CH. Cerebral energy metabolism during transient hyperglycemia in patients with severe brain trauma. Intensive Care Med. 2003;29:544–50.
29. Aronson D. Hyperglycemia and the pathobiology of diabetic complications. Adv Cardiol. 2008;45:1–16.
30. Sperry JL, Frankel HL, Vanek SL, Nathens AB, Moore EE, Maier RV, Minei JP. Early hyperglycemia predicts multiple organ failure and mortality but not infection. J Trauma. 2007;63:487–93.
31. Vespa P, Boonyaputthikul R, McArthur DL, Miller C, Etchepare M, Bergsneider M, Glenn T, Martin N, Hovda D. Intensive insulin therapy reduces microdialysis glucose values without altering glucose utilization or improving the lactate/pyruvate ratio after traumatic brain injury. Crit Care Med. 2006;34:850–6.
32. Strong AJ, Hartings JA, Dreier JP. Cortical spreading depression: an adverse but treatable factor in intensive care? Curr Opin Crit Care. 2007;13:126–33.
33. Perel P, Yanagawa T, Bunn F, Roberts I, Wentz R, Pierro A. Nutritional support for head-injured patients. Cochrane Database Syst Rev. 2006;(4):CD001530.
34. Boateng AA, Sriram K, Meguid MM, Crook M. Refeeding syndrome: treatment considerations based on collective analysis of literature case reports. Nutrition. 2010;26:156–67.
35. Hartl R, Gerber LM, Ni Q, Ghajar J. Effect of early nutrition on deaths due to severe traumatic brain injury. J Neurosurg. 2008;109:50–6.
36. Badjatia N. Nutrition and metabolism. 2013 Neurocritical Care Society Practice Update.
37. Davalos A, Ricart W, Gonzalez-Huix F, Solers S, Marrugat J, Molins A, Suner R, Genis D. Effect of malnutrition after stroke on clinical outcome. Stroke. 1996;27:1028–32.
38. Dennis MS, Lewis SC, Warlow C, FOOD Trial Collaboration. Effect of timing and method of enteral tube feeding for dysphagic stroke patients (FOOD): a multicentre randomised controlled trial. Lancet. 2005;365:764–72.
39. Dennis MS, Lewis SC, Warlow C, FOOD Trial Collaboration. Routine oral nutritional supplementation for stroke patients in hospital (FOOD): a multicentre randomised controlled trial. Lancet. 2005;365:755–63.
40. Esper DH, Coplin WM, Carhuapoma JR. Energy expenditure in patients with nontraumatic intracranial hemorrhage. JPEN J Parenter Enteral Nutr. 2006;30:71–5.
41. Dhall SS, Hadley MN, Aarabi B, Gelb DE, Hurlbert RJ, Rozzelle CJ, Ryken TC. Nutritional support after spinal cord injury. Neurosurgery. 2013;72 Suppl 2:255–9.
42. Rodriguez DJ, Benzel EC, Clevenger FW. The metabolic response to spinal cord injury. Spinal Cord. 1997;35(9):599–604.
43. Kirmani JF, Yahia AM, Qureshi AI. Myasthenic crisis. Curr Treat Op Neurol. 2004;6:3–15.
44. Varelas PN, Chua HC, Natterman J, Barmadia L, Zimmerman P, Ulatowski J, Bhardwaj A, Williams MA, Hanley DF. Ventilatory care in myasthenia gravis crisis: assessing the baseline adverse event rate. Crit Care Med. 2002;30:2663–8.
45. Roubenoff RA, Borel CO, Hanley DF. Hypermetabolism and hypercatabolism in Guillain-Barré syndrome. J Parenter Enteral Nutr. 1992;16(5):464–72.
46. Harms M. Inpatient management of Guillain-Barré syndrome. Neurohospitalist. 2011;1: 78–84.

Chapter 5
Monitoring in the Neurocritical Care Unit

Said Hachimi-Idrissi

Introduction

Besides the continuous monitoring and assessment of cardiorespiratory functions common to all critically ill patients, monitoring of critically ill brain-injured patients includes neurological examination, neuroimaging modalities and other techniques that allow global and regional brain monitoring. These specialized monitoring techniques provide early warning of impending brain ischemia and guide therapeutic interventions in brain-injured patients.

Continuous neurological evaluations such as control of the pupils, the reflexes, the muscle tone and search for neurological deficits are somewhat unreliable [1]. Computed tomography (CT) scan, magnetic resonance imaging (MRI) and other radiological and angiographic investigations are valuable but are non-continuous, and not available at the bedside. Other neurological monitoring old and new, invasive and non-invasive have emerged or been revived lately, and led to a trend toward development of new strategies for the management of acute brain injury. This review describes current neuromonitoring techniques used during the intensive care management of severely brain-injured ICU patients. Interpretation of the data from these monitors depends on a thorough knowledge of the clinical and technical aspects of the modality in use. A list of neuromonitors that are currently available is given in Table 5.1.

None of the following neuromonitoring modalities have demonstrated its superiority compared to others in terms of improving the outcome, but it is helpful to detect potential harmful events that may cause secondary brain damage if not earlier detected and appropriately managed. Different non-invasive and invasive

S. Hachimi-Idrissi, MD, PhD, FCCM, FAAP
Critical Care Department and Cerebral Resuscitation Research Group,
Universiteit Ziekenhuis, Ghent, Belgium
e-mail: said.hachimiidrissi@uzgent.be; said.hachimiidrissi@ugent.be

© Springer International Publishing Switzerland 2015
K.E. Wartenberg et al. (eds.), *Neurointensive Care: A Clinical Guide to Patient Safety*, DOI 10.1007/978-3-319-17293-4_5

Table 5.1 Neurological monitoring techniques

General systemic monitoring
Blood pressure, respiratory rate, heart rate, body temperature, laboratory test, blood gas analysis, cardiac output, systemic vascular resistance
Neurological examination
Pupils, reflexes, neurological deficits, Glasgow Coma Scale, National Institute of Health Stroke Scale, Barthel index, modified Rankin scale
Neuroimaging
Computer tomography scan or magnetic resonance imaging with angiography and perfusion imaging, magnetic resonance spectroscopy, positron emission tomography
Monitoring intracranial pressure, blood flow dynamics, oxygen, and metabolism
Intracranial pressure monitor, transcranial Doppler sonography, jugular venous oxygen saturation, brain tissue oxygen tension monitor, near-infrared spectroscopy, cerebral microdialysis, cerebral blood flow monitor
Monitoring brain electrical activity
Electroencephalography, evoked potentials, *cortical and intracortical electrodes*
Multimodal monitoring

methods are indispensable to detect changes in stuporous or comatose patients that would otherwise be unnoticed. The following provides a detailed insight into the management of neuromonitoring.

Intracranial Pressure (ICP)

ICP is defined as the pressure inside the lateral ventricles/lumbar subarachnoid space in supine position. The normal value for ICP is 10–15 mmHg in adults and 2–4 mmHg in neonates and infants. ICP is a reflection of the relationship between intracranial contents and the available intracranial volume. The purpose of ICP monitoring is to identify a potential increase in ICP that may cause cerebral ischemia or herniation of the brain structures [2].

The oversimplified understanding that increased ICP >20 mmHg is pathologic lead to the current misconception that normal ICP guarantees absence of pathologic processes. Extended neuromonitoring, however, shows that this is incorrect [3]. Metabolic and functional alterations even precede increases in ICP following TBI [4]. It is important to remember that this threshold of 20 mmHg stems from the period where other neuromonitoring tools such as jugular venous oxygen saturation, brain tissue oxygen tension monitoring, cerebral microdialysis, and Transcranial Doppler sonography were not yet integrated into daily routine. A very simple measure to indirectly estimate global cerebral perfusion is to calculate cerebral perfusion pressure (CPP): CPP=mean arterial pressure (MAP) − ICP.

A "normal" CPP, however, does not guarantee sufficient cerebral perfusion and oxygenation. To define an optimal CPP, other parameters such as partial pressure of brain tissue oxygen (PtO_2), jugular venous saturation of oxygen ($SjvO_2$), cerebral metabolism and blood flow velocities are helpful. Direct ICP measurement requires a surgical intervention that is associated with certain risks (e.g., bleeding, additional brain damage, and infections) [5]. Augmentation of CPP helps to avoid both global and regional ischemia in brain trauma. The Brain Trauma Foundation suggests a CPP>60 mmHg as an option in the management of severe TBI [6].

Indications for ICP Monitoring

Head trauma provided the largest volume of experience with ICP monitoring, though it has also been used in various other neurological conditions. Recommendations for ICP monitoring in some of the common neurological conditions are as follows.

Traumatic Brain Injury

About two-thirds of patients with traumatic brain injury (TBI) have intracranial hypertension (ICP>20 mmHg). Aggressive maintenance of ICP below 15 mmHg has been suggested to improve the outcome [2], however this contested by some recent evidence [7]. The Brain Trauma Foundation and American Association of Neurological Surgeons have recommended that for ICP monitoring is appropriate in TBI in the following situation [6, 8]:

1. In patients with severe head injury (Glasgow Coma Scale (GCS) 3–8 after cardiopulmonary resuscitation) with an abnormal CT scan on admission.
2. In patients with severe TBI with a normal CT scan and displaying on admission at least two of the following features: age over 40 years, unilateral or bilateral motor posturing, systolic blood pressure<90 mmHg.
3. ICP monitoring is not routinely indicated in patients with mild or moderate TBI. However, a physician may choose to monitor ICP in certain conscious patients with traumatic mass lesions such as hematomas and contusions.

Hydrocephalus

Patients with hydrocephalus require placement of an intraventricular catheter which also provides ICP monitoring. This condition is frequently encountered in subarachnoid hemorrhage, intraventricular hemorrhage, obstructive mass lesions, severe bacterial meningitis, etc.

Other Conditions

In patients undergoing surgical or interventional neuroradiological procedures for arteriovenous malformations (AVM), ICP monitoring helps to detect potential complications that follow acute embolization or ablation of a high flow AVM. ICP monitoring has also been used in Reye's syndrome, hepatic encephalopathy, and encephalitis associated with raised ICP though the indications are not clearly established. In patients with ischemic stroke, intracerebral hemorrhage, and other cerebrovascular conditions, the indication for ICP monitoring depends on the amount and the location of mass effect, the presence of intraventricular hemorrhage and of hydrocephalus.

Techniques of ICP Monitoring

Intraventricular Catheter

Percutaneous intraventricular pressure monitoring is the gold standard against which all other ICP monitors are evaluated. The transducer is zeroed at the level of the external auditory meatus. This intraventricular monitoring is reliable, can be used for the measurement of intracranial compliance and for drainage of cerebrospinal fluid (CSF) to decrease the ICP. However, it is an invasive procedure associated with definite risks of infection and trauma to the brain during cannulation. Ventricular collapse in patients with brain edema may render placement of the catheter difficult and also interfere with actual pressure recordings, even if the catheter is in place.

Subdural Bolt

A subdural bolt is a hollow bolt threaded through a twist drill hole into the skull and dura mater until the inner surface of the bolt lies along with the arachnoid membrane. The advantage of this system is a low potential for brain injury during insertion. Its disadvantages include inability to draw CSF, risk of infection, and malfunction.

Fiberoptic Devices

Miniature fiberoptic catheters can be placed into the ventricles, epidural or subdural space or even into the brain parenchyma. Since it is a self-enclosed electronic system, problems associated with fluid-filled systems such as leaking, drift, and infection are minimized.

Transcranial Doppler (TCD)

Since its introduction into clinical routine, TCD sonography has been helpful in diagnosing conditions of low flow, vasospasm, and hyperemia states that require appropriate therapeutic interventions [9]. TCD measures cerebral blood flow velocity within the large basal cerebral arteries and regional cerebral perfusion, cerebral autoregulation, as well as CO_2 reactivity under normal and pathological conditions [10].

In addition to measures such as absolute flow velocities, calculated values such as the pulsatility index (PI) and resistance index (RI), TCD allows for non-invasive estimation of ICP and CPP [11]. This approach is helpful if an ICP probe cannot be inserted due to a coagulation disorder or if an ICP probe is damaged or malfunctioning and a new probe cannot be inserted right away. However, this non-invasive assessment of ICP is not a substitute for continuously measured ICP at present.

Jugular Venous Oxygen Saturation (SjvO$_2$)

Cannulation of the internal jugular vein with a venous catheter allows for analysis of jugular venous oxygen saturation (SjvO$_2$). It reflects changes in global cerebral oxygen supply, cerebral perfusion and cerebral oxygen consumption as SjvO$_2$ correlates directly with perfusion and correlates inversely with cerebral oxygen consumption. Thus, an increase in MAP with subsequent amelioration of CPP as well as reduced hyperventilation will improve cerebral oxygen supply due to pressure-dependent and vasodilation-mediated increased perfusion. Reducing cerebral oxygen consumption due to pharmacological inhibition of neuronal activity during sedation or by reducing brain temperature will also elevate SjvO$_2$ due to reduced oxygen consumption [12]. Global cerebral changes as reflected by SjvO$_2$ correlate well with local measurements using ptO$_2$ [13]. SjvO2 ≤ 50 % reflects cerebral ischemia and should be avoided. Immediate correction is important [14] since hypoxic/ischemic SjvO$_2$ values are associated with metabolic perturbation reflected by increased lactate and glutamate levels [15] as well as sustained mortality and morbidity [16].

SjvO2 values >80 % reflect underlying hyperemia or luxury perfusion, an increase in inspired oxygen, or decreased consumption due to decreased metabolic demand. The treating clinician should take more clinical variables in account in order to identify the problem and implement the correct treatment.

Cannulation of the jugular vein is associated with certain risks such as, for example, puncture of the carotid artery followed by hemorrhage. This risk can be reduced by using sonographic guidance. Thrombosis formation and catheter-related infections are other complications. In addition, the side of insertion relative to the location of the traumatic lesions has been discussed controversially.

Brain Tissue Oxygen Tension Monitoring (PTO$_2$)

Direct measurement of PtO$_2$ is growing into the gold standard bedside monitor of cerebral oxygenation [17]. Assessing PtO$_2$ helps to detect both local changes and the cerebral consequences of systemic influences [13, 18].

Similar to changes in SjvO$_2$, PtO$_2$ values indirectly reflect alterations of cerebral perfusion and oxygenation. Low SjvO$_2$ and PtO$_2$ values reveal reduced cerebral perfusion due to, for example, systemic hypotension or local cerebral vasoconstriction caused by hyperventilation or vasospasm, reduced supply (low inspired fraction of oxygen, anemia, low cardiac output) or increased cerebral consumption. Sustained high oxygen consumption may be due to increased neuronal activity secondary to insufficient analgesia/sedation or seizures. Thus, assessing global as well as local changes reflected by $SjvO_2$ and $PtiO_2$ permits detailed and controlled therapeutic corrections [19].

Validation studies have shown that PtO_2 values <10 mmHg (Licox®, Integra Neurosciences, Plainsboro, New Jersey, USA) reflecting tissue hypoxia are associated with increased extracellular glutamate accumulation if not corrected within 30 min [20, 21]. In addition, these ischemic values correlate with neuropsychological deficits in survivors of brain trauma [22]. As stated by Maloney-Wilensky et al., PtO_2<10 mmHg longer than 15 min is associated with worse outcome and increased mortality after traumatic brain injury [23].

Near-Infrared Spectroscopy (NIRS)

NIRS is a non-invasive technique based on the transmission and absorption of near infrared (NIR) light (700–950 nm) as it passes through tissue. Oxygenated and deoxygenated hemoglobin have characteristic and different absorption spectra in the NIR and their relative concentrations in tissue can be determined by their relative absorption of light at these wavelengths. It is now possible to measure changes in the concentration of oxidized cytochrome c oxidase (CCO), the terminal complex of the mitochondrial electron transfer chain responsible for over 95 % of oxygen metabolism. NIRS-derived CCO concentration measurement therefore offers the potential to assess cerebral cellular energy status as well as oxygenation and hemodynamics, in multiple regions of interest [24].

The "normal" range lies between 60 and 75 %, with a coefficient of variation for absolute baseline values of around 10 % because of NIRS signal contamination from extracranial tissue. Thus, NIRS is best used as a trend monitor without application of absolute thresholds for cerebral ischemia or hypoxia, as there is a wide intra- and inter-individual variability.

Cerebral Microdialysis (CM)

CM provides detailed insight into metabolic alterations by measuring changes in glucose, lactate, pyruvate, glycerol, glutamate and calculating the lactate to pyruvate ratio [25, 26]. Due to the duration of dialysis of the cerebral metabolites up to 60 min, clinical decisions are based on metabolic changes, which have previously occurred. Consequently, the metabolic alterations measured by CM should always be analyzed in conjunction with other continuous parameters such as PtO_2, $SjvO_2$, CPP and ICP.

Signs of impaired cerebral metabolism (decrease in glucose, increase of the lactate to pyruvate ratio, increase in glutamate) are found even in regions without obvious signs of structural damage. This functional impairment can result from increased ICP due to local changes and can be induced by systemic influences due to hypotension, hyperemia, vasospasm, hyperventilation, fever, seizures, hypoglycemia, or anemia. In addition, improvement of signs of metabolic deterioration may reflect positive therapeutic effects [27]. Integration of CM allowed reduction of CPP in a controlled manner to 50 mmHg as practiced utilizing the "LUND-concept" [28]. In addition to assessing relative changes of the different metabolic parameters over time, calculating lactate to pyruvate ratio reflects the severity of underlying metabolic impairment [29]. Pathologically increased lactate to pyruvate ratio is associated with subsequent chronic frontal lobe atrophy after traumatic brain injury [29].

Excessive neuronal excitations or signs of severe cell damage result in elevated extracellular glutamate secondary to the release of intracellularly stored glutamate. Increased lactate levels exhibit an energetic deficit secondary to an increased cellular uptake and metabolism and/or insufficient supply due to systemic hypoglycemia, impaired perfusion, or insufficient expression of glucose transporters. Elevated glycerol values reflect membrane damage. Overall, CM can be used to detect pathological changes and guide therapeutic interventions (e.g., hyperventilation, oxygenation, sedation, CPP level). Low glucose and elevated lactate to pyruvate ratios are significant independent predictors of mortality after brain trauma [30]. Metabolic changes determined by CM can even be used as a warning system as early as 12 h prior to an increase in ICP [4, 21].

Integrating monitoring of CM into daily routine could be valuable in the detection of functional deterioration with subsequent edema formation and increase in ICP or due to delayed cerebral ischemia after subarachnoid hemorrhage.

Electroencephalography (EEG)

EEG can be applied to monitor the depth of sedation in brain-injured patients and to diagnose and guide therapy in those suffering from seizures or status epilepticus. Continuous electroencephalogram (c EEG) monitoring has the benefit of providing real-time information about seizures, level of consciousness, and evolution of global and focal insults. Still, it is a labor-intensive prospect since a dedicated team of technicians and physicians is needed constantly to maintain the equipment and to interpret the EEG data. Moreover, artifacts from the other ICU equipment make EEG interpretation burdensome [31]. The introduction of quantitative analysis and spectral power arrays may facilitate the use of continuous EEG monitoring in the ICU in the future. Moreover, intracortical EEG electrodes may provide more sensitive recordings.

Evoked Potentials (EPs)

EPs are the electrical responses generated in the nervous system in response to a stimulus. Unlike EEG, which records random electrical activity, evoked potentials are event-related. After appropriate stimulation, the EP responses are recorded from surface electrodes placed on the scalp at the area of interest. They are pathway-specific. They have a much lower amplitude than the normally recorded EEG activity and therefore require computer-averaging techniques to filter artifacts and noises from the signal. There are two broad categories of evoked potentials: the sensory evoked potentials (SEPs) and the motor evoked potentials (MEPs).

These EP investigations, whether sensory or motor evoked potentials, require specialized and well-trained personnel. Changes in their recording can be influenced by lesions of the pathway as well as concomitant sedation/analgesia and inhalation anesthetics [32–35]. Apart from their role in the diagnosis of neurological conditions, they are also used to assess the integrity of neural tracts and prognostication.

SEP

SEPs are the electrical potentials generated in response to stimulation of a peripheral sensory nerve. The individual modalities of evoked potentials are named after the sensory fibers stimulated: somatosensory evoked potentials (SSEPs) are obtained by stimulation of somatic sensory nerve fibers, visual evoked potentials (VEPs) by stimulation of visual pathways, and auditory evoked potentials (AEPs) by auditory pathway stimulation. Once the nerves are stimulated, the responses are generally recorded from the scalp by surface electrodes. Interpretation of an evoked potential recording consists of identification of specific peaks representing specific neural originators and quantification of the latencies and amplitudes of the individual peaks. Changes in the amplitudes and latencies of specific peaks indicate injury to their corresponding neural originators.

A number of physiological parameters can affect the latencies and the amplitudes of the various peaks in evoked potential recordings. It is essential to ensure that these parameters do not fluctuate widely during the course of EP monitoring in order to obtain reliable information on intraoperative neurological injury. Different parameters influence EP responses such as cerebral blood flow, systemic blood pressure, hematocrit, ICP, $PtiO_2$, temperature, and carbon dioxide tension among others. Complete absence of SSEP is a reliable prognosticator of no recovery of function [34, 36].

MEP

Monitoring the motor tracts is very important during spinal procedures. EPs generated by transcranial stimulation of the motor cortex have been used for this purpose.

The stimulation may be electric or magnetic. The wave of depolarization generated by the stimulation of corticospinal neurons descends through the corticospinal tracts and causes compound muscle action potentials. Responses to transcranial stimulation can be recorded in the epidural space, over the peripheral nerves or from evoked muscle activity (compound muscle action potentials, CAMP).

Multimodal Monitoring

In reality, no monitoring is perfect when used in isolation. Combining data from multiple modalities overcomes many of the limitations of individual techniques. However, the term "multimodal monitoring" is used to describe real-time data processing of combinations of monitoring techniques, which produce voluminous data, often requiring the use of integrated bedside computer systems. This allows simultaneous access to different measured variables, and hence improves real-time clinical information [37]. Investment in and maintenance of infrastructure are key factors [38]. At the end, the success or failure of multimodal monitoring depends on the judgment of clinical team, because they should interpret the data and act appropriately in timely fashion (Fig. 5.1).

Case Scenario

A 45-year-old construction worker fell from a 3 m height down to the street. On admission, he was unconscious and barely breathing with a Glasgow Coma Scale of 4. Hemodynamic stabilization was followed by surgical removal of a large subdural hematoma with midline shift. An intraventricular catheter was placed, and ICP and CPP were continuously monitored along with other ICU physiological parameters. Forty eight hours after ICU admission, he developed a sudden increase in ICP to 35 mmHg and CPP has declined down to 52 mmHg. On examination the patient showed dilated pupils. An urgent CT scan demonstrated severe global cerebral edema, and a subsequent MRI displayed severe brain edema and diffuse axonal injury. Despite aggressive pharmacological treatment of brain edema, the patient died 5 days after admission.

Is ICP/CPP monitoring adequate in patients with severe TBI, or are there other parameters that might influence the outcome?

ICP monitoring has become an integral part in the management of TBI, but is not enough to prevent brain damage even if an ICP crisis can be managed sufficiently. Metabolic and functional alterations even precede increases in ICP following TBI [4]. Thus ICP/CPP monitoring by itself will not provide metabolic and/or functional alterations preceding an ICP crisis, and therefore critical therapeutic interventions that might improve the outcome will occur too late.

Monitoring $SjvO_2$ might be of use if the jugular catheter is in place, because it might detect changes in global cerebral oxygen delivery and utilization prior to an

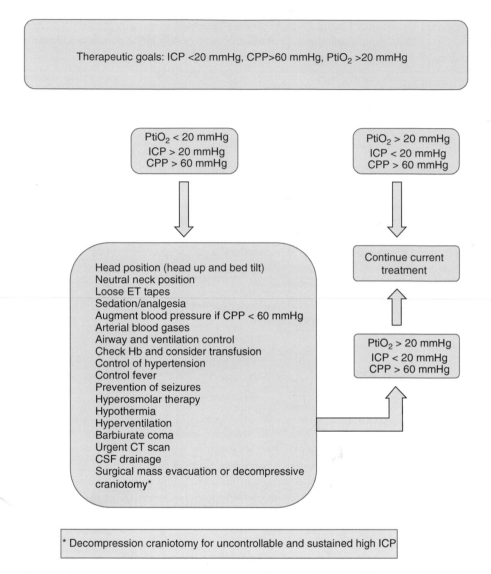

Fig. 5.1 Brain tissue oxygen-guided management. *ET* endotracheal tube, *CSF* cerebrospinal fluid, *ICP* intracranial pressure, *CPP* cerebral perfusion pressure, *Hb* hemoglobin

ICP crisis. Reduction of SjvO$_2$ to <55 % indicates that cerebral oxygen delivery is inadequate to meet the demand or oxygen supply is not sufficient. Reduction of SjVO$_2$ to <50 % in TBI is associated with poor outcome [39].

Other monitoring modalities such as PtO$_2$ inserted either on the injured side or the non-injured side but not directly into the lesion could be an integral part of neuromonitoring. PtO$_2$ detects hypoxic episodes prior to intracranial hypertension and is considered an independent predictor of unfavorable outcome and death.

Treatments to maintain PtO_2 within the normal range were associated with more favorable patient outcomes in traumatic brain injury [40]. Implementation of protocols using PtO_2 monitoring among other parameters such as ICP, CPP and appropriate treatment algorithms are associated with improved resource utilization, improved patient care, reduced duration of mechanical ventilation, and increased ICU hospital discharge [41].

Dos and Don'ts

Dos

- Recognize the intracranial variables that can be monitored at the bedside
- Recognize the advantages and limitations of different monitoring techniques
- Integrate data from different monitoring devices
- Correlate data obtained from multimodal neuromonitoring with the clinical situation of the patient
- Establish therapeutic strategies based on multimodal monitoring
- Evaluate, implement change, reassess

Don'ts

- Don't focus on one monitoring device
- Don't treat just one abnormal value without taking into account the entire situation
- Don't treat a single abnormal reading without checking the device or the patient

References

1. Shimoda M, Takeuchi M, Tominaga J, et al. Asymptomatic versus symptomatic infarcts from vasospasm in patients with subarachnoid hemorrhage; serial magnetic resonance imaging. Neurosurgery. 2001;49:1341–8.
2. Marshall LF, Smith RW, Shapiro HM. The outcome with aggressive treatment in severe head injuries Part I. Significance of intracranial pressure monitoring. J Neurosurg. 1979;50:20–5.
3. Smith M. Monitoring intracranial pressure in traumatic brain injury. Anesth Analg. 2008; 106(1):240–8.
4. Belli A, Sen J, Petzold A, Russo S, Kitchen N, Smith M. Metabolic failure precedes intracranial pressure rises in traumatic brain injury: a microdialysis study. Acta Neurochir. 2008;150(5): 461–9.
5. Sahuquillo J, Poca MA, Arribas M, Garnacho A, Rubio E. Interhemispheric supratentorial intracranial pressure gradients in head-injured patients: are they clinically important? J Neurosurg. 1999;90(1):16–26.

6. Bratton SL, Chestnut RM, Ghajar J, McConnell Hammond FF, Harris OA, Hartl R, et al. Guidelines for the management of severe traumatic brain injury. J Neurotrauma. 2007;24: s1–106.
7. Resnick DK, Marion DW, Carlier P. Outcome analysis of patients with severe head injury and prolonged intracranial hypertension. J Trauma. 1997;42:1108–11.
8. The Brain Trauma Foundation. The American Association of Neurological Surgeons. The joint section on neurotrauma and critical care. Indications for intracranial pressure monitoring. J Neurotrauma. 2000;17:479–91.
9. van Santbrink H, Schouten JW, Steyerberg EW, Avezaat CJ, Maas AI. Serial transcranial Doppler measurements in traumatic brain injury with special focus on the early posttraumatic period. Acta Neurochir. 2002;144(11):1141–9.
10. Rasulo FA, De Peri E, Lavinio A. Transcranial Doppler ultrasonography in intensive care. Eur J Anaesthesiol Suppl. 2008;42:167–73.
11. Moppett IK, Mahajan RP. Transcranial Doppler ultrasonography in an- aesthesia and intensive care. Br J Anaesth. 2004;93(5):710–24.
12. Holbein M, Béchir M, Ludwig S, Sommerfeld J, Cottini SR, Keel M, et al. Differential influence of arterial blood glucose on cerebral metabolism following severe traumatic brain injury. Crit Care. 2009;13(1):R13.
13. Kiening KL, Unterberg AW, Bardt TF, Schneider GH, Lanksch WR. Monitoring of cerebral oxygenation in patients with severe head in- juries: brain tissue PO2 versus jugular vein oxygen saturation. J Neurosurg. 1996;85(5):751–7.
14. Vigué B, Ract C, Benayed M, Zlotine N, Leblanc PE, et al. Early SjvO2 monitoring in patients with severe brain trauma. Intensive Care Med. 1999;25(5):445–51.
15. Chan MT, Ng SC, Lam JM, Poon WS, Gin T. Re-defining the ischemic threshold for jugular venous oxygen saturation – a microdialysis study in patients with severe head injury. Acta Neurochir Suppl. 2005;95:63–6.
16. Gopinath SP, Robertson CS, Contant CF, Hayes C, Feldman Z, Narayan RK, et al. Jugular venous desaturation and outcome after head injury. J Neurol Neurosurg Psychiatry. 1994;57(6):717–23.
17. Nortje J, Gupta AK. The role of tissue oxygen monitoring in patients with acute brain injury. Br J Anaesth. 2006;97:95e106.
18. Rosenthal G, Hemphill 3rd JC, Sorani M, Martin C, Morabito D, Obrist WD, et al. Brain tissue oxygen tension is more indicative of oxygen diffusion than oxygen delivery and metabolism in patients with traumatic brain injury. Crit Care Med. 2008;36(6):1917–24.
19. Jaeger M, Soehle M, Schuhmann MU, Winkler D, Meixensberger J. Correlation of continu- ously monitored regional cerebral blood flow and brain tissue oxygen. Acta Neurochir. 2005;147(1):51–6.
20. Sarrafzadeh AS, Sakowitz OW, Callsen TA, Lanksch WR, Unterberg AW. Bedside microdialy- sis for early detection of cerebral hypoxia in traumatic brain injury. Neurosurg Focus. 2000;9(5):e2.
21. Meixensberger J, Kunze E, Barcsay E, Vaeth A, Roosen K. Clinical cerebral microdialysis: brain metabolism and brain tissue oxygenation after acute brain injury. Neurol Res. 2001;23(8):801–6.
22. Meixensberger J, Renner C, Simanowski R, Schmidtke A, Dings J, Roosen K. Influence of cerebral oxygenation following severe head injury on neuropsychological testing. Neurol Res. 2004;26(4):414–7.
23. Maloney-Wilensky E, Gracias V, Itkin A, Hoffman K, Bloom S, Yang W, et al. Brain tissue oxygen and outcome after severe traumatic brain injury: a systematic review. Crit Care Med. 2009;37(6):2057–63.
24. Highton D, Elwell C, Smith M. Noninvasive cerebral oximetry: is there light at the end of the tunnel? Curr Opin Anaesthesiol. 2010;23:576e81.
25. Tisdall MM, Smith M. Cerebral microdialysis: research technique or clinical tool. Br J Anaesth. 2006;97(1):18–25.

26. Vespa P, Bergsneider M, Hattori N, Wu HM, Huang SC, Martin NA, et al. Metabolic crisis without brain ischemia is common after traumatic brain injury: a combined microdialysis and positron emission tomography study. J Cereb Blood Flow Metab. 2005;25(6):763–74.
27. Reinert M, Barth A, Rothen HU, Schaller B, Takala J, Seiler RW. Effects of cerebral perfusion pressure and increased fraction of inspired oxygen on brain tissue oxygen, lactate and glucose in patients with severe head injury. Acta Neurochir. 2003;145(5):341–9.
28. Nordström CH, Reinstrup P, Xu W, Gärdenfors A, Ungerstedt U. Assessment of the lower limit for cerebral perfusion pressure in severe head injuries by bedside monitoring of regional energy metabolism. Anesthesiology. 2003;98(4):809–14.
29. Marcoux J, McArthur DA, Miller C, Glenn TC, Villablanca P, Martin NA, et al. Persistent metabolic crisis as measured by elevated cerebral microdialysis lactate-pyruvate ratio predicts chronic frontal lobe brain atrophy after traumatic brain injury. Crit Care Med. 2008;36(10): 2871–7.
30. Timofeev I, Carpenter KL, Nortje J, Al-Rawi PG, O'Connell MT, Czosnyka M, et al. Cerebral extracellular chemistry and outcome following traumatic brain injury: a microdialysis study of 223 patients. Brain. 2011;134:484–94.
31. Friedman D, Claassen J. Continuous electroencephalogram monitoring in the intensive care unit. Anesth Analg. 2009;109:506e23.
32. Zentner J, Albrecht T, Heuser D. Influence of halothane, enflurane and isoflurane on motor evoked potentials. Neurosurgery. 1992;32:298–305.
33. Glassman SD, Shields CB, Linden RD. Anesthetic effects on motor evoked potentials in dogs. Spine. 1993;18:1083–9.
34. Kalkman CJ, Drummond JC, Ribberink AA. Effects of propofol, etomidate, midazolam, and fentanyl on motor evoked responses to trascranial electrical or magnetic stimulation in humans. Anesthesiology. 1992;76:502–9.
35. Sloan TB. Evoked potentials. In: Cottrell JE, Smith DS, editors. Anesthesia and neurosurgery. St. Louis: Mosby; 2001. p. 183–200.
36. Carter BG, Butt W. Are somatosensory evoked potentials the best predictor of outcome after severe brain injury? A systematic review. Intensive Care Med. 2005;31(6):765–75.
37. Wright WL. Multimodal monitoring in the ICU: when could it be useful? J Neurol Sci. 2007;261:10–5.
38. De Georgia MA, Deogaonkar A. Multimodal monitoring in the neurological intensive care unit. Neurologist. 2005;11:45–54.
39. Robertson CS, Gopinath SP, Goodman JC, et al. SjvO2 monitoring in head injured patients. J Neurotrauma. 1995;12:891–6.
40. Valadka A, Gopinath S, Contant CF, Uzura M, Robertson CS. Relationship of brain tissue PO$_2$ to outcome after severe head injury. Crit Care Med. 1998;26:1576–81.
41. Coles JP, Fryer TD, Smielewski P, et al. Incidence and mechanism of cerebral ischemia in early clinical head injury. J Cereb Blood Flow Metab. 2004;24:202–11.

Chapter 6
Intracranial Pressure Monitoring

Othman Solaiman and Faisal Al-Otaibi

Introduction

Intracranial pressure (ICP) is a pressure within the cranium that is derived from circulation of cerebral blood, cerebrospinal fluid (CSF), and brain matter. Normal ICP in a supine healthy adult ranges between 7 and 15 mmHg [1]. The ICP increases when compensatory mechanisms that control ICP, such as changes in CSF dynamic, cerebral blood flow (CBF), and cerebral blood volume (CBV), are exhausted. The definition of intracranial hypertension depends on age, body position, and specific pathology; in general, an ICP over 15 mmHg is considered abnormal, and an ICP over 20 mmHg is considered pathological [1]. Most centers use an ICP value of 20 mmHg as the upper limit at which the treatment should be initiated [2].

The most reliable method of ICP monitoring is the use of ventricular catheters [3, 4]. Intraparenchymal, subarachnoid, subdural, and epidural devices can also be used, but these alternatives are less accurate. The advantages of the ventricular catheter are continuous measurement of global ICP, therapeutic drainage of CSF, and administration of drugs such as antibiotics [5]. Sometimes insertion of a ventricular catheter may be difficult due to displacement or compression of ventricles because of brain edema. The potential risks of EVD insertion are increased risk of catheter-related hemorrhage, infection, catheter occlusion from clotted blood, and system malfunction [5].

Although ICP monitoring may not affect the survival rate in traumatic brain injury cases, it was found that ICP monitoring is helpful in guiding ICP-targeted

O. Solaiman, MD, SB-IM, AB-IM (✉)
Department of Critical Care Medicine, King Faisal Specialist
Hospital and Research Centre, Riyadh, Saudi Arabia
e-mail: Omsmd@yahoo.com

F. Al-Otaibi, MD
Division of Neurological Surgery, Department of Neuroscience,
King Faisal Specialist Hospital and Research Centre, Riyadh, Saudi Arabia

© Springer International Publishing Switzerland 2015
K.E. Wartenberg et al. (eds.), *Neurointensive Care: A Clinical Guide
to Patient Safety*, DOI 10.1007/978-3-319-17293-4_6

87

therapy in intensive care units (ICU) [3]. ICP monitoring is used for different disorders associated with increased ICP such as traumatic brain injury, metabolic brain edema, and intracranial hemorrhage; however, it is not without its risks. In this chapter, we shed light on the challenges and pitfalls of ICP monitoring.

Case Scenario

A 30-year-old female was admitted to a Neurocritical care unit with a Fisher 3 grade aneurysmal (anterior communicating artery) subarachnoid hemorrhage. An external ventricular drain (EVD) was inserted due to the presence of communicating hydro-cephalus and brain edema and for ICP management. Afterward, the ICP was ranging between 14 and 18 mmHg with good ICP waves. The following day the patient underwent coil occlusion of the anterior communicating artery aneurysm. Upon arrival at the ICU after the aneurysmal coiling, the ICP was found to be 1 mmHg and some time below zero without evidence of any ICP waves. However, the patient was maintained on sedation without any changes in treatment strategies. The EVD was not opened to drainage because the ICP reading was not high. Fourteen hours later, the patient developed hypertension (BP: 180/100 mmHg) and bilateral dilated pupils. Nevertheless, the ICP ranged between 1 and 5 mmHg. The patient received multiple boluses of 20 % mannitol, hyperventilation, and more intravenous sedation. An emergent cerebral computed tomography (CT) angiogram revealed no vaso-spasm but showed hydrocephalus with diffuse brain edema and effacement of basal cisterns. Immediately, the EVD patency was checked and was found to be blocked. The EVD started to drain CSF after the catheter was irrigated. Afterward, the pupils' size normalized and the ICP was ranging between 8 and 16 mmHg. The patient showed some improvement in her neurological state after 1 week.

On the tenth day of ICU admission, the patient developed high fever (40 °C), and CSF was obtained from the EVD showing 1,500 cells (95 % polymorphonuclear cells). A culture revealed Klebsiella pneumonia. The ventriculitis was treated with intravenous *ceftazidime* and intraventricular *gentamicin* for 14 days. In addition, the catheter was replaced. Subsequently, the fever subsided. Repeated CSF cultures were negative and remained so till the course of antibiotics finished. The patient's clinical symptoms and ICP gradually improved, and the EVD was removed. The patient required placement of a tracheostomy and percutaneous gastrostomy tube during her course in the ICU, and neurological improvement was gradual over 4 months of rehabilitation.

Risks of Patient Safety

Persistent intracranial hypertension causes a significant reduction in cerebral perfu-sion pressure (CPP) and CBF and may lead to secondary brain ischemia and hernia-tion through the tentorial hiatus (the incisura tentorii) or foramen magnum. Many studies reported that an ICP greater than 20 mmHg is strongly associated with a poor outcome in brain injury, particularly if the duration of increased ICP is prolonged [6, 7]. Treggiari et al. reported in a systematic review that, relative to normal ICP (<20 mmHg), raised ICP was associated with an elevated odds ratio (OR) of death: 3.5 (95 % CI: 1.7, 7.3) for ICP 20–40 mmHg, and 6.9 (95 % CI: 3.9, 12.4) for ICP >40 mmHg [8]. Higher but reducible ICP was associated with a three- to four-fold increase in OR of death or poor neurological outcome. A refractory ICP pattern was associated with a dramatic increase in the relative risk of death (OR = 114.3; 95 % CI: 40.5, 322.3). On other hand, outcomes tend to be good in patients with normal ICP [8]. Based on the above, aggressive treatment of high ICP may result in a better overall outcome [9].

Certain clinical trials reported that monitoring of ICP under situations in which ICP may be high either facilitates better outcome or promotes aggressive management [6, 10]. Ventriculostomy coupled with a pressure transducer remains the gold standard for monitoring ICP because of its accuracy and ease of calibration. Access to CSF for dynamic testing and drainage to control ICP are additional benefits. Disadvantages are that catheter placement can be difficult when the ventricles are compressed or shifted from the midline, and the risk of infection rises in ventriculostomies after 5–10 days. Current estimates have associated intraventricular monitoring with less than 2 % hemorrhagic complications and less than 10 % infective complications [11]. In one study, changing the catheter at regular intervals did not appear to reduce the infection rate [12]. Parenchymal monitors, by contrast, have less than 1 % infective complications [13].

Monitoring ICP presents its own challenges, including EVD blockage that may result in inaccurate ICP readings. This particular ICP monitoring of troubleshooting needs to be noted once there is no ICP waveform that is associated with an unusual ICP reading. Similar problems can happen with any other methods of ICP monitoring and can also mislead patient caregivers if not detected early.

Safety Barriers

There are several disorders that require monitoring of ICP, such as severe traumatic brain injury, fulminant hepatic failure, certain cases of intracerebral bleeding, and subarachnoid hemorrhage. The role of monitoring in metabolic encephalopathies, cerebral infarction, or diffuse cerebritis is less clear [14]. CSF can be removed to lower pressure by external drainage through an EVD. This method can be followed by reducing the bulk of the brain by removal of extracellular fluid by the use of osmotherapy such as mannitol. During this type of therapy, serum osmolality must be monitored. In certain groups of patients, vasopressors, hypothermia, and barbiturates may be required.

Despite the benefits of ICP monitoring in guiding the overall management of intracranial hypertension, it is not without risks and practical challenges. The use of EVDs as the gold standard method of monitoring ICP is associated with procedure-related risks. During EVD insertion, hemorrhage might occur at the point of insertion or at the catheter tract [11, 14]. This risk increases in patients with coagulopathy or on anticoagulation agents. ICP monitoring through EVD is considered a closed system that minimizes the chance of infections, but CSF sampling is required for analysis to rule out ongoing EVD-related infections. Theoretically, opening this closed system might be a source of infection. In addition, the length of the EVD use may play a role in increasing the infection rate [15].

There are many types of ICP monitoring technology and methods in addition to EVDs, such as intraparenchymal sensors and subdural sensors. Some ICP monitoring machines can assess brain oxygenation and temperature at the same time. Therefore, optimal knowledge is required and familiarity with all device troubleshooting and practical problems. In any ICP monitoring method, the ICP waves should be seen on the monitor in addition to the reading (Table 6.1, Fig. 6.1). In certain cases EVD blockage can give a false reading without ICP waves. Intraparenchymal sensors are also prone to kinks in the cable that may cause errors in ICP level readings (Table 6.2) [14, 16]. All aforementioned troubleshooting should be noted by the intensivist and coordinated with the neurosurgeons.

Table 6.1 Summary of EVD-ICP monitor troubleshooting in abnormal waves and readings

Assess system for air bubbles
Check system setting
Recalibration
Assess monitor scale
Assess catheter patency
Assess EVD patency by lowering draining system down
Assess for response to jugular vein compression

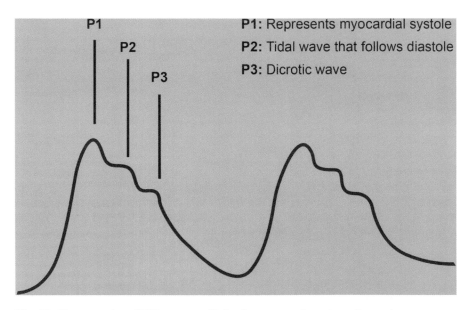

Fig. 6.1 Demonstration of ICP waves oscillation in correspondence to cardiac cycle

Table 6.2 Summary of the main ICP monitoring devices and its advantages and disadvantages

Device	Advantages	Disadvantages
External ventricular drain (EVD)	High accuracy, allows CSF drainage to control ICP "Gold standard"	More invasive than other methods, Difficult to insert in case of severe brain edema and compressed ventricle, Dependent on head level and position, Risk of infection
Intraparenchymal sensor	Less infection rate Not dependent on head position Less bleeding risk	Probe kink Less reliable than EVD High cost Does not allow CSF drainage
Subdural/epidural	Least invasive Quick placement	Less accuracy Low reliability
Subarachnoid bolt	Quick placement ? Less infection rate	Low reliability Frequent recalibration

Discussion of Risk–Benefit Ratio

Monitoring of the ICP is an integral part of Neurocritical care. It is used for the management of patients with severe traumatic brain injury, cerebral infection, fulminant hepatic failure, brain tumors, hydrocephalus, subarachnoid hemorrhage, and stroke [1]. There has been a significant effort in the past 50 years to establish the safety and efficacy of ICP monitoring technology and techniques [17]. In carrying out ICP monitoring, doctors should make sure there is minimal intracranial tissue injury during placement and no CSF leak. ICP monitoring is easy to use, offers a reliable recording of ICP, and can be used continuously during patient transfer for any therapeutic or diagnostic procedure. Based on guidelines for ICP monitoring technology, the maximum error during ICP recording should not exceed 10 %; for example, in a range of 0–20, the recording error should not exceed 2 [18].

Over time, EVD use has remained the gold standard for measuring ICP and the most popular one [1, 18, 19]. The EVD is inserted using an external landmark targeting the anterior lateral ventricle with the tip of the catheter toward the foramen of Monro. The tube is then tunneled under the skin away from the wound to minimize CSF leakage and infection [20]. Ventricular fluid pressure represents ICP. In turn, CSF is transmitted via the fluid-filled EVD to an external transducer that can be connected to many standard ICU monitoring systems. ICP waves are usually seen with monitored heart rate and oxygen saturation. EVDs have the therapeutic advantage of draining CSF and lowering ICP, and they are low-cost and reliable [4]. The complications of EVD placement include malposition, blockage, intracranial bleeding, and infection [14]. Malposition of EVD occurs in 4–20 % of cases [21, 22]. Occlusion of EVD occurs more frequently with cases of subarachnoid hemorrhage and intraventricular hemorrhage [22]. The chance of bleeding from EVD placement is around 1.1 % [23]. The incidence of significant intracranial hemorrhage that requires surgical removal is less than 0.5 % and is related to abnormal coagulation [24]. The most frequent complication of EVD is infection. Lozier and coworkers, in their extensive review of the literature, found an infection range of 0–22 % with a cumulative incidence of 8.8 % [5]. The use of post-EVD implantation prophylactic antibiotics is not recommended by the guidelines for severe traumatic brain injury [25]. Prolonged prophylactic antibiotic use appears to be associated with more aggressive pathogens such as candida and gram negative organisms. Most studies showed that the infection rate increases significantly after 10 days of EVD placement [12]. The location of EVD implantation, whether in the ICU or an operating room, did not affect infection incidence [26]. The use of antibiotic-impregnated EVDs was found to reduce the infection rate from 9.4 to 1.3 % [27]. Intraparenchymal ICP monitoring is an alternative to EVDs that can give high reliability and a low risk rate [28].

Although there is a risk from the use of intracranial monitoring, there is cumulative evidence that high ICP is associated with poor outcomes [7]. In this context, ICP monitoring can guide the treatment of patients with high ICPs [4].

Solutions

ICP monitoring needs to be coordinated between the intensivist and the neurosurgeon to choose the optimal method, whether an EVD or an intraparenchymal-based monitor. To minimize the risk of intracranial bleeding during EVD insertion, coagulation abnormalities need to be corrected [22]. Tunneling the EVD under the scalp away from the entry point wound is a factor that has been found to reduce infection rate [5]. Although there is no strong evidence, replacement of the EVD at day 10 is recommended to minimize infection incidence [12, 25]. Based on a pool of studies, the prolonged use of prophylactic antibiotics is not recommended; instead, using an antibiotic-impregnated EVD is a better solution that may reduce the risk of infection [28]. Moreover, the use of new noninvasive ICP monitoring could be the future way to overcome all invasive ICP monitoring morbidity [29].

The treatment team should be familiar with ICP waves and troubleshooting problems that may arise for technical reasons (Table 6.1). A misleading result can occur due to a blockage or kink in the EVD tube that can be noted and managed by careful assessment of the device. Intensive care nurses need to be familiar with the ICP monitoring device in use to give early alerts so the intensivist can take appropriate action. The intensivist should observe any error in the ICP recording and waves and try to identify the cause of any abnormalities and involve neurosurgeon to solve the problem. Table 6.2 summarizes various ICP monitoring methods and devices.

Summary

Persistent intracranial hypertension causes a significant reduction in CPP and CBF and may lead to secondary brain ischemia and herniation through the tentorial hiatus or foramen magnum. Many studies reported that an ICP greater than 20 mmHg is strongly associated with poor outcomes in brain injury cases, particularly if the duration of increased ICP is prolonged [6]. Knowledge of the ICP monitoring method and devices being used is mandatory to optimize patient safety and minimize risks. The infection rate from ICP monitoring can be reduced by using an antibiotic-impregnated EVD and following the recommended technique during implantation. Furthermore, the use of noninvasive ICP monitoring might prove to be the method that will minimize potential morbidity.

Dos and Don'ts

Dos

- Involve neurosurgery early and coordinate which ICP method and technology will be applied.
- Be familiar with the ICP monitoring device being utilized and how to trouble-shoot it.
- Use an antibiotic-impregnated EVD to reduce the chance of infection.
- Replace EVD at 10 days to help reduce incidence of infection.
- Check for and resolve possible system malfunction indicated by the absence of ICP waves.
- Correct coagulopathy before ICP monitor implantation.
- Noninvasive ICP monitoring can be used.

Don'ts

- Don't rely on the ICP reading when the monitor shows an ICP that is lower than expected, and the monitor does not show an ICP wave.
- Don't use prophylactic antibiotics for a prolonged period after EVD implantation.
- Don't keep an EVD inserted for a prolonged period without replacement.

References

1. Andrews PJ, Citerio G. Intracranial pressure. Part one: historical overview and basic concepts. Intensive Care Med. 2004;30(9):1730–3.
2. Bullock MR, Povlishock JT. Guidelines for the management of severe traumatic brain injury. Editor's Commentary. J Neurotrauma. 2007;24 Suppl 1:2 p preceding S1.
3. Mendelson AA, et al. Intracranial pressure monitors in traumatic brain injury: a systematic review. Can J Neurol Sci. 2012;39(5):571–6.
4. Citerio G, Andrews PJ. Intracranial pressure. Part two: clinical applications and technology. Intensive Care Med. 2004;30(10):1882–5.

5. Lozier AP, et al. Ventriculostomy-related infections: a critical review of the literature. Neurosurgery. 2002;51(1):170–81; discussion 181–2.
6. Saul TG, Ducker TB. Effect of intracranial pressure monitoring and aggressive treatment on mortality in severe head injury. J Neurosurg. 1982;56(4):498–503.
7. Balestreri M, et al. Impact of intracranial pressure and cerebral perfusion pressure on severe disability and mortality after head injury. Neurocrit Care. 2006;4(1):8–13.
8. Treggiari MM, et al. Role of intracranial pressure values and patterns in predicting outcome in traumatic brain injury: a systematic review. Neurocrit Care. 2007;6(2):104–12.
9. Eide PK, et al. A randomized and blinded single-center trial comparing the effect of intracranial pressure and intracranial pressure wave amplitude-guided intensive care management on early clinical state and 12-month outcome in patients with aneurysmal subarachnoid hemorrhage. Neurosurgery. 2011;69(5):1105–15.
10. Schwab S, et al. The value of intracranial pressure monitoring in acute hemispheric stroke. Neurology. 1996;47(2):393–8.
11. Clark WC, et al. Complications of intracranial pressure monitoring in trauma patients. Neurosurgery. 1989;25(1):20–4.
12. Holloway KL, et al. Ventriculostomy infections: the effect of monitoring duration and catheter exchange in 584 patients. J Neurosurg. 1996;85(3):419–24.
13. Pople IK, et al. Results and complications of intracranial pressure monitoring in 303 children. Pediatr Neurosurg. 1995;23(2):64–7.
14. Blei AT, et al. Complications of intracranial pressure monitoring in fulminant hepatic failure. Lancet. 1993;341(8838):157–8.
15. Mayhall CG, et al. Ventriculostomy-related infections. A prospective epidemiologic study. N Engl J Med. 1984;310(9):553–9.
16. Zhong J, et al. Advances in ICP monitoring techniques. Neurol Res. 2003;25(4):339–50.
17. Lundberg N, Troupp H, Lorin H. Continuous recording of the ventricular-fluid pressure in patients with severe acute traumatic brain injury. A preliminary report. J Neurosurg. 1965;22(6): 581–90.
18. Bratton SL, et al. Guidelines for the management of severe traumatic brain injury. VII. Intracranial pressure monitoring technology. J Neurotrauma. 2007;24 Suppl 1:S45–54.
19. O'Neill BR, et al. A survey of ventriculostomy and intracranial pressure monitor placement practices. Surg Neurol. 2008;70(3):268–73; discussion 273.
20. Friedman WA, Vries JK. Percutaneous tunnel ventriculostomy. Summary of 100 procedures. J Neurosurg. 1980;53(5):662–5.
21. Bogdahn U, et al. Continuous-pressure controlled, external ventricular drainage for treatment of acute hydrocephalus–evaluation of risk factors. Neurosurgery. 1992;31(5):898–903; discussion 903–4.
22. Kakarla UK, et al. Safety and accuracy of bedside external ventricular drain placement. Neurosurgery. 2008;63(1 Suppl 1):ONS162-6; discussion ONS166-7.
23. Paramore CG, Turner DA. Relative risks of ventriculostomy infection and morbidity. Acta Neurochir. 1994;127(1–2):79–84.
24. Davis JW, et al. Placement of intracranial pressure monitors: are "normal" coagulation parameters necessary? J Trauma. 2004;57(6):1173–7.
25. Bratton SL, et al. Guidelines for the management of severe traumatic brain injury. IV. Infection prophylaxis. J Neurotrauma. 2007;24 Suppl 1:S26–31.
26. Poon WS, Ng S, Wai S. CSF antibiotic prophylaxis for neurosurgical patients with ventriculostomy: a randomised study. Acta Neurochir Suppl. 1998;71:146–8.
27. Zabramski JM, et al. Efficacy of antimicrobial-impregnated external ventricular drain catheters: a prospective, randomized, controlled trial. J Neurosurg. 2003;98(4):725–30.
28. Munch E, et al. The Camino intracranial pressure device in clinical practice: reliability, handling characteristics and complications. Acta Neurochir. 1998;140(11):1113–9; discussion 1119–20.
29. Ragauskas A, et al. Innovative non-invasive method for absolute intracranial pressure measurement without calibration. Acta Neurochir Suppl. 2005;95:357–61.

Chapter 7
Postoperative Care in Neurooncology

Konstantin A. Popugaev and Andrew Yu Lubnin

Introduction

Almost 41,000 procedures were performed for the treatment of intracranial neoplasms in 2009 in the United States [1]. In spite of the progress in neurosurgery, neurooncology, neuroanesthesiology, and neurocritical care, morbidity and mortality (M&M) remains high [2]. Although morbidity rates range from 9 to 40 % and mortality rates from 1.5 to 16 %, there are no available guidelines for postoperative care after brain tumor (BT) resection [3–5]. This chapter addresses the most common postoperative complications in neurooncology patients and their intensive care. The contemporary approach for choosing optimal tactics for postoperative patient care is provided. The presented material is based on both literature data and our own Burdenko Neurosurgical Research Institute experience with more than 7,000 annual neurosurgical operations and manipulations in patients with BT.

Case Scenario

A patient underwent transsphenoidal resection of giant pituitary adenoma and was successfully extubated after regaining consciousness and adequate spontaneous breathing. Patient received polyhormonal substitutional therapy,

K.A. Popugaev, MD, PhD (✉)
Department of Neurocritical Care, Burdenko Neurosurgical Research Institute, Moscow, Russia
e-mail: Stan.Popugaev@yahoo.com

A.Y. Lubnin, MD, PhD
Department of Neuroanesthesia, Burdenko Neurosurgical Research Institute, Moscow, Russia

© Springer International Publishing Switzerland 2015
K.E. Wartenberg et al. (eds.), *Neurointensive Care: A Clinical Guide to Patient Safety*, DOI 10.1007/978-3-319-17293-4_7

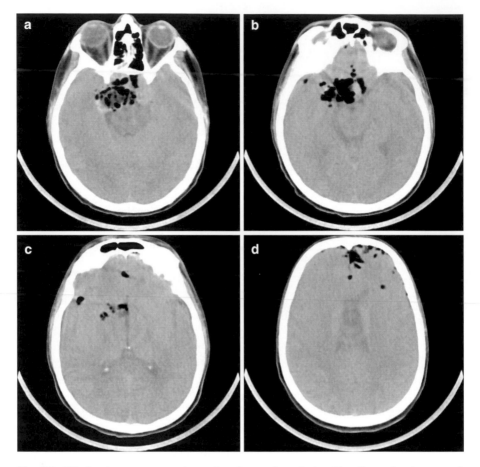

Fig. 7.1 CT, showing common postoperative changes in patients with sellar region tumors and transsphenoidal surgery (Courtesy of Drs. Pavel L. Kalinin and Maxim A. Kutin)

dexamethasone, proton pump inhibitors, antiemetics, analgetics, 24-h of periop-erative prophylactic antibiotic therapy, infusion therapy, and antiepileptic pro-phylactic therapy with valproat at a dose of 20 mg/kg/day. Mean arterial blood pressure (BP) was strictly maintained between 85 and 110 mmHg. Water–electrolyte balance was controlled. He was stable during the next postoperative day; 36 h after the operation he developed drowsiness and respiratory insuffi-ciency (RI). After reintubation, an emergent computerized tomography (CT) was performed and demonstrated only common postoperative changes (cavity after tumor resection, no ischemia, no hematoma, no hydrocephalus) (Fig. 7.1). The electroencephalogram (EEG) showed prolonged generalized epileptiform activ-ity. The plasma valproat level was 53 μg/mL. Emergent initial therapy of noncon-vulsive status epilepticus included intramuscular midazolam (10 mg), and urgent control therapy included increase the valproats dose up to 30 mg/kg/day, and levetiracetam administration at a dose of 25 mg/kg/day. This led to EEG normalization and regain of consciousness. The patient was extubated for the next 3 days and then transferred to the ward.

The presented case raises the question regarding the necessity of prophylactic antiepileptic therapy in patients after BT resection and emphasizes the complexity of managing specific neurocritical care patients with sellar region tumors (SRT). Below we present the most important topics on postoperative care of patients with BTs in different localizations.

Location for Postoperative Care for Neurooncology Patients: Neurocritical Care Unit Versus Recovery Room (RR)

Historically, after elective neurosurgical intervention patients almost always required intensive care [6]. A neurocritical intensive care unit (NICU) is better and safer compared to a non-specialized intensive care unit (ICU) [7, 8]. Therefore, if the patient after BT resection requires intensive care, he should be transferred to an NICU. With the termination of era of dominating conception of postoperative sedation and prolonged mechanical ventilation (MV), the question of whether or not the patients really need to be admitted to an NICU after elective neurosurgery became relevant. If extubated early, many patients remain stable enough to be transferred to the ward after several hours of surveillance. Economic aspects support the idea of early patient discharge from NICU as well. Advanced age, high anesthetic risk, prolonged operation time, extensive blood loss, and other severe intraoperative complications are important factors, which should define patient admission to the NICU [9]. Tumor localization did not directly influence the decision; however, patients with infratentorial resection frequently required NICU hospitalization [9]. It is very important to keep the balance between benefits from short patient stay in the NICU and patient safety. Recovery room (RR) creation became a cornerstone in keeping such a balance [10]. The vast majority of cases of intracerebral hemispheric convexital tumors, neoplasms resected with transsphenoidal approach in the absence of factors, such as prolonged operation time, extensive blood loss, high anesthetic risk, and advanced age do not require an NICU admission. They can be safely transferred to the RR. Surveillance by both the anesthesiologist and neurosurgeon during several postoperative hours allows for a safe decision to transfer patient to the ward. Patients with posterior fossa (PF) tumors, large tumors of any localization, SRT after transcranial resection, and risk factors indicated above need admission to the NICU after tumor resection. NICU admission is required if patient does not wake up sufficiently and cannot be extubated safely in the RR [11].

A complicated postoperative period for which NICU admission is absolutely needed is discussed below. Stable neurooncology patients without postoperative deterioration, who can be safely cared for in the RR and transferred to the ward, are beyond the scope of the chapter.

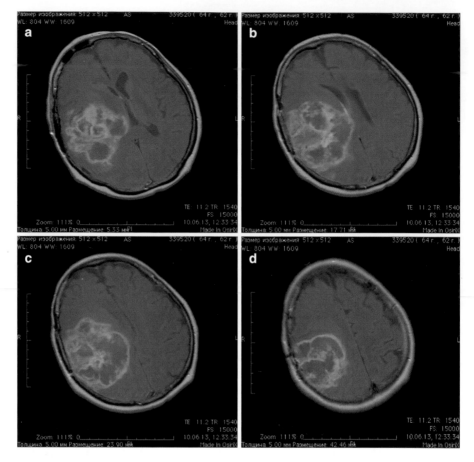

Fig. 7.2 Preoperative MRI of glioblastoma (Courtesy of Dr. Anton G. Gavrilov)

Intracerebral Hemispheric and Convexital Tumors

Almost any type of primary BT and metastasis may be localized in cerebral hemispheres, but glioma, brain metastasis, and convexital meningioma are most frequent types of BT (Fig. 7.2). Typical postoperative complications include new neurologic deficits (NNDs) and seizures [12–14].

Postoperative New Neurologic Deficit (NND)

Delayed awakening, hemiparesis, and aphasia are the forms of NND in patients with intracerebral hemispheric and convexital tumors [13, 14]. NND appearance should be diagnosed as early as possible. In the light of this concept, prolonged postoperative sedation is contraindicated in patients with BT. NND occurrence is a direct indication for an emergency brain CT. Possible causes of NND are direct

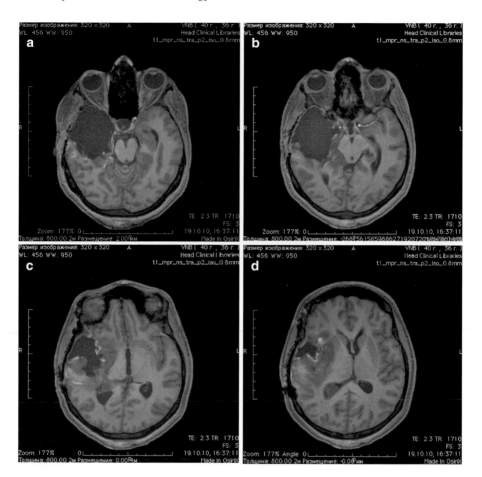

Fig. 7.3 Postoperative MRI of glioma (Courtesy of Dr. Anton G. Gavrilov)

surgical damage of the brain tissue, ischemia, intracranial hemorrhage, or peritumoral edema.

Direct Surgical Damage of the Brain Tissue

Direct surgical damage of the brain tissue in functionally active zones leads to hemiparesis or aphasia. Emergent CT reveals a postoperative defect in the resected tumor bed (Fig. 7.3). Peritumoral edema cannot be distinctly differentiated from the postoperative defects. Discrimination between the direct surgical damage of the brain tissue and brain ischemia due to microcirculation disturbance is very difficult and almost impossible without magnetic resonance imaging (MRI) [13]. Although postoperative ischemia is more likely to be the cause of motor NND, both direct surgical damage of the brain tissue and microcirculation disturbances can also be present, but differentiation between them does not influence the intensivist management. The patient can be safely extubated and discharged to the neurosurgical ward. Active rehabilitation can improve functional outcomes in these patients [15].

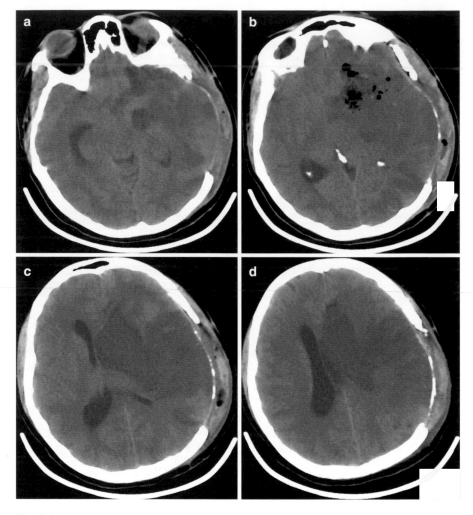

Fig. 7.4 Postoperative CT, showing ischemic infarction after glioma resection (Courtesy of Dr. Anton G. Gavrilov)

Brain Ischemia

Brain ischemia due to perioperative damage of perforating arteries, arteries of Willis circle, deep veins, venous sinuses, and paradoxical venous air embolism (PVAE) disturbance results in much more severe deficits compared to impaired microcirculation.

Perioperative damage of the arteries leads to an acute ischemic stroke (Fig. 7.4). Combination of the nature of postoperative NND with the intraoperative data about surgical damage of the arteries should result in a conclusion about the etiology of the ischemia, even if the emergency CT does not reveal any zones of ischemia. Otherwise, inadequate delay in the intensive care leads to an irreversible brain damage of the penumbra [16]. Main therapy should be performed in accordance to the recent guidelines for early management of patients with ischemic stroke, published in 2013 [17]. However, there are some important concerns dictated by the specific patients' characteristics in the early period after BT resection. Invasive BP monitoring should be started immediately. In neurosurgical intensive care, mean BP is preferable as a monitored goalpost, because it is required for the calculation of such a cornerstone parameter as cerebral perfusion pressure (CPP) (difference between mean BP and intracranial pressure (ICP)). During three postoperative days, mean BP should be maintained above 75 mmHg [18]. On the other hand, postoperative arterial hypertension is an established cause of the intracranial hemorrhage, especially if it occurs during first six postoperative hours [19]. It seems that 90–100 mmHg is a maximally safe level for mean BP, depending on other clinical conditions; however, studies dedicated to this topic do not exist. Another concern is the administration of anticoagulants and antiplatelet agents. As opposed to the acute ischemic stroke guidelines, both antiplatelet agents and low-molecular-weight heparins (LMWH) are contraindicated during 48 h after the surgery. Antiplatelet agents are not routinely used in the neurosurgical practice during the whole duration of the early postoperative period [20]. LMWH can be used 48 h after the surgery in the prophylactic dose, because the patients with BT are at high risk for thromboembolism [20].

In cases of the malignant ischemia with severe edema, midline shift and axial dislocation effective intensive care are impossible without ICP monitoring. General principles of the intracranial hypertension correction are not different from the wide-accepted Columbia step-wise protocol [21].

Venous Cerebral Infarction

Venous cerebral infarction due to the perioperative occlusion of deep veins or venous sinuses is a much less frequent complication in patients with BT (Fig. 7.5). If secondary hemorrhage into the ischemia zone does not occur, CT would reveal brain edema [22]. ICP monitoring shows intracranial hypertension, usually resistant to first line therapy conducted in accordance with the step-wise Columbia protocol. In such cases, only hypothermia, decompressive craniotomy, or both can stabilize intracranial hypertension and save the patient's life [23].

Paradoxical Venous Air Embolism (PVAE)

Paradoxical venous air embolism (PVAE) is a rare complication, which requires a special discussion, because only prompt and correct therapeutic strategy can improve the patient's outcome. Venous air embolism (VAE) is an intraoperative complication, and outcome is usually favorable if the air does not pass through the pulmonary vasculature into the systemic circulation [24, 25]. If this occurs, PVAE develops. There are two main causes of PVAE: a patent foramen ovale, which is described in almost 25 % of the adults [26], and the transpulmonary air passage via bronchial arterial anastomoses, if its volume exceeds 50 mL per minute [27]. Massive cerebral air embolism leads to the diffuse ischemic brain injury, because cerebral arterioles are blocked by the air bubbles (Fig. 7.6). Postoperative NND develops. An emergent CT several hours after the surgery can miss these abnormalities, because the formation of CT signs of ischemia is a time-dependent process. There are only two effective therapeutic modalities: hyperbaric oxygenation and hypothermia [28]. These methods should be performed as early as possible. Delayed initiation or failure to implement these methods leads to irreversible ischemic brain

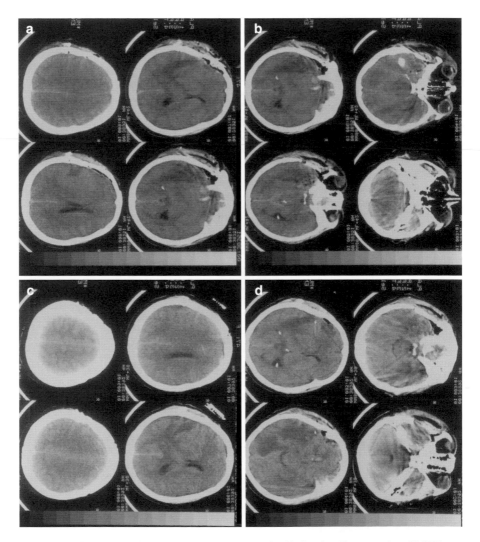

Fig. 7.5 Early postoperative CT, showing venous cerebral infarction (four scans) and MRV, performed 6 weeks thereafter showing absence of blood flow in the left transverse and sigmoid sinuses (last scan)

Fig. 7.5 (continued)

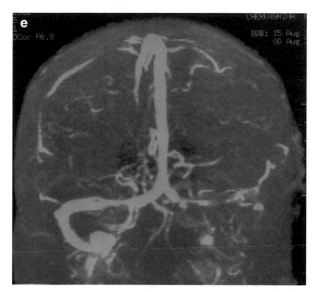

damage, severe resistant NND, and poor outcomes [28]. Therefore, only intensivist awareness of PVAE in combination with thorough analysis of the clinical picture, the data of neurovisualization, the surgical protocol, and the anesthesiologist report can help to suspect this complication and to make a correct decision.

Intracranial Hemorrhage

Epidural and subdural hematomas, hemorrhage into a bed of the resected tumor, or intracerebral hemorrhage far from the resected tumor bed should be diagnosed as early as possible with an emergent CT (Fig. 7.7). In the majority of these cases, the development of the intracranial hemorrhage is a direct indication for revision and hematoma evacuation. An exception can be made for a hematoma in the resected tumor bed, when it is lesser in volume than the resected tumor and peritumoral edema is not larger compared to the preoperative state. Usually ICP monitoring is not needed, if hematoma evacuation was successfully performed and the patient is awake after the revision.

Peritumoral Brain Edema

Severe edema usually develops around both the malignant BTs (glioblastoma, metastasis) and the meningioma [12]. In practice, peritumoral edema does not lead to postoperative NND or intracranial hypertension due to two main reasons [29]. First is the performed inner decompression due to the tumor resection. Second is the usage of dexamethasone, which is effective in decreasing the amount of edema in

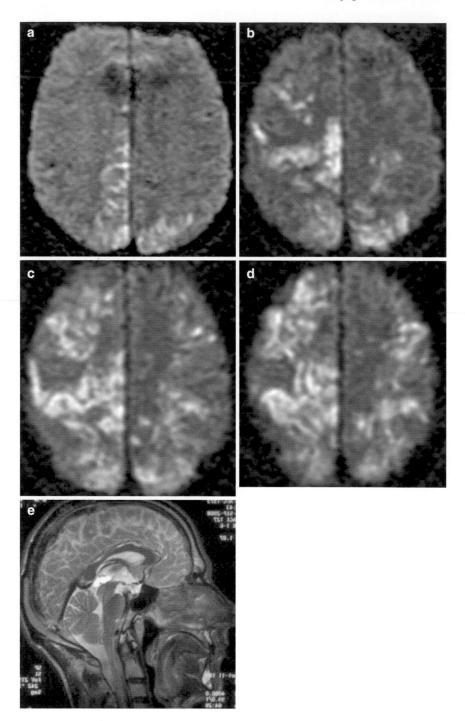

Fig. 7.6 Postoperative MRI (DWI) of a patient with paradoxical venous air embolism (four scans), developed during pineal cyst resection (last scan – preoperative MRI) (Courtesy of Dr. David I. Pitshelauri)

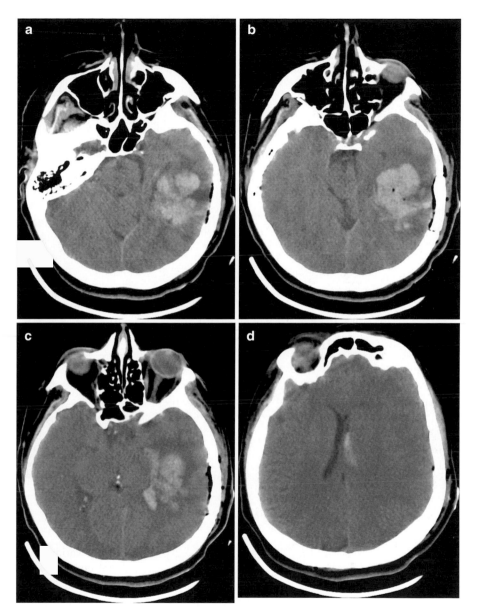

Fig. 7.7 Postoperative CT, showing hematoma of tumor bed (Courtesy of Drs. David I. Pitshelauri and Anton G. Gavrilov)

cases with malignant tumors. The dose of dexamethasone differs from case to case and ranges from 4 to 40 or even 100 mg per day intravenously [30]. Proton pump inhibitors and blood glucose control should be always administered as an obligatory medication together with dexamethasone.

Seizures

Patients with preoperative epilepsy must receive their anti-epileptic drugs (AEDs) postoperatively in the effective doses [14]. Typical preoperative AEDs are phenytoin, carbamazepine, valproate, or their combination [12]. Receiving an AED therapy does not guarantee the absence of postoperative seizures [14]. Therefore, continuous EEG monitoring should be performed immediately along with an emergent CT every time when seizures or decreased level of consciousness occur postoperatively. Postoperative seizures, including convulsive and non-convulsive status epilepticus, develop in 13–60 % of patients with BT [31, 32]. Early seizure verification and implementation of treatment improves the treatment results [12], and should be performed in the strict accordance with the recent guidelines [33].

The question of prophylactic use of AED postoperatively in patients without preoperative epilepsy remains unanswered. There are a lot of studies which advocate both strategies [34–36]. Pathophysiological studies with microdialysis revealed high glutamate concentration in peritumoral edema fluid, which triggered epileptogenesis and represented a predisposing factor for the occurrence of postoperative seizures [37, 38]. Clinical studies concluded that the patient needs prophylactic AED administration if the tumor has invaded the cortex and is located in the areas of high epileptogenicity [12]. In reality, the majority of neurosurgeons administrate prophylactic AED [35]. This strategy seems quite reasonable, especially in the light of the presence of AEDs with few side effects, such as levetiracetam [39]. Important concern applies to the adequate dosing of any AEDs [40]. The best way to select the appropriate, individualized dose of AED is the measurement of the plasma level of the medication [41]. The duration of prophylactic AED therapy is another disputable question. Five or seven days of prophylactic postoperative AED treatment in patients with intracerebral hemispheric and convexital tumors is a reasonable approach, based on the experience in patients with severe subarachnoid hemorrhage (SAH) or traumatic brain injury (TBI) [36, 42, 43]. Early postoperative seizures are a significant risk factor for the late postoperative seizures, which considerably worsen the quality of life and the outcome [14]. Therefore, prophylactic therapy of early seizures may not only improve the patient's safety during the early postoperative period but also lead to the improvement of patient's quality of life during the late postoperative period.

Posterior Fossa Tumors

Almost any type of primary BT and metastasis may be localized in the PF, but acoustic neuroma, meningioma, glioma, ependymoma, and medulloblastoma are the most frequent histological types (Fig. 7.8). A tumor may grow from the cerebellum, cerebellopontine angle, or from any layer of the brain stem – tectum, tegmentum, basis, as well. It also may spread to the PF from the spinal cord, thalamus, pineal, or sellar region. There are several anatomical factors which influence the

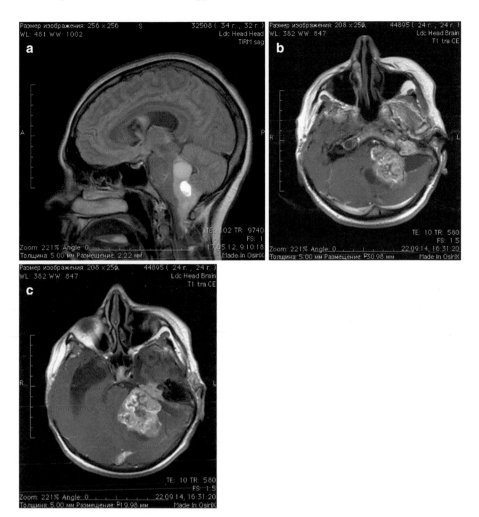

Fig. 7.8 Posterior fossa tumors. (**a**) Ependymoma. (**b, c**) acoustic neuroma (Courtesy of Dr. Anton G. Gavrilov)

development of the postoperative complications. The PF contains the brain stem – a unique structure, which holds ascending and descending sensorimotor pathways, nuclei of all the cranial nerves, the reticular activating system, the neural networks sustaining extremely important reflexes as coughing, swallowing, and cardiorespiratory regulatory centers in a very narrow cavity with limited volume surrounded by bones and the tentorium. The PF contains the narrowest parts of the ventricular system – the forth ventricle and the cerebral aqueduct. Keeping in mind all these factors allows intensivists to provide maximum safety for patients with PF tumors during the postoperative care.

PF contains the brain stem, which is a unique structure. This fact found an interesting clinical reflection in a recent study, published in 2014, which showed that infratentorial neurosurgery is an independent risk factor for RI and death in patients undergoing tumor resection [44]. It clearly demonstrates extremely high importance of the problem of RI and timely reintubation in patients with PF tumors in the postoperative period. Possible causes of RI are direct surgical, ischemic, or hemorrhagic damage of the brainstem [45]. Every time when RI, dysphagia, or decreased level of consciousness develops in the postoperative period, emergent CT should be performed immediately after securing airway and breathing, because inadequate spontaneous breathing is a very reliable sign of perioperative brainstem damage. Even small hematomas in the PF need to be surgically evacuated. Regardless of the cause of RI, incorrect airway management is one of the most significant factors that define M&M in patients with PF tumors [44]. In other words, the correct airway management would considerably increase patient's safety and improve outcome.

Possible causes of RI are (a) bulbar palsy with swallowing and coughing disturbances (damage of nuclei or IX–XII nerves' roots or corticobulbar tracts), (b) damage of the respiratory center, (c) reticular formation injury with decline of consciousness, (d) a combination of these reasons [46]. Thorough evaluation of the intubated patient for assessment of their readiness for spontaneous breathing is impossible because (1) intubated patients are usually sedated and the true level of consciousness is not always clear; (2) they are not able to swallow adequately due to the pain and the discomfort; (3) the cough reflex is impaired by the ET tube, which impedes the glottic closure, the so-called "cough without glottic closure" [47, 48]. On the other hand, the patient should be extubated as early as possible, immediately after meeting the criteria for extubation [49]. Otherwise the length of time on MV and the ICU stay might extend, the rates of pneumonia might increase, and the outcome could worsen. There are no criteria or scales that reliably predict the success of extubation [50]. The rate of extubation failures remains high, especially in the neurocritical care population which emphasizes the inability of correct prognostication of the extubation success or failure [51]. Therefore, the main concern about patient's safety shifts to the postextubation period when the correct decision should be made – to reintubate or not to reintubate. For this purpose, the Burdenko Respiratory Insufficiency Scale (BRIS) was developed [52] (Table 7.1). It can objectify the patient's status and help to make a correct decision.

BRIS consists of three parts: (1) assessment of the mental status with Richmond agitation sedation scale (RASS); (2) evaluation of the swallowing, cough, and airway patency based on the previously reported protocols [53]; (3) measurement of pO_2/FiO_2 index. Each part gets an independent score from 0 to 4, and then the scores of each individual section are added to a sum. Scoring is increased by 1 point with obesity because it has negative impact on the respiratory function [54]. Minimal total score is 0 (healthy person), maximal total score is 12 in a patient with normal weight and 13 in an obese patient. BRIS parts begin with a normal criterion (normal consciousness, independent swallowing, effective cough, preserved airway patency, and normal pO_2/FiO_2 index) and ends with criteria of the extreme degree of pathology: comatose state or deep sedation, severe lung injury with index pO_2/FiO_2 less 200, impaired airway patency with ineffective cough, and aspiration for two or more food consistencies. Every condition taken separately is a standard indication for the

Table 7.1 BRIS: Burdenko Respiratory Insufficiency Scale

	Score 0	Score 1	Score 2	Score 3	Score 4
Mental status	RASS 0 or consciousness	RASS −1/+1 or hypersomnia	RASS −2/+2 or obtundation	RASS −3-4/+3 + 4 or stupor	RASS −5 or coma
Swallowing, cough, airway patency	Independent swallowing, effective cough, normal airway patency	Independent swallowing, ineffective cough, normal airway patency	Slight aspiration of liquids, effective cough, normal airway patency	Aspiration for 2 or more food constituents, ineffective cough, normal airway patency	Aspiration for 2 or more food constituents, ineffective cough, impaired airway patency
Index pO_2/FiO_2	>300	250–300	220–250	200–220	<200

Scoring is increased by 1 in patients with obesity (body mass index >30)

RASS Richmond Agitation Sedation Scale

intubation and MV. Therefore, if the patient has 4 in any part of BRIS, he must be intubated and ventilated immediately. However, there are a lot of intermediate clinical situations when patients have different combinations of the alteration of consciousness, swallowing disorders, cough impairment, loss of airway control, and lung injury. In this situation, intubation is based on the expert opinion of the intensivist. BRIS has been developed for the standardization of indications for intubation. A BRIS score of 3 or less means that the patient can breathe spontaneously, however, enteral feeding via nasogastric tube may be needed if cough and swallowing are impaired. A BRIS score of 4 as sum points of all three parts of BRIS, but not as a point of any part of BRIS, is still a grey zone. Some patients with a BRIS score of 4 require intubation and MV, but some patients will successfully keep adequate spontaneous breathing during their stay in intensive care and will be discharged to the ward. Perhaps there are some additional factors which determine the patient's ability to breathe spontaneously which BRIS does not take into consideration.

PF is a small cavity with the limited volume surrounded by bones and the tentorium. Even small hematomas or not very pronounced edema due to ischemia or intraoperative brain retraction may lead to intracranial hypertension in the PF compartment. Routinely monitored supratentorial ICP is usually normal. If there is blockage of the aqueduct or forth ventricle, a transtentorial ICP gradient will occur [55, 56]. Consequently, the patients will develop neurological deficits such as consciousness decline and focal brainstem symptoms. Those appear in spite of normal supratentorial ICP. A decision in management based on supratentorial ICP monitoring is incorrect and leads to wrong decisions and patient management.

PF has the narrowest parts of ventricular system. Small additional volume in PF easily leads to ventricular system occlusion and rapid development of hydrocephalus. The clinical picture includes signs of the intracranial hypertension as severe headache, nausea, vomiting, head extension forced position, decerebrate posturing, and declined consciousness. After prompt neuroimaging, emergent external ventriculostomy must be done [57]. Fast and excessive cerebrospinal fluid (CSF) diversion can be a cause of another serious and vitally dangerous complication – brain dislocation and upward tentorial herniation [58]. Controlled CSF diversion is the only method for the effective prophylaxis of this complication [59].

Sellar Region Tumors (SRT)

Pituitary adenoma, craniopharyngioma, and parasellar meningioma are the most frequent tumors of this localization (Fig. 7.9). The sellar region is difficult to approach [60, 61]. With the development of the endoscopic transsphenoidal surgery, the number of approach-related complications has considerably decreased. Nowadays, almost all histological types of SRT can be successfully resected using the transsphenoidal approach [62, 63]. Thus, SRT surgery became much safer during the last two decades. This statement is absolutely true for the small-to-medium-size tumors with infrasellar, laterosellar, and anterosellar growth. However, surgery

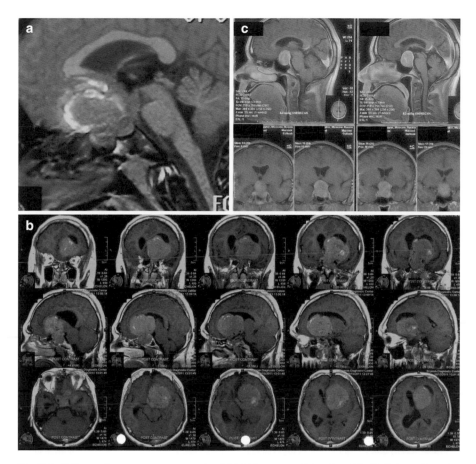

Fig. 7.9 Sellar region tumors, preoperative MRI (Courtesy of Drs. Pavel L. Kalinin and Maxim A. Kutin)

of the large tumors which are invading the suprasellar structures and the resection of craniopharyngiomas, which almost always are extending to the suprasellar region, still demonstrate the high risk of postoperative complications due to the damage of the diencephalon [64, 65]. Another serious problem for the patients with SRT is postoperative meningitis [65].

Damage of the Diencephalon

The diencephalon consists of the thalamus, hypothalamus, epithalamus, subthalamus, and the pituitary gland [66]. The thalamus as part of the diencephalon provides the primary precortical analysis of the information accepted by all the sensitive analyzers except the olfactory system. The hypothalamus is the highest center of the

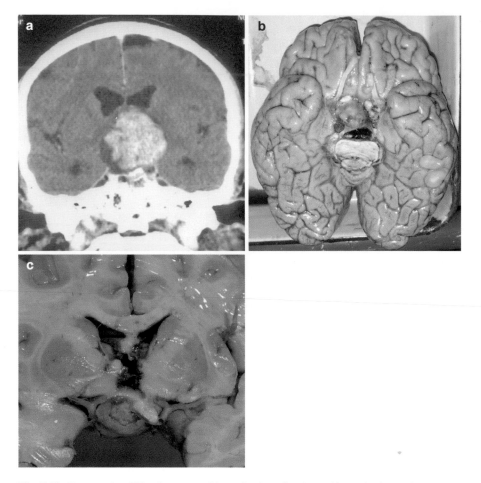

Fig. 7.10 Preoperative CT and postmortal investigation of patient with craniopharyngioma, postoperative diencephalon damage, and postoperative severe diencephalon dysfunction syndrome (Courtesy of Dr. Maxim A. Kutin)

autonomic nervous system and the endocrine regulation. It provides the homeostasis, regulates the vital organ functions, and coordinates the endocrine, nervous, and immune systems. The epithalamus controls the autonomic functions, emotions, and the sleep–wake cycle. The subthalamus takes part in the extrapyramidal regulation of movements. The pituitary gland secrets all tropic hormones, contains vasopressin, oxytocin, and melatonin. Therefore, the diencephalon is a relatively small area with the highest concentration of vitally important centers of the entire brain. Therefore, any type of local perioperative damage, such as a direct surgical injury of diencephalon, ischemic or hemorrhagic lesions, or intraoperative traction and coagulation during the SRT resection, leads to the diencephalic dysfunction (Fig. 7.10). Conception of the diencephalon dysfunction syndrome (DDS) in patients with SRT was recently created [67]. DDS consists of dysnatremia, alterations of consciousness, and at least one somatic organ dysfunction (OD).

Dysnatremia

Dysnatremia is the most typical and widely discussed complication of the SRT surgery [64, 65, 68]. All patients with SRT and a complicated postoperative period, who need intensive care longer than 24 h, have dysnatremia [67]. The perioperative impairment of hypothalamus and pituitary gland function in patients with SRT defines the rates of dysnatremia. Postoperative hypernatremia (Na > 145 mmol/L) develops in up to 75–90 % of patients [69, 70]. The main cause of hypernatremia is diabetes insipidus (DI), which leads to the excessive fluid loss and hypovolemia. Therefore, the patients with DI require timely and adequately substantial usage of desmopressin acetate and sodium-free fluid replacement according to their free water deficit. Otherwise, hypovolemia leads to arterial hypotension and hypoperfusion of the peritumoral zone in the early postoperative period. Postoperative hyponatremia (Na < 135 mmol/L) develops in up to 35 % of patients [71–73]. It can be moderate (Na = 134–125 mmol/L) or severe (Na < 125 mmol/L); acute, which develops with 72 h postoperatively, or late, more than 72 h postoperatively [74]. Severe hyponatremia may result in coma, seizures, and unfavorable outcome. Sodium correction rates must be limited by 6–8 mmol/L per day for late hyponatremia because rapid sodium increase leads to a severe and potentially lethal complication – pontine or extrapontine myelinolysis [74]. The differential diagnosis of hyponatremia encompasses the syndrome of inappropriate secretion of antidiuretic hormone (SIADH), the cerebral salt wasting syndrome (CSWS), or adrenal insufficiency (AI). Their main pathophysiological difference is the volume status. SIADH leads to hyper- or normovolemia, whereas both CSWS and AI are causes of hypovolemia [68, 71]. This discrepancy defines the management. In SIADH, the fluids should be restricted, and vaptans are cardinally indicated, whereas the infusion for fluid replacement and glucocorticoids and mineralocorticoids are needed for the patients with CSWS and AI. Hypertonic solutions are indicated for CSWS and AI, but should be avoided in SIADH. Only severe hyponatremia in comatose or epileptic patients with SIADH should be treated with hypertonic saline.

Postoperative Glucocorticoid Therapy

The combination of intravenous dexamethasone and hydrocortisone is advocated in patients with SRT [75]. Dexamethasone, an anti-edema drug, should be tapered relatively fast, during 5–7 postoperative days [12, 76]. This strategy can maximally protect the patient from the adrenal depression and development of primary AI. The opposite approach is recommended for hydrocortisone. The postoperative dose should be at least 150–200 mg per day [76]. Unstable patient conditions require higher doses of hydrocortisone. The hydrocortisone dose can be increased up to 1,200 mg per day [77]. The correct dose of hydrocortisone should be chosen on the individual basis in accordance with sodium, potassium, and glucose levels as well as BP, temperature, and several other clinical and laboratory parameters [75]. The correct hydrocortisone dose is one of the cornerstone issues of postoperative care in patients with SRT and a complicated postoperative period. Incorrect hydrocortisone usage in these patients makes a successful recovery almost impossible.

Consciousness Alterations (CA)

Consciousness alterations develop in all patients with SRT and a complicated postoperative period [67]. Coma develops rarely, but delirium is the prevailed disorder of consciousness. Like in other groups of critical care patients, hypoactive and mixed types of delirium are the most frequent types [78]. However, the most common complication of SRT patients is the high rate of the convulsive and nonconvulsive seizures [67]. Aggressive anticonvulsant therapy may improve consciousness and the outcome.

Organ Dysfunction

Since the hypothalamus is the highest center of the autonomic nervous system which regulates the function of almost all vital organs, perioperative diencephalic damage may lead to multi-OD. In spite of the clearness of this fact, an extremely small amount of studies dedicated to postoperative OD in patients with SRT are available [79]. Cardiovascular, RI, and ileus are the most frequent types of OD.

Postoperative Cardiovascular Insufficiency

Postoperative cardiovascular insufficiency in patients with SRT may have several reasons, among which the commonest are acute adrenal or thyroid insufficiency, hypopituitarism, hypovolemia in cases with the decompensated DI, or direct diencephalic injury [80]. SRT is the cause for the endocrine pathology, and postoperative polyhormonal substitutional therapy is always needed in all cases with a complicated postoperative period, even the in the absence of endocrine disturbances before the surgery. Hydrocortisone, levothyroxine, and desmopressin acetate are the obligate medications. Hydrocortisone doses were discussed above. Levothyroxine should be administrated intravenously at a dose of 2–3 mcg/kg per day [76]. Desmopressin is used in accordance with the fluid balance and the sodium plasma level. Thereby, the combination of hydrocortisone, levothyroxine, and desmopressin in adequate doses is able to prevent the cardiovascular instability due to adrenal, thyroid insufficiency, hypopituitarism, and hypovolemia. Ignorance of postoperative polyhormonal substitutional therapy is dangerous for patients with SRT and complicated postoperative period.

Cardiovascular insufficiency due to the perioperative direct diencephalic injury is a rarely discussed issue. Diencephalic damage can be a real and immediate cause of arterial hypotension due to severe decrease of vascular resistance [80]. The verified mechanism of the arterial hypotension led to the recommendation of administration of alpha-adrenomimetics (norepinephrine, phenylephrine) as vasoactive agents of choice. The occurrence of bradycardia during the infusion of alpha-adrenomimetics may be secondary to a non-compensated thyroid insufficiency [80]. Both thyroid hormones dose increase and temporal administration of beta-sympathomimetics increase the heart rate. Gradual beta-sympathomimetics tapering is possible after thyroid saturation and correction of thyroid insufficiency [80].

Another important issue for patient's safety is the level of optimal BP. This topic is widely discussed in the wide spectrum of neurocritical care patients except SRT patients. The optimal BP in patients with SRT and the complicated postoperative period can be selected using jugular vein oxygen saturation monitoring. Otherwise, mean BP should be maintained at the upper level of normal, which is between 95 and 110 mmHg [81].

Respiratory Insufficiency (RI)

Respiratory insufficiency is another important complication in patients with SRT. Neurogenic pulmonary edema is hypothetically a possible complication for the patients with diencephalic injury following a sympathetic surge, given the fact that the diencephalon is the highest autonomic center. However, practically this particular complication is extremely rare. *Ileus* is a serious clinical problem for neurocritical care patients, but there are no available studies dedicated to the problem in patients with SRT. In spite of the adequate thyroid replacement dose, ileus is a common complication and a significant risk factor for intraabdominal hypertension [82]. Intraabdominal hypertension and abdominal compartment syndrome should be treated as an emergency [83]. Thoracic epidural anesthesia seems to be a reliable method for intraabdominal pressure correction in patients with SRT, if conservative intensive care methods have failed [82].

Therefore, DDS that consists of dysnatremia, CA, and, at least, one OD is a severe condition that requires a multimodal approach for its successful correction. The amount of OD defines the severity of DDS and the outcome.

Postoperative Meningitis

Postoperative meningitis is another serious problem for SRT patients. Transsphenoidal surgery is a relatively sterile surgery associated with many risk factors for meningitis: intraoperative and postoperative CSF leak, spinal and ventricular external drainages, revision of the postoperative wound for defects of the skull-base plastics with the postoperative CSF leaks [64, 65, 84, 85]. Frequent disconnection of the CSF diversion system and intraventricular injections of medications are other significant risk factors for meningitis [86]. There is no effective prophylactic antibiotic regimen available to decrease meningitis rates. Several prophylactic measures may be effective: durable intraoperative skull-base plastics, prevention of postoperative CSF leaks, shortage of the duration of CSF drainage, aseptic approach to the drainage management with decreased number of the system disconnection for obtaining CSF samples or injection of medications [our own unpublished data]. In patients with transcranial resection of suprasellar tumors, postoperative meningitis is a rare phenomenon. CSF collection under the cutaneous flap in the area of the surgical approach is the only significant risk factor for meningitis [our own unpublished data].

Special Issues of Postoperative Care

Pain, postoperative nausea, and vomiting (PONV), and residual neuromuscular blockade (RNMB) are the important issues, which should be kept in mind during postoperative intensive care management. All these conditions can lead to the arterial hypertension, which contributes to the development of early postoperative hematomas [87].

There are no generally accepted protocols for postoperative analgesia in neurosurgical practice. Pain assessment is the cornerstone and is very difficult in unconscious, aphasic, delirious, or disoriented patients, in whom the pain intensity numeric rating scale cannot be applied, which is a gold standard in pain assessment [88]. Therefore, in neurocritical care settings, pain can be precisely evaluated in consciousness patients only. Local and regional anesthetics applied to the incision site are the reliable methods of postoperative pain control [89]. These kinds of anesthesia are a part of the so-called "pre-emptive analgesia," which may be effective. This management principle also includes the usage of non-steroidal anti-inflammatory drugs (NSAID) and NMDA antagonists [90]. At the same time, NSAIDs and acetaminophen alone as well as codeine-based analgesia are ineffective [91, 92]. Systemic opioids provide effective analgesia, but cannot be recognized as the optimal analgetics for the patients with BT and a complicated postoperative period due to a lot of side effects: nausea, vomiting, cognitive impairment, respiratory depression, urinary retention, constipation, dependence, and tolerance [93]. Dexmedetomidine as a continuous and titratable infusion modulates the pain perception and can be suitable for postoperative sedation.

Postoperative nausea and vomiting (PONV) after craniotomy develops in up to 70 % of patients, and does not only cause discomfort, arterial hypertension and increased risk of aspiration, but also intracranial hypertension, fluid–electrolytes disturbances, and acid–base imbalance [94, 95]. The combination of dexamethasone and $5HT_3$ or Neurokinin (NK)-1 receptors antagonists reduces the rates of PONV [96]. Additional administration of metoclopramide, droperidol, or gabapentin can be effective as well [95, 97]. These strategies decrease the incidence of PONV, but do not eliminate it completely. PONV has a specific significance for the neurosurgical patients, because it can be a clinical sign of intracranial hypertension with dislocation of brain structures, especially in the PF. Combination of PONV and delayed arousal with or without posturing and focal neurologic symptoms such as anisocoria and mydriasis are indications for an emergent CT.

Non-depolarizing muscle relaxants (RNMB) are routinely used during BT resection to ensure optimal surgical conditions. RNMB leads to delayed awakening, which may be caused by a number of reasons as well [98]. Unnecessary transportation to CT during the early postoperative period is undesirable, because even short intrahospital transport of the neurosurgical patient increases the risk of different complications [99]. Therefore, intensivists should be aware of RNMB and apply train of four (TOF) monitoring in the perioperative period in order to assess the depth of neuromuscular blockade.

Summary

Patients with BT and a complicated postoperative period constitute a very specific neurocritical care population. Some diagnostic, therapeutic, and prognostic approaches can be fully accepted from the guidelines and principles, which are used in other neurocritical care cohorts. However, there are some unique groups, like patients with SRT or PF tumors, who urgently need specific guidlines for management of tumor surgery specific complications. Cases with BT and a complicated postoperative period present the so-called "mono-level brain injury model." Thorough investigation of these models not only helps to better understand the patients with multi-level brain injury, like patients with TBI and SAH, but also enforces the creation of new concepts.

Dos and Don'ts

Dos

- If the patient after BT resection needs intensive care, he should be cared for in a neurocritical care unit.
- New neurologic deficit occurrence is a direct indication for emergency CT.
- During the early postoperative period, mean BP should be maintained between 75 and 100 mmHg.
- Peritumoral edema should be treated with dexamethasone.
- EEG monitoring should be performed if postoperative consciousness alterations occur.

- Start prophylactic antiepileptic drugs if the tumor invaded the cortex or is localized in epileptogenic areas.
- Pay maximum attention on airway management in patients after resection of posterior fossa tumors.
- Use Burdenko Respiratory Insufficiency Scale for making decisions about the need for reintubation.
- Perform emergent external ventriculostomy in occlusive hydrocephalus that can be developed due to an even small additional volume in the posterior fossa.
- Use a combination of dexamethasone and hydrocortisone in patients with sellar region tumors and a complicated postoperative period.
- Recognize the diencephalon dysfunction syndrome for patients with sellar region tumors and a complicated postoperative period.
- Use thoracic epidural anesthesia for severe ileus in patients with sellar region tumors.

Don'ts

- Routine prolonged postoperative sedation should be avoided.
- Avoid both arterial hypotension and hypertension in patients with a complicated postoperative period.
- Avoid both antiplatelet agents and low-molecular-weight heparins during 48 h after the surgery.
- Avoid risk of aspiration in patients with dysphagia after resection of fossa posterior tumors.
- Supratentorial pressure does not correlate with infratentorial pressure in patients with infratentorial hematoma or edema. Don't assume the absence of intracranial hypertension in patients after posterior fossa tumor surgery and normal supratentoral ICP.
- Avoid fast and excessive cerebral spinal fluid diversion in patients with occlusive hydrocephalus.
- Avoid fast correction of hyponatremia, especially in the cases with late hyponatremia (6–8 mmol per day).
- Avoid pain, postoperative nausea, and vomiting during the early postoperative period.

References

1. http://hcupnet.ahrq.gov 2009.
2. Liu CY, Apuzzo MLJ. The genesis of neurosurgery and the evolution of the neurosurgical operative environment: part I-prehistory to 2003. Neurosurgery. 2003;52:3–19.
3. Black P, Kathiresan S, Chung W. Meningioma surgery in the elderly: a case-control study assessing morbidity and mortality. Acta Neurochir. 1998;140:1013–7.

4. Solheim O, Jakola AS, Gulati S, et al. Incidence and causes of perioperative mortality after primary surgery for intracranial tumors: a national, population-based study. J Neurosurg. 2012;116:825–34.
5. Chang SM, Parney IF, McDermott M, et al. Perioperative complications and neurological outcomes of first and second craniotomies among patients enrolled in the Glioma Outcome Project. J Neurosurg. 2003;98:1175–81.
6. Rincon F, Mayer SA. Neurocritical care: a distinct discipline? Curr Opin Crit Care. 2007;13:115–21.
7. Diringer MN, Edwards DF. Admission to a neurologic/neurosurgical intensive care unit is associated with reduced mortality rate after intracerebral hemorrhage. Crit Care Med. 2001;29:635–40.
8. Varelas PN, Eastwood D, Yun HJ, et al. Impact of a neurointensivist on outcomes in patients with head trauma treated in a neurosciences intensive care unit. J Neurosurg. 2006;104:713–9.
9. Bui JQH, Mendis RL, van Gelder JM, et al. Is postoperative intensive care unit admission a prerequisite for elective craniotomy? J Neurosurg. 2011;115:1236–41.
10. Herman MA, Gravenstein N, Gravenstein D. Postoperative neurosurgical care: recovery room misadventures and immediate concerns. In: Layon AJ, editor. Textbook of neurointensive care. London: Springer; 2013. p. 863–97.
11. Lubnin AY, Tseitlin AM, Gromova VV, et al. Waking-up anesthesiology ward at a neurosurgery clinic: annual report. Anesteziol Reanimatol. 2004;2:61–4.
12. Wen PY, Schiff D, Kesari S, et al. Medical management of patients with brain tumors. J Neurooncol. 2006;80:313–32.
13. Gempt J, Krieg SM, Hüttinger S, et al. Postoperative ischemic changes after glioma resection identified by diffusion-weighted magnetic resonance imaging and their association with intraoperative motor evoked potentials. J Neurosurg. 2013;119:829–36.
14. Zheng Z, Chen P, Fu W, et al. Early and late postoperative seizure outcome in 97 patients with supratentorial meningioma and preoperative seizures: a retrospective study. J Neurooncol. 2013;114:101–9.
15. Mukand JA, Blackinton DD, Crincoli MG, et al. Incidence of neurologic deficits and rehabilitation of patients with brain tumors. Am J Phys Med Rehabil. 2001;80:346–50.
16. Coplin WM. Critical care management of acute ischemic stroke. Continuum Lifelong Learning Neurol. 2012;18:547–59.
17. Jauch EC, Saver JL, Adams Jr HP, et al. Guidelines for the early management of patients with acute ischemic stroke a guideline for healthcare professionals from the American Heart Association/American Stroke Association. Stroke. 2013;44:870–947.
18. Rodrigue T, Selman WR. Postoperative management in the neurosciences critical care unit. In: Suarez J, editor. Critical care neurology and neurosurgery. Totowa: Humana Press; 2004. p. 433–48.
19. Taylor WA, Thomas NW, Wellings JA, et al. Timing of postoperative intracranial hematoma development and implications for the best use of neurosurgical intensive care. J Nerosurg. 1995;82:48–50.
20. Gerlach R, Krause M, Seifert V, et al. Hemostatic and hemorrhagic problems in neurosurgical patients. Acta Neurochir. 2009;151:873–900.
21. Dennis LJ, Mayer SA. Diagnosis and management of increased intracranial pressure. Neurol India. 2001;49:S37–50.
22. Ferro JM, Crassard I, Coutinho JM, et al. Decompressive surgery in cerebrovenous thrombosis: a multicenter registry and a systematic review of individual patient data. Stroke. 2011;42:2825–31.
23. Popugaev KA, Savin IA, Goriachev AS, et al. Atypical course of cerebral edema developing after basal tumor removal. Anesteziol Reanimatol. 2008;2:91–4.
24. Black S, Ockert DB, Oliver Jr WC, et al. Outcome following posterior fossa craniectomy in patients in the sitting or horizontal positions. Anesthesiology. 1988;69:49–56.
25. Ooba H, Abe T, Momii Y, et al. Venous air embolism (VAE) associated with stereotactic biopsies. Acta Neurochir. 2014;156:433–7.

26. Hagen PT, Scholz DG, Edwards WD. Incidence and size of patent foramen ovale during the first 10 decades of life: an autopsy study of 965 normal hearts. Mayo Clin Proc. 1984;59:17–20.
27. Bedell EA, Berge KH, Losasso TJ. Paradoxic air embolism during venous air embolism: trans-esophageal echocardiographic evidence of transpulmonary air passage. Anesthesiology. 1994;80(4):947–50.
28. Tekle WG, Adkinson CD, Chaudhry SA, et al. Factors associated with favorable response to hyperbaric oxygen therapy among patients presenting with iatrogenic cerebral arterial gas embolism. Neurocrit Care. 2013;18:228–33.
29. Raiten J, Thiele RH, Nemergut EC. Anesthesia and intensive care management of patients with brain tumors. In: Kaye AH, Laws ER, editors. Brain tumors. An encyclopedic approach. 3rd ed. Edinburgh/New York: Saunders, Elsevier; 2012. p. 249–81.
30. Kaal EC, Vecht CJ. The management of brain edema in brain tumors. Curr Opin Oncol. 2004;16:593–600.
31. Chaichana KL, Pendleton C, Zaidi H, et al. Seizure control for patients undergoing meningioma surgery. World Neurosurg. 2012;79:515–24.
32. Cavaliere R, Schiff D. Clinical implications of status epilepticus on patients with cancer. Neuro Oncol. 2003;5:331.
33. Brophy GM, Bell R, Claassen J, et al. Guidelines for the evaluation and management of status epilepticus. Neurocrit Care. 2012;17:3–23.
34. Wu A, Trinh V, Suki D, et al. A prospective randomized trial of perioperative seizure prophylaxis in patients with intraparenchymal brain tumors. J Neurosurg. 2013;118:873–83.
35. Glantz MJ, Cole BF, Friedberg MH, et al. A randomized, blinded, placebo-controlled trial of divalproex sodium prophylaxis in adults with newly diagnosed brain tumors. Neurology. 1996;46:985–91.
36. Sughrue ME, Rutkowski MJ, Chang EF, et al. Postoperative seizures following the resection of convexity meningiomas: are prophylactic anticonvulsants indicated? J Neurosurg. 2011;114:705–9.
37. Chan PH, Fishman RA, Lee JL, et al. Effects of excitatory neurotransmitter amino acid on edema induction in rat brain cortical slices. J Neurochem. 1979;33:1309–15.
38. Yuen TI, Morokoff AP, Bjorksten A, et al. Glutamate is associated with a higher risk of seizures in patients with gliomas. Neurology. 2012;79:883–9.
39. Maschio M, Dinapoli L, Sperati F, et al. Levetiracetam monotherapy in patients with brain tumor-related epilepsy: seizure control, safety, and quality of life. J Neurooncol. 2011;104:205–14.
40. Leppik IE. Compliance during treatment of epilepsy. Epilepsia. 1988;29:S79–84.
41. Forsyth PA, Weaver S, Fulton D, et al. Prophylactic anticonvulsants in patients with brain tumour. Can J Neurol Sci. 2003;30:106–12.
42. Temkin NR. Preventing and treating posttraumatic seizures: the human experience. Epilepsia. 2009;50:S10–3.
43. Zubkov AY, Wijdicks EF. Antiepileptic drugs in aneurysmal subarachnoid hemorrhage. Rev Neurol Dis. 2008;5:178–81.
44. Flexman AM, Merriman B, Griesdale DE, et al. Infratentorial neurosurgery is an independent risk factor for respiratory failure and death in patients undergoing intracranial tumor resection. J Neurosurg Anesthesiol. 2014;26(3):198–294.
45. Ito E, Ichikawa M, Itakura T, et al. Motor evoked potential monitoring of the vagus nerve with transcranial electrical stimulation during skull base surgeries. J Neurosurg. 2013;118:195–201.
46. Mayer SA, Fink ME. Respiratory care: diagnosis and management. In: Rowland LP, editor. Merritt's neurology. Philadelphia: Lippincott Williams & Wilkins; 2001.
47. Salam A, Tilluckdharry L, Amoateng-Adjepong Y, et al. Neurologic status, cough, secretions and extubation outcomes. Intensive Care Med. 2004;30:1334–9.

48. Ko R, Ramos L, Chalela JA. Conventional weaning parameters do not predict extubation failure in neurocritical care patients. Neurocrit Care. 2009;10:269–73.
49. Coplin WM, Pierson DJ, Cooley KD, et al. Implications of extubation delay in brain-injured patients meeting standard weaning criteria. Am J Respir Crit Care Med. 2000;161:1530–6.
50. Epstein SK. Decision to extubate. Intensive Care Med. 2002;28:535–46.
51. Navalesi P, Frigerio P, Moretti MP. Rate of reintubation in mechanically ventilated neurosurgical and neurologic patients: evaluation of a systemic approach to weaning and extubation. Crit Care Med. 2008;36:2986–92.
52. Popugaev KA, Savin IA, Goriachev AS, et al. A respiratory failure rating scale in neurosurgical patients. Anesteziol Reanimatol. 2010;4:42–50.
53. O'Neil KH, Purdy M, Falk J, et al. The dysphagia outcome and severity scale. Dysphagia. 1999;14:139–45.
54. Hamad GG, Peitzman AB. Morbid obesity and chronic intra-abdominal hypertension. In: Ivatury RR, Cheatham M, Malbrain ML, et al., editors. Abdominal compartment syndrome. Texas: Landes Bioscience; 2006. p. 189–96.
55. Oshorov AV, Savin IA, Goriachev AS, et al. Monitoring of intracranial pressure difference between supra- and infratentorial spaces after posterior fossa tumor removal (case report). Anesteziol Reanimatol. 2011;4:74–7.
56. Slavin KV, Misra M. Infratentorial intracranial pressure monitoring in neurosurgical intensive care unit. Neurol Res. 2003;25:880–4.
57. Roberson Jr JB, William DE, Hitselberger E, et al. Acute postoperative hydrocephalus following translabyrinthine craniotomy for acoustic neuroma resection. Skull Base Surg. 1995;5:143–8.
58. Cuneo RA, Caronna JJ, Pitts LH, et al. Upward transtentorial herniation: seven cases and literature review. Arch Neurol. 1979;36:618–23.
59. Rappaport ZH, Shalit MN. Perioperative external ventricular drainage in obstructive hydrocephalus secondary to infratentorial brain tumours. Acta Neurochir. 1989;96:118–21.
60. Kaltsas GA, Evanson J, Chrisoulidou A. The diagnosis and management of parasellar tumours of the pituitary. Endocr Relat Cancer. 2008;15:885–903.
61. Ruscalleda J. Imaging of parasellar lesions. Eur Radiol. 2005;15:549–59.
62. Cavallo LM, Messina A, Cappabianca P, et al. Endoscopic endonasal surgery of the midline skull base: anatomical study and clinical considerations. Neurosurg Focus. 2005;19:E2.
63. Koutourousiou M, Gardner PA, Fernandez-Miranda JC, et al. Endoscopic endonasal surgery for giant pituitary adenomas: advantages and limitations. J Neurosurg. 2013;118:621–31.
64. Koutourousiou M, Gardner P, Fernandez-Miranda J, et al. Endoscopic endonasal surgery for craniopharyngiomas: surgical outcome in 64 patients. J Neurosurg. 2013;119:1194–207.
65. Berker M, Hazer DB, Yücel T, et al. Complications of endoscopic surgery of the pituitary adenomas: analysis of 570 patients and review of the literature. Pituitary. 2012;15:288–300.
66. Brodal P. Autonomic nervous system. In: Broadal P, editor. The central nervous system. Structure and function. 4th ed. New York: Oxford University Press; 2010. p. 409–58.
67. Popugaev KA, Savin IA, Lubnin AU, et al. Structure and severity of acute diencephalon dysfunction syndrome. Neurocrit Care. 2012;17:S1.
68. Abla AA, Wait SD, Forbes JA, et al. Syndrome of alternating hypernatremia and hyponatremia after hypothalamic hamartoma surgery. Neurosurg Focus. 2011;30:E6.
69. Freeman JL, Zacharin M, Rosenfeld JV, et al. The endocrinology of hypothalamic hamartoma surgery for intractable epilepsy. Epileptic Disord. 2003;5:239–47.
70. Wait SD, Garrett MP, Little AS, et al. Endocrinopathy, vision, headache, and recurrence after transsphenoidal surgery for Rathke cleft cysts. Neurosurgery. 2010;67:837–43.
71. Palmer BF. Hyponatremia in patients with central nervous system disease: SIADH versus CSW. Trends Endocrinol Metab. 2003;14:182–7.
72. Sane T, Rantakari K, Poranen A, et al. Hyponatremia after transsphenoidal surgery for pituitary tumors. J Clin Endocrinol Metab. 1994;79:1395–8.

73. Sata A, Hizuka N, Kawamata T, et al. Hyponatremia after transsphenoidal surgery for hypothalamo-pituitary tumors. Neuroendocrinology. 2006;83:117–22.
74. Brown WD. Osmotic demyelination disorders: central pontine and extrapontine myelinolysis. Curr Opin Neurol. 2000;13:691–7.
75. Gomes JA, Stevens RD, Lewin 3rd JJ, et al. Glucocorticoid therapy in neurologic critical care. Crit Care Med. 2005;33:1214–24.
76. Sakharova OV, Inzucchi SI. Endocrine assessment during critical illness. Crit Care Clin. 2007;23:467–90.
77. Moro N, Katayama Y, Kojima J, et al. Prophylactic management of excessive natriuresis with hydrocortisone for efficient hypervolemic therapy after subarachnoid hemorrhage. Stroke. 2003;34:2807–11.
78. Peterson JF, Pun BT, Dittus RS, et al. Delirium and its motoric subtypes: a study of 614 critically ill patients. J Am Geriatr Soc. 2006;54:479–84.
79. Fernandez-Miranda JC, Gardner PA, Snyderman CH, et al. Craniopharyngioma: a pathologic, clinical, and surgical review. Head Neck. 2012;34:1036–44.
80. Popugaev KA, Savin IA, Goriachev AS, et al. Hypothalamic injury as a cause of refractory hypotension after sellar region tumor surgery. Neurocrit Care. 2008;8:366–73.
81. Popugaev KA, Savin IA, Goriachev AS, et al. Optimizing blood pressure in patients with sellar region tumors during complicated postoperative period. Zh Vopr Neirokhir Im N N Burdenko. 2012;76:20–7.
82. Popugaev KA, Savin IA, Lubnin AU, et al. Intra-abdominal hypertension in patients with sellar region tumors. Ann Intensive Care. 2012;2:S2.
83. Malbrain ML, Cheatham ML, Kirkpatrick A, et al. Results from the international conference of experts on intra-abdominal hypertension and abdominal compartment syndrome. II. Recommendations. Intensive Care Med. 2007;33:951–62.
84. Popugaev KA, Savin IA, Lubnin AU, et al. Unusual cause of cerebral vasospasm after pituitary surgery. Neurol Sci. 2011;32:673–80.
85. Nishioka H, Haraoka J, Ikeda Y. Risk factors of cerebrospinal fluid rhinorrhea following transsphenoidal surgery. Acta Neurochir. 2005;147:1163–6.
86. Beer R, Lackner P, Pfausler B, et al. Nosocomial ventriculitis and meningitis in neurocritical care patients. J Neurol. 2008;255:1617–24.
87. Basali A, Mascha EJ, Kalfas I, et al. Relation between perioperative hypertension and intracranial haemorrhage after craniotomy. Anesthesiology. 2000;93:48–54.
88. Breivik H, Borchgrevink PC, Allen SM, et al. Assessment of pain. Br J Anaesth. 2008;101(1):17–24.
89. Nguyen A, Girard F, Boudreault D, et al. Scalp nerve blocks decrease the severity of pain after craniotomy. Anesth Analg. 2001;93(5):1272–6.
90. Gottschalk A, Ochroch EA. Is preemptive analgesia clinically effective? In: Fleisher L, editor. Evidence-based practice of anesthesia. Philadelphia: Saunders; 2008.
91. Dolmatova EV, Imaev AA, Lubnin AY. 'Scheduled' dosing of lornoxicam provides analgesia superior to that provided by 'on request' dosing following craniotomy. Eur J Anaesthesiol. 2009;26:633–7.
92. De Gray LC, Matta BF. Acute and chronic pain following craniotomy: a review. Anaesthesia. 2005;60:693–704.
93. Yaster M, Kost-Byerly S, Maxwell LG. Opiod agonists and antagonists. In: Schechter NL, Berde CB, Yaster M, editors. Pain in infants, children, and adolescents. Philadelphia: Lippincott Williams and Wilkins; 2003. p. 181–224.
94. Pugh SC, Jones NC, Barsoum LZ. A comparison of prophylactic ondansetron and metoclopramide administration in patients undergoing major neurosurgical procedures. Anaesthesia. 1996;51:1162–4.
95. Apfel CC, Korttila K, Abdalla M, et al. A factorial trial of 6 interventions for the prevention of postoperative nausea and vomiting. N Engl J Med. 2004;350:2441–51.

96. Habib AS, Keifer JC, Borel CO, et al. A comparison of the combination of aprepitant and dexamethasone versus the combination of ondansetron and dexamethasone for the prevention of postoperative nausea and vomiting in patients undergoing craniotomy. Anesth Analg. 2011;112:813–8.
97. Leslie K, Williams DL. Postoperative pain, nausea and vomiting in neurosurgical patients. Curr Opin Anaesthesiol. 2005;18:461–5.
98. Murphy GS. Residual neuromuscular blockade: incidence, assessment, and relevance in the postoperative period. Minerva Anestesiol. 2006;72:97–109.
99. Warren J, Fromm RE, Orr RA, et al. Guidelines for the inter- and intrahospital transport of critically ill patients. Crit Care Med. 2004;32:256–62.

Chapter 8
Subarachnoid Hemorrhage

Edgar Avalos Herrera and Corina Puppo

Introduction

Patient's safety can be defined as "The avoidance, prevention and amelioration of adverse outcomes or injuries stemming from the process of healthcare" [1]. It is considered one of the essential components of high-quality health care [2]. "Safety resides in systems as well as people, and safety has to be actively pursued and promoted. Simply trying to avoid damage is not enough" [3].

Aneurysmal subarachnoid hemorrhage (SAH) is associated with significant morbidity and mortality [4]. The lack of clinical trials regarding safety issues in neurocritical care of SAH has to be highlighted. Literature addressing this point is scant [5]. This chapter refers to the patient's safety issues after having experienced a spontaneous SAH.

Case Scenario

A 43-year-old female experienced a sudden onset of severe headache followed by a syncopal episode at work. She was transported to the emergency department (ED) and arrived within one hour of the event. The patient had no past medical history and was not on any medications. On exam, she was vigilant, without motor deficit, her pupils were symmetrical and reactive. Her head exam was atraumatic, cervical

E. Avalos Herrera, MD, MsC (✉)
Department of Neurology and Neurophysiology,
Hospital General San Juan de Dios, Guatemala City, Gautemala
e-mail: edgar@avalosherrera.me

C. Puppo, MD
Department of Emergency and Critical Care, Clinics Hospital,
Universidad de la República School of Medicine, Montevideo, Uruguay

© Springer International Publishing Switzerland 2015   125
K.E. Wartenberg et al. (eds.), *Neurointensive Care: A Clinical Guide to Patient Safety*, DOI 10.1007/978-3-319-17293-4_8

Fig. 8.1 Computed
tomography showing
modified Fisher 2 grade
subarachnoid hemorrhage in
the basal cisterns

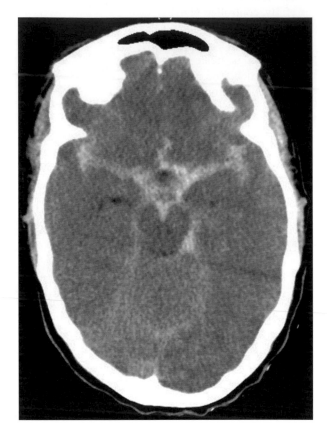

spine non-tender, heart and lungs were normal. She was alert. No cranial nerve
deficits were noted and the rest of the neurologic exam was normal. Her electrocardiogram (EKG) showed II, III, and a VF T-wave inversions. Computed tomography
(CT) showed SAH modified Fisher grade 2 (see Fig. 8.1). Blood pressure (BP) on
admission was 240/110 mmHg and continuous intravenous infusion of nitroprusside was started while waiting for a bed in the ICU. At shift change to night time,
she was expecting her transfer to the ICU and felt sleepy. On the next day she was
still in the ED. Deterioration of awareness was noted, her BP was 80/50 mmHg but
there was no record of BP measurements over the last 2 h and a trend to lower BP
was noted in the preceding hours. There was a complete lack of response to stimuli
and a final diagnosis of brain death was made.

Risks of Patient's Safety

The risks of patient's safety are many; we can broadly classify them in pitfalls in
diagnosis and pitfalls in treatment.

Pitfalls in diagnosis could result in failure to recognize the presence of a disease and send the patient home which would require re-admission to the hospital, or a wrong diagnosis could result in unnecessary or unsafe treatments. SAH is missed in 20–50 % of patients at first presentation [6, 7]. This can be due to several conditions:

The clinical presentation of the patients covers a wide range of syndromes, which have been divided as minor, focal, major, and catastrophic presentation [8]. Patients with good clinical grade are sometimes at a higher risk of misdiagnosis, especially when headache is not characteristic.

The different clinical scenarios include headache, with or without stiff neck, confusion, seizures, coma of sudden onset, focal deficits in a patient who presented with a headache one week earlier, etc.

Each of these different clinical presentations can be erroneously diagnosed. The risks of misdiagnosing SAH include

1. Not performing a CT. In this case, the emergency physician has been misled by the headache [9]
2. Inaccurate reading of the CT
3. Stopping the diagnostic workup without performing a lumbar puncture (LP) after obtaining a normal CT when the suspicion of SAH is high

Headache Characteristics

The classic description of the headache that accompanies SAH is thunderclap headache (TCH). It is a sudden severe headache that peaks to maximum intensity within 1 min. SAH is the most commonly identified etiology for this headache [10]. However, not every patient with a subarachnoid bleed presents with a headache described as "the worst of my life" nor has the patient experienced a rapid increase in headache intensity. Headache is a common presenting symptom in the ED, representing the 3.1 % of ED visits [11]. Most of these patients have primary headache disorders, such as migraine or tension headaches as well as other self-limited processes. Therefore, extensive, urgent evaluation for SAH is inappropriate for the entire group [12]. The emergency physician can be misled and a high grade of suspicion is needed.

Several Frequent Misdiagnoses Have to Be Underlined

- The most important cause of delay in diagnosis is not a misdiagnosis, but the delay in the patient to seek consultation [13]. The only way to overcome this problem is public education.
- The patient with headache, low fever, and nuchal rigidity can be misdiagnosed as meningitis.

- Headache with severe nausea and vomiting can be interpreted as of digestive origin.
- EKG changes can draw attention to an ischemic cardiac origin.
- Severe hypertension can be attributed to a hypertensive encephalopathy.
- Severe neck pain can be misdiagnosed as arthritis originated cervical contracture.

SAH is the underlying diagnosis in about 1 of 4 headaches with an acute onset. Patients with sudden severe headache lasting 1 h or more, even if there are no other symptoms, need investigation [14].

Similarly, increased efforts at educating general practitioners and emergency physicians about the signs and symptoms of aneurysmal hemorrhage may decrease the likelihood of misdiagnosis.

The initial test of choice is a noncontrast CT of the brain. Only 10 % of the patients with a TCH will eventually show SAH in the CT. The CT sensitivity is a function of time from the onset of the headache as well as severity of the hemorrhage. If there is a small amount of blood it can be rapidly washed away from the subarachnoid space, and it can be also washed away if enough time has passed since the bleeding. Even with the newest scanners, CT by itself is insufficient to exclude SAH. There is one exception. The time limit from headache onset to CT has been set to be 6 h by some experts, after reviewing the results of trials with new generation CT scanners [15–17] which showed that the sensitivity of CT within 6 h from ictus is 100 %. Therefore, in a patient with a TCH without neurologic signs and with a CT without subarachnoid blood performed in less than 6 h from the start of the headache, an LP does not need to be performed [18, 19]. There are two exceptions that have to be underlined: (1) The CT has to be interpreted by an experienced physician, and (2) if the pain is localized in the neck, without a diffuse headache, a normal CT does not rule out a spinal SAH.

In all other cases, if there is no visible blood in the CT, an LP is mandatory. The characteristics of the cerebrospinal fluid (CSF) to be looked for are [20] hemorrhagic appearance, supernatant xantochromia, opening pressure. Red blood cells give the spinal fluid a hemorrhagic appearance. CSF supernatant from an SAH patient is yellowish (xantochromic) depending on the time from onset. Xantochromia is the result of the metabolism of heme to bilirubin, and it suggests that the blood has been in the subarachnoid space for a considerable period of time (>12 h), which has allowed metabolic changes to occur. Xantochromic changes are proportional to the time spent between the bleeding and the CSF procurement. However, there are often concerns about the possibility that these blood cells originate from trauma by the needle causing bleeding into the subarachnoid space, known as a traumatic tap. The three methods/characteristics that help to differentiate traumatic LP from real SAH are the three tubes test, aperture pressure, and the visual inspection for xantochromia. Guidelines on CSF study in suspected SAH have been published [21]. Crenated red blood cells, which were once considered markers of a long period of blood accumulation in the subarachnoid space, have now been abandoned as criteria of importance [22, 23]. Table 8.1 shows the different criteria and their relative importance.

Table 8.1 Criteria of CSF finding in SAH

CSF finding	Traumatic LP	True SAH	Index
Opening pressure	Normal	Elevated or normal	A
3 tube tests	Initially bloody, gradually clearing	Persistently bloody	B
Xantochromia	No xantochromia	Xantochromia if more than 6–12 h from onset	C
Spectrophotometry for xantochromia	No hemoglobin breakdown products	Hemoglobin breakdown products	C
RBC count	Diminishing in sequential tubes	Does not diminish (there is not a diagnostic threshold number)	B
WBC count	Maintains the proportion of peripheral blood	Proportional to peripheral blood initially, then relatively increased later	B
Crenated RBC	Absent	Present	D

Modified from Shah and Edlow [20] with permission
A: should be routinely conducted in adults; useful when positive and also helps in differential diagnosis
B: should be routinely conducted; can be false positive but very helpful when the count in the last tube is zero
C: should be routinely conducted
D: not recommended to be performed routinely; usually not helpful

Pitfalls in treatment could result in serious undesired effects and impact outcomes unfavorably. Patient's safety measures should be a part of every ICU protocol, since adverse events are encountered in about 20 % of patients of ICU and half of them could be preventable, about 10 % are life-threatening or fatal; most serious medical errors occur during the ordering or execution of treatments, especially medications [24, 25]. Up to one preventable error for every five doses of medication administered was reported in a tertiary care academic medical center [25].

Errors and adverse events occur more frequently in ICU than elsewhere because of high frequency decision making. The likelihood of adverse events in critical care increases with severity of illness and greater complexity of the care provided. Approaches to studying medical errors had been described elsewhere [26].

Safety Barriers

The case scenario at the beginning of this chapter is a good example taken from real life where everything that could go wrong actually went wrong. The first safety barrier is a correct diagnosis and that requires an appropriate training in neurological emergencies and constant supervision from senior medical staff. Otherwise, a brain CT probably would not have been ordered in this patient and the headache would have been considered a result of BP elevation. After initial brain CT, an LP was performed. This implies a second safety barrier, the correct interpretation of LP results. After these initial steps, a diagnosis is made and a third safety barrier becomes activated: the treatment protocols. At this point, if protocols are not continuously updated and based on the best evidence available, then bad outcomes will be the result of a wrong approach from those who wrote the protocols. It has been demonstrated that just a change in medical treatment protocols can result in better outcomes in SAH patients [27]. When resource limitations in medications or equipment preclude following every step of a protocol, the management will not be considered a medical error. However, in our case scenario there was a tremendous gap in patient's safety at the moment of being transferred to ICU and that was a result of a wrong process. Examples of deteriorating patients during transfers can be found even in textbooks because this is a time where the department or hospital that is sending the patient begins to de-escalate neuromonitoring and neurotherapeutics until the patient reaches the next department or hospital [28]. As in this case, an ineffective shift handover may endanger patient's safety [29].

Other safety barriers that are becoming more prevalent in clinical practice are checklists. They offer a code that represents a fast bedside translation of extensive and detailed clinical guidelines [30]. Checklists can be used to prevent secondary insults in neurointensive care [31] and could have an impact in mortality or saving costs to hospitals [32]. Basically, checklists could be tailored to each desired goal of treatment as aids in the correct application of protocols and as an inexpensive and easy way to overcome patient's safety barriers.

Discussion of Risk–Benefit Ratios in Management of SAH

A recent detailed and comprehensive review that covers all of the aspects related to neurocritical management of SAH patients will be of interest for the reader [33]. Here we present only the main aspects to bear in mind regarding BP, elevated intracranial pressure, prevention of rebleeding, deep vein thrombosis and gastrointestinal bleeding, seizure prophylaxis, prevention and treatment of cerebral vasospasm, delayed cerebral ischemia (DCI), and early aneurysm repair among other relevant complications which could arise as a result of undertaken approaches.

Rebleeding

The risk of rebleeding during the first 6 h after the initial bleeding can reach 15 % of patients and increase mortality to nearly 50 %. To prevent this severe complication, three different kinds of treatment are available: (a) antifibrinolytic medication as a bridge to definite (b) aneurysm repair through (c) endovascular coiling or surgical clipping.

Antifibrinolytic therapy can be applied during the first hours before the patient can undergo definitive securement of the aneurysm. It prevents the intrinsic fibrinolytic system to act and lyse the clot inside the aneurysm which prevents it from rebleeding. There are several publications supporting the use of antifibrinolytic therapy administered from the time of e-diagnosis until the aneurysm is secured or for a maximum of 72 h [34–38]. Although antifibrinolytic therapy use (tranexamic acid, aminocaproic acid) had been associated to an increased risk of hydrocephalus, deep venous thrombosis (DVT), pulmonary emboli (PE), myocardial infarction, as well as myopathy earlier [39, 40], this paradigm has changed at present. Ischemic events were described during the first period of antifibrinolytic therapy, when the use of dehydration was a common part of management and administration of antifibrinolytic medication was prolonged into the vasospasm phase. A Cochrane review has not found enough evidence for its use, but this review included several publications from the time during which antifibrinolytics were administered for weeks, and along with dehydration. The prolonged or delayed antifibrinolytic drug administration would expose the patient to unnecessary adverse effects [38].

The aneurysm repair should be attempted during the first hours after ictus [41] using detachable-coil treatment or microsurgical clipping. Nevertheless, the choice between the available techniques depends on multiple factors. A multidisciplinary team, including neurointensivists, interventional radiologists, and neurosurgeons, should discuss all treatment options with a focus on patient's safety and long-term results [38, 42]. The repair of the aneurysm responsible for the ictus is not without significant risks. Whenever possible, patients should be transferred to centers of high patient volume (more than 60 cases per year) that have a multidisciplinary team including neurointensivists, vascular neurosurgeons, and interventional neuroradiologists. The main risk of endovascular techniques includes a low rate of late rebleeding [38].

Endovascular coiling is the preferred option due to a reduction in death and disability compared to surgical clipping [43]. The main risk of endovascular techniques is revascularization of the aneurysm associated with a high risk of rerupture. Clipping should be considered especially in SAH patients with large intraparenchymal hematomas and middle cerebral artery aneurysms. Endovascular coiling may be the treatment of choice in the elderly, in poor clinical grade cases, and in those with aneurysms of the posterior circulation [42].

Blood Pressure

Blood pressure management is difficult in every neurocritical patient. In SAH patients different difficulties arise at different stages. Before the aneurysm is secured, the rebleeding risk is a major concern. During the DCI phase, the best BP to perfuse the brain without endangering other organs or systems has to be found for each case. Existing guidelines recommend safest BP levels; however, each case has to be individualized. Therapeutic options to manage BP have to be taken into account: the patient's previous BP, clinical status, phase of the disease, state (secured or not secured) of the aneurysm. The response to each modification has to be analyzed before taking a new step. These steps, however, have to be fast and the neurointensivist taking care of these patients has to be prepared not only to continue with the next step but also to go back when treatment does not work as expected.

One of the most important variables to be taken into account when targeting BP treatment in a specific patient is the repair status of the responsible aneurysm. If the aneurysm repair is delayed, the use of antihypertensive medications is not recommended if BP values are lower than 160 mmHg systolic BP, or 110 mmHg mean BP. At this stage of treatment, pharmacologic interventions are only required when there are extreme BP increases [38]. In the same line, the main objective is to attain a systolic BP lower than 160 mmHg to diminish the rebleeding risk [42].

Intracranial Pressure

General measures include management of increased intracranial pressure with the head of bed elevated at 30° as well as treating hyperglycemia and fever.

Acute hydrocephalus occurs in 10–87 % of patients with an SAH [35]. Hydrocephalus can already be present at the initial evaluation in ED or may be delayed. Hydrocephalus after SAH frequently requires emergency treatment, and should respond to external ventricular drainage (EVD) [44]. Three to 48 % of patients with SAH require permanent CSF diversion for hydrocephalus [35]. Acute hydrocephalus may be asymptomatic or associated with intracranial hypertension with alteration of consciousness, herniation, and brain death, therefore, it is important to maintain a high index of suspicion when a patient deteriorates. Factors associated with shunt-dependent hydrocephalus include increasing age, poor grade in Hunt and Hess scale at admission, thick SAH on admission CT, intraventricular hemorrhage, hydrocephalus at the time of admission, post-surgery meningitis, posterior circulation location of the ruptured aneurysm, clinical vasospasm, and endovascular treatment [40]. However, the presence of intracerebral hemorrhage, multiple aneurysms, vasospasm, and gender did not influence the development of shunt-dependent chronic hydrocephalus.

When placing an EVD, care should be taken not to dramatically reduce ICP at insertion as this may favor aneurysm rebleeding because of the pressure gradient [45].

Adequate sedation and analgesia should be provided when required, and the use of anesthetics could be considered in rare situations. Hyperventilation to a goal of PCO_2 to 30–35 mmHg should only be a transient measure. Hypertonic solutions can also reduce intracranial pressure and increase cerebral perfusion pressure and cerebral blood flow. Mannitol could result in hypovolemia if fluid reposition is not adequately performed. The fluid goal is euvolemia [38]. Failure to accomplish these general measures could be not only unsafe but detrimental.

In cases of intracranial pressure crisis, administration of 30 mL of hypertonic saline as bolus over 20 min via a central line could be required. This leads to changes in blood viscosity and cerebral blood flow that are accompanied by the augmentation of brain tissue oxygenation causing a compensatory vasoconstriction and decreased cerebral blood volume resulting in a decrease of intracranial pressure. Gradually an osmotic gradient is created and extravascular free water moves into the intravascular space [46]. Adverse effects of hypertonic saline administration include acute renal failure, myelinolysis, metabolic acidosis or metabolic alkalosis, rebound hyponatremia, hypokalemia, infection, coagulopathy, phlebitis, and rebound increased intracranial pressure. Decompressive craniectomy must be considered in selected cases of life-threatening cerebral edema.

Delayed Cerebral Ischemia

Delayed cerebral ischemia (DCI) is one of the causes of delayed neurological deterioration (DND) and should be considered as a clinical manifestation secondary to an ischemic process that may or may not be associated with vasospasm demonstrated by imaging or sonography. Neurological deterioration accompanying vasospasm or DCI may go unnoticed especially in patients under sedation or in coma so that continuous monitoring in a neurointensive unit is vital for early detection. For prophylaxis, the role of statin is currently unclear. The STASH trial did not detect any benefit in the use of simvastatin for long-term or short-term outcome in patients with aneurysmal SAH. Despite demonstrating no safety concerns, investigators concluded that patients with SAH should not be treated routinely with simvastatin during the acute stage [47].

Fever and glycemic control as well as adequate oxygenation are general basic measures for the prevention and treatment of DCI.

A practical method for monitoring vasospasm is transcranial Doppler sonography (TCD) which should include calculation of the Lindegaard index (LI). An LI greater than 6 should trigger a vascular imaging study. Invasive monitoring methods can provide more information. However, they must be applied by personnel widely experienced in the interpretation of the different techniques to maintain an optimal risk–benefit balance.

Nimodipine should be given up to 60 mg every 4 h to all patients until day 21 after bleeding since its neuroprotective effects can be used to prevent DCI [38]. The treatment of DCI involves hemodynamic and endovascular management. Main safety risks of prevention and treatment of DCI involve cardiac arrhythmias and hemodynamic disturbances including cardiopulmonary failure, pulmonary edema, and myocardial ischemia, especially in older SAH patients or in those with past medical history of cardiovascular disease. Cardiac adverse events could result in brain tissue hypoperfusion and aggravation of DCI. Patients with increased cardiovascular risk require more intense monitoring.

Hyperdynamic therapy, also referred as hemodynamic augmentation, is the main therapeutic aid to manage delayed cerebral ischemia (DCI). Its objective is to increase cerebral blood flow (CBF) and to reverse neurological deficits. It is not safe in the setting of an unrepaired aneurysm because of an unpredictable risk of rebleeding. Inotropics or vasopressors could be used. Drug selection has to be based on cardiac function. A decreased cardiac function will guide the physician toward inotropic drugs, while vasopressors are preferred in patients with a normal ejection fraction. The infusion rate will be slowly increased with simultaneous monitoring of blood pressure and patient's clinical status. A safe way to start is a moderate (around 10%) increase and to evaluate the clinical response in 30 min. If the clinical status improves, this level of BP is maintained. The objective would be not to surpass a systolic BP of 240 mmHg, or a mean BP of 140 mmHg [48, 49]. The preferred agent is norepinephrine, but the local availability of medications commands the choice; initial clinical variables like heart rate and cardiac function are safe clinical guides when starting to titrate the selected agent. Hemodynamic augmentation has to be maintained until there is evidence or clinical suspicion that the neurological decline is overcome. Some authors recommend continuing until TCD measured cerebral blood flow velocities (CBFV) progressively decrease for 48–72 h [37]. However, the decrease in CBFV does not always correspond to the improvement of DCI. A decrease in CBFV can also be due to a low regional perfusion pressure which has reached the lower limit of cerebral autoregulation and CBF is decreasing. In these cases, when hypertensive treatment is installed, there is a CBFV increase parallel to the increase in CBF due to the improvement in regional cerebral perfusion pressure [50]. The Lindegaard Index can help to elucidate the meaning of these changes in CBFV.

When there is a consensus on terminating the hemodynamic augmentation, the continuous infusion of vasopressors or inotropes has to be weaned slowly. It is judicious to decrease BP not more than 10% in 24 h to prevent a new ischemic deficit generated by a rapid change in the presence of residual vasospasm. At this point it can be helpful to reevaluate the patient clinically and by neuroimaging or TCD examination. If vasospasm persists, hemodynamic augmentation has to be maintained. The use of intraventricular tissue plasminogen activator, lumbar drainage, or microsurgical fenestration of the lamina terminalis for the prevention of vasospasm or hydrocephalus after aneurysmal SAH still requires more evidence before its use in appropriately selected patients could be recommended [51–53].

Medical Complications

The risk of DVT in SAH patients is estimated to be lower than 20 %, and the risk of PE is lower than 5 %. Significant independent predictors of DVT include increasing age, male sex, congestive heart failure, coagulopathy, paralysis, fluid and electrolyte disorders, obesity, smoking, race, and length of stay [48, 54]. Based on these factors, patients should be screened with increased awareness. DVT prevention is recommended in all SAH patients. Sequential compression devices (SCDs) do not increase the risk of hemorrhagic complications during the initial first hours and therefore they can be used from the first hours of admission and continuously. Intermittent pneumatic compression devices are inexpensive and could even improve survival [49]. After the aneurysm has been secured and at least 24 h after ictus, unfractionated heparin or low-molecular-weight heparin can be administered until the patient is fully mobilized [38]. Low-dose intravenous heparin infusion has been recently tried as DVT prophylaxis starting 12 h after surgical clipping and was shown to be superior to subcutaneous heparin twice daily [55]. The safety of subcutaneous unfractionated heparin within 24 h of a neurosurgical procedure had formerly been demonstrated in patients with SAH, intracerebral hemorrhage, subdural or epidural hemorrhage [56].

The incidence of gastrointestinal bleeding in SAH patients is approximately 4 %. In the patient receiving enteral nutrition, no prophylaxis is needed. However, in mechanically ventilated patients or in those with a history of peptic ulcer disease, the use of gastric prophylaxis is recommended. Antacids use could result in metabolic or electrolyte disorders. Ranitidine and sucralfate could interact with medications frequently used in SAH patients [57]. Some authors suggested an increased risk of pneumonia, hypotension, or thrombocytopenia through ranitidine [58, 59], while sucralfate was found to be inferior to ranitidine regarding the expected prophylactic activity [60]. When proton pump inhibitors (PPI) were compared to histamine-2 receptor antagonists (H2 blockers), no difference was found on delayed neurological deficits or delayed infarction, however PPI use was associated to a lower favorable functional outcome [61]. It has been observed recently that PPIs are associated with greater GI hemorrhage, pneumonia, and Clostridium difficile infection risks than histamine-2 receptor antagonists in mechanically ventilated patients [62]. The final choice is determined by local medication availability or institution preferences [63]. A decrease in hemoglobin concentration, or thrombocyte count, or an unexplained increase in blood urea nitrogen can suggest GI bleeding and should prompt for an endoscopic evaluation [57, 64].

Among electrolyte disorders, sodium disturbances are particularly deleterious to the injured brain. Hyponatremia can be found in 9 % of SAH patients and hypernatremia in 6 %. Hypertonic saline is used to correct hyponatremia but a fast rate of sodium correction (>6–8 mEq/L in 24 h) carries the risk of development of central pontine myelinolysis. To avoid this side effect the rate of correction should not exceed 0.5 mEq/L hourly and no more than 6–8 mEq/L over the first 24 h.

Seizures

Seizures are common after SAH. The frequency reported ranges from 4 to 9 % after the initial bleed, most of them were triggered by a focal clot. In comatose patients, non-convulsive seizures range from 10 to 19 % [65]. Seizures may occur during or soon after rupture of an intracranial aneurysm. The risk and implications of seizures associated with SAH are not well defined, nor the need for and efficacy of routinely administered anticonvulsants after SAH. The prophylactic use of antiepileptic drugs (AEDs) in patients with SAH is controversial. In poor grade patients, even one seizure can worsen the clinical situation. However, long-term AED use was associated with worse outcome. A retrospective study investigated the impact of the use of prophylactic anticonvulsants (phenytoin) on cognitive outcome and found that phenytoin burden was independently associated with worse cognitive function at 3 months after hemorrhage [66]. Phenytoin or levetiracetam can be used for seizure prophylaxis for a short term (<7 days) [38]. Early studies show that levetiracetam may have neuroprotective effects in animal models of closed head injury and SAH [67]. Electroencephalographic monitoring may be helpful in making the decision to proceed with AED treatment in patients with SAH.

Sedation

Main objectives of sedation in neurocritical care patients include treatment of anxiety and pain, collaboration with neurologic evaluation, facilitation of mechanical ventilation, and prevention of intracranial hypertension. Benzodiazepines and propofol are the sedative agents most frequently administered. Promotion of sleep should also be taken into account as part of treatment goals and the use of adjunctive hypnotics as well as non-pharmacologic measures is required. Pain management is mandatory, options include fentanyl, morphine (with the associated risk of constipation, ileus, and vomiting), and acetaminophen or non-steroidal anti-inflammatory drugs (NSAIDs) [68, 69]. CoX inhibitors were found to decrease platelet aggregation associated with the risk of rebleeding and DCI [70].

Solutions to Potential Risks

Neurocritical care is an emerging field and therefore one of the most rapidly evolving specialties. A safe neurocritical intensive care unit (NICU) is one that promotes continuing neurocritical care education not only to its own staff of nurses and physicians but also to other specialties. The NICU should nurture itself from its own mistakes and be open to learning from the multidisciplinary team which would provide the highest level of care. In an established and functional ICU devoted to neurological care or integrated in a general ICU, local protocols to treat the neurological emergencies should exist, be continuously revised and updated taking into account the local resources of equipment, medications, and medical staff. These protocols are shared with all of the members of the multidisciplinary team and reflect the most recent evidence-based knowledge. We will focus on a single aspect that will have greater impact on outcomes.

When finding solutions to patient's safety risks, each institution should investigate their local issues and have an error detection team in charge of auditing selected cases to diagnose aspects that could be improved (i.e., action slips, lapses, mistakes, protocol violations) [24]. A section that must be included in every diagnostic and therapeutic protocol of patients with SAH is the neurological examination utilizing clinical scales. We recommend hourly evaluations using Glasgow Coma Scale (GCS), Full Outline of UnResponsiveness (FOUR) score, and World Federation of Neurological Surgeons (WFNS) grading scale or Hunt and Hess scale on admission and once a day until patient becomes clinically stable. These scales should be recorded while admitting the patient to hospital, no matter which department is currently taking care of the patient and during the NICU stay [71].

Along with these scales, vital signs should be recorded. The BP goal should be adjusted to the clinical situation. It has to be underlined that hypotension and a negative fluid balance are deleterious for the patient; oxygen saturation should be maintained >95 %, core temperature ≤37 °C, and the fluid goal is euvolemia [33, 39]. But just measuring and recording clinical data are not enough; physicians must be immediately alerted when treatment goals for neuromonitoring are not being reached [72, 73]. These clinical variables are used to set thresholds of alarms and alert physicians of an impending deteriorating condition. However, the high number of false alarms can lead to alarm fatigue, a "sensory overload when clinicians are exposed to an excessive number of alarms, which can result in desensitization to alarms and missed alarms" [74].

There are newer techniques designed to facilitate the analysis of various clinical variables and support critical decisions. A bedside computer-based system coupled to neuromonitoring is feasible and could elevate the alertness for avoiding secondary insults and helps in the evaluation of patients [31]. Recently, a model of prediction of vasospasm using automated features of existing ICU data was proposed as a new monitoring technique after SAH that could be useful as early warning or decision support system without increasing human workload [75]. Even a fully automatic method for SAH volume and density quantification had been described with the potential to provide important determinants in clinical practice and research [76].

Finally, miscommunication between nurses or between nurses and physicians will result in delay or lack of urgent changes in therapy or diagnostic techniques followed by clinical deterioration [29, 77]. The other relevant gap in communication is among physicians from different specialties, especially regarding the timing of intervention of each next level of specialization. One way to solve this gap would be the creation of an SAH code that must be activated at the moment of diagnosis of SAH. This special code is a call to the entire SAH multidisciplinary team at the same time, not just the neuroradiologist to obtain and interpret the first images or just the neurointensivist to start the neuromonitoring and neuroresuscitation of the injured brain but also the neurosurgeon to start evaluating for urgent EVD placement or consider decompressive craniectomy for massive hemispheric edema if appropriate, and the neurointerventional expert to start planning the approach of the aneurysm repair in consensus with the remainder of the team.

Summary

In summary, every institution must develop its own diagnostic and treatment protocols tailored according to local human and therapeutic resources. Better results will be achieved by a multidisciplinary team headed by a neurointensivist taking care of patients in a high volume center. Checklists can be designed as an aid to remember main critical points that will guide therapy at every step of the local protocols. With every undesired or unexpected clinical change in the neurological status of the patient, a reaction to the situation should be followed by the appropriate diagnostic test and management with a broad differential diagnosis for the numerous complications after SAH taking into account medical errors.

Dos and Don'ts

Dos

- Do administer nimodipine up to 60 mg each 4 h for 21 days
- Do keep target hemoglobin at >10 g/dL
- Do perform daily TCD as a part of the neurological evaluation and more frequently to evaluate response of the hyperdynamic therapy in DCI
- Do maintain euvolemia with isotonic crystalloids
- Do apply continuous surface electroencephalogram if available or perform standard surface EEGs in alternate days to screen for non-convulsive seizures especially in poor grade patients
- Do prevent DVT in all SAH patients using sequential compression devices in the first 24 h
- Do attempt aneurysm repair in the first 72 h of ictus
- Do maintain systolic BP less than 160 mmHg to prevent rebleeding in the patient with an unsecured aneurysm
- Do manage SAH patients in a multidisciplinary medical environment at high volume centers
- Do involve patient's family at each relevant stage of therapy

Don'ts

- Don't administer high dose corticosteroids
- Don't allow preventable increase of ICP attributed to pain or anxiety
- Don't pursue hemodilution or hypervolemia as a treatment of DCI
- Don't allow negative fluid balance or hypovolemia
- Don't consider hyperventilation as a prolonged therapy for brain edema

- Don't use antihypertensives if systolic BP does not exceed 160 mmHg or mean BP is not above 110 mmHg when the aneurysm has not been secured
- Don't intubate unless GCS is less than 9 (excluding pulmonary indications)

References

1. Vincent C. Patient safety. Edinburgh: Elsevier Churchill Livingstone; 2006.
2. Institute of Medicine, Committee on Quality of Health Care in America. Crossing the quality chasm: a new health system for the 21st century. Washington, DC: National Academy Press; 2001.
3. Vincent C. Integrating safety and quality. In: Patient safety. 2nd ed. Chichester, West Sussex: Wiley-Blackwell, 2010.
4. van Gijn J, Kerr RS, Rinkel GJE. Subarachnoid haemorrhage. Lancet. 2007;369(9558):306–18.
5. Manno EM. Safety issues and concerns for the neurological patient in the emergency department. Neurocrit Care. 2008;9:259–64.
6. Kassell NF, Kongable GL, Torner JC, Adams Jr HP, Mazuz H. Delay in referral of patients with ruptured aneurysms to neurosurgical attention. Stroke. 1985;16:587–90.
7. Kowalski RG, Claassen J, Kreiter KT, Bates JE, Ostapkovich ND, Connolly ES, Mayer SA. Initial misdiagnosis and outcome after subarachnoid hemorrhage. JAMA. 2004;291: 866–9.
8. Van Gent MW, Kuiper MA, Manschot T, Jerzewsky A, Rommes JH, Spronk PE. Subarachnoid haemorrhage presenting clinically as circulatory arrest in acute myocardial infarction. Ned Tijdschr Geneeskd. 2008;152:331–6.
9. Malatt C, Zawaideh M, Chao C, Hesselink JR, Lee RR, Chen JY. Head computed tomography in the emergency department: a collection of easily missed findings that are life-threatening or life-changing. J Emerg Med. 2014;47(6):646–59. pii: S0736-4679(14)00743-4.
10. Dilli E. Thunderclap headache. Curr Neurol Neurosci Rep. 2014;14:437.
11. National Hospital Ambulatory Medical Care Survey: 2010 emergency department summary table. Available at: http://www.cdc.gov/nchs/data/ahcd/nhamcs_emergency/2010_ed_web_ tables.pdf.
12. Edlow JA. Diagnosis of subarachnoid hemorrhage. Neurocrit Care. 2005;2:99–109.
13. Wang MY, Gianotta SL. Delays in the treatment of patients with aneurysmal subarachnoid hemorrhage: experience at a county hospital. J Stroke Cerebrovasc Dis. 2000;9:282–6.
14. Linn FH, Wijdicks EF, van der Graaf Y, Weerdesteyn-van Vliet FA, Bartelds AI, van Gijn J. Prospective study of sentinel headache in aneurysmal subarachnoid haemorrhage. Lancet. 1994;344(8922):590–3.
15. Perry JJ, Stiell IG, Sivilotti ML, Bullard MJ, Emond M, Symington C, Sutherland J, Worster A, Hohl C, Lee JS, Eisenhauer MA, Mortensen M, Mackey D, Pauls M, Lesiuk H, Wells GA. Sensitivity of computed tomography performed within six hours of onset of headache for diagnosis of subarachnoid haemorrhage: prospective cohort study. BMJ. 2011;343:d4277.
16. Cortnum S, Sorensen P, Jorgensen J. Determining the sensitivity of computed tomography scanning in early detection of subarachnoid hemorrhage. Neurosurgery. 2010;66:900–2.
17. Backes D, Rinkel GJ, Kemperman H, Linn FH, Vergouwen MD. Time-dependent test characteristics of head computed tomography in patients suspected of nontraumatic subarachnoid hemorrhage. Stroke. 2012;43:2115–9.
18. Edlow JA, Fisher J. Diagnosis of subarachnoid hemorrhage: time to change the guidelines? Stroke. 2012;43:2031–2.
19. Perry JJ, Stiell IG, Sivilotti ML, Bullard MJ, Hohl CM, Sutherland J, Émond M, Worster A, Lee JS, Mackey D, Pauls M, Lesiuk H, Symington C, Wells GA. Clinical decision rules to rule out subarachnoid hemorrhage for acute headache. JAMA. 2013;310:1248–55.

20. Shah KH, Edlow JA. Distinguishing traumatic lumbar puncture from true subarachnoid hemorrhage. J Emerg Med. 2002;23(1):67–74.
21. UK National External Quality Assessment Scheme for Immuno- chemistry Working Group. National guidelines for analysis of cerebro- spinal fluid for bilirubin in suspected subarachnoid haemorrhage. Ann Clin Biochem. 2003;40:481–8.
22. Veuger AJ, Kortbeek LH, Booij AC. Siderophages in differentiation of blood in cerebrospinal fluid. Clin Neurol Neurosurg. 1977;80:46–56.
23. Mauer AM. Crenated red cells in spinal fluid. Am J Dis Child. 1964;108:451.
24. Drews FA, Musters A, Samore MH. Error producing conditions in the intensive care unit. In: Henriksen K, Battles JB, Keyes MA, et al. editors. Advances in patient safety: new directions and alternative approaches. Vol. 3: Performance and Tools. Rockville: Agency for Healthcare Research and Quality (US); 2008. Available from: http://www.ncbi.nlm.nih.gov/books/NBK43691/.
25. Rothschild JM, Landrigan CP, Cronin JW, Kaushal R, Lockley SW, Burdick E, Stone PH, Lilly CM, Katz JT, Czeisler CA, Bates DW. The Critical Care Safety Study: The incidence and nature of adverse events and serious medical errors in intensive care. Crit Care Med. 2005;33:1694–700.
26. Bucknall TK. Medical error and decision making: learning from the past and present in intensive care. Aust Crit Care. 2010;23:150–6.
27. Lerch C, Yonekawa Y, Muroi C, Bjeljac M, Keller E. Specialized neurocritical care, severity grade, and outcome of patients with aneurysmal subarachnoid hemorrhage. Neurocrit Care. 2006;5:85–92.
28. Lee K. The neuro ICU book. New York: McGraw-Hill Companies, Inc; 2012. p. 01–34.
29. Malekzadeh J, Mazluom SR, Etezadi T, Tasseri A. A standardized shift handover protocol: improving nurses' safe practice in intensive care units. J Caring Sci. 2013;2:177–85.
30. Rosen MA, Pronovost PJ. Advancing the use of checklists for evaluating performance in health care. Acad Med. 2014;89:963–5.
31. Nyholm L, Lewén A, Fröjd C, Howells T, Nilsson P, Enblad P. The use of nurse checklists in a bedside computer-based information system to focus on avoiding secondary insults in neurointensive care. ISRN Neurol. 2012;2012:903954.
32. Lee JC, Horst M, Rogers A, Rogers FB, Wu D, Evans T, Edavettal M. Checklist-styled daily sign-out rounds improve hospital throughput in a major trauma center. Am Surg. 2014;80:434–40.
33. Wartenberg KE. Acute treatment in subarachnoid haemorrhage. In: Norrving B, editor. Oxford textbook of stroke and cerebrovascular disease. Oxford; New York: Oxford University Press, 2014. p. 139–52.
34. Diringer MN, Bleck TP, Hemphill 3rd CJ, Menon D, Shutter L, Vespa P, Bruder N, Connolly Jr ES, Citerio G, Gress D, Hanggi D, Hoh BL, Lanzino G, Le Roux P, Rabinstein A, Schmutzhard E, Stocchetti N, Suarez JI, Treggiari M, Tseng MY, Vergouwen MD, Wolf S, Zipfel G, Neurocritical Care Society. Critical care management of patients following aneurysmal subarachnoid hemorrhage: recommendations from the Neurocritical Care Society's Multidisciplinary Consensus Conference. Neurocrit Care. 2011;15:211–40.
35. Connolly Jr ES, Rabinstein AA, Carhuapoma JR, Derdeyn CP, Dion J, Higashida RT, Hoh BL, Kirkness CJ, Naidech AM, Ogilvy CS, Patel AB, Thompson BG, Vespa P, American Heart Association Stroke Council, Council on Cardiovascular Radiology and Intervention, Council on Cardiovascular Nursing, Council on Cardiovascular Surgery and Anesthesia, Council on Clinical Cardiology. Guidelines for the management of aneurysmal subarachnoid hemorrhage: a guideline for healthcare professionals from the American Heart Association/American Stroke Association. Stroke. 2012;43:1711–37.
36. Aiyagari V, Cross 3rd DT, Deibert E, Dacey Jr RG, Diringer MN. Safety of hemodynamic augmentation in patients treated with Guglielmi detachable coils after acute aneurysmal subarachnoid hemorrhage. Stroke. 2001;32:1994–7.
37. Koenig MA. Management of delayed cerebral ischemia after subarachnoid hemorrhage. Continuum (Minneap Minn). 2012;18:579–97.

38. Schuette AJ, Hui FK, Obuchowski NA, Walkup RR, Cawley CM, Barrow DL, Samuels OB. An examination of aneurysm rerupture rates with epsilon aminocaproic acid. Neurocrit Care. 2013;19:48–55.
39. Aaslid R. Transcranial Doppler assessment of cerebral vasospasm. Eur J Ultrasound. 2002;16:3–10.
40. Chwajol M, Starke RM, Kim GH, Mayer SA, Connolly ES. Antifibrinolytic therapy to prevent early rebleeding after subarachnoid hemorrhage. Neurocrit Care. 2008;8:418–26.
41. Tseng MY, Al-Rawi PG, Pickard JD, Rasulo FA, Kirkpatrick PJ. Effect of hypertonic saline on cerebral blood flow in poor-grade patients with subarachnoid hemorrhage. Stroke. 2003;34:1389–96.
42. Starke RM, Kim GH, Fernandez A, Komotar RJ, Hickman ZL, Otten ML, Ducruet AF, Kellner CP, Hahn DK, Chwajol M, Mayer SA, Connolly Jr ES. Impact of a protocol for acute antifibrinolytic therapy on aneurysm rebleeding after subarachnoid hemorrhage. Stroke. 2008;39(9):2617–21.
43. Hillman J, Fridriksson S, Nilsson O, Yu Z, Saveland H, Jakobsson KE. Immediate administration of tranexamic acid and reduced incidence of early rebleeding after aneurysmal subarachnoid hemorrhage: a prospective randomized study. J Neurosurg. 2002;97:771–8.
44. Baharoglu MI, Germans MR, Rinkel GJ, Algra A, Vermeulen M, van Gijn J, Roos YB. Antifibrinolytic therapy for aneurysmal subarachnoid haemorrhage. Cochrane Database Syst Rev. 2013;(8):CD001245.
45. Oudshoorn SC, Rinkel GJ, Molyneux AJ, Kerr RS, Dorhout Mees SM, Backes D, Algra A, Vergouwen MD. Aneurysm treatment <24 versus 24–72 h after subarachnoid hemorrhage. Neurocrit Care. 2014;21:4–13.
46. Molyneux AJ, Kerr RS, Yu LM, Clarke M, Sneade M, Yarnold JA, Sandercock P, International Subarachnoid Aneurysm Trial (ISAT) Collaborative Group. International subarachnoid aneurysm trial (ISAT) of neurosurgical clipping versus endovascular coiling in 2143 patients with ruptured intracranial aneurysms: a randomised comparison of effects on survival, dependency, seizures, rebleeding, subgroups, and aneurysm occlusion. Lancet. 2005;366:809–17.
47. Serrone JC, Wash EM, Hartings JA, Andaluz N, Zuccarello M. Venous thromboembolism in subarachnoid hemorrhage. World Neurosurg. 2013;80:859–63.
48. Simard JM, Aldrich EF, Schreibman D, James RF, Polifka A, Beaty N. Low-dose intravenous heparin infusion in patients with aneurysmal subarachnoid hemorrhage: a preliminary assessment. J Neurosurg. 2013;119:1611–9.
49. CLOTS (Clots in Legs Or sTockings after Stroke) Trials Collaboration. Effect of intermittent pneumatic compression on disability, living circumstances, quality of life, and hospital costs after stroke: secondary analyses from CLOTS 3, a randomised trial. Lancet Neurol. 2014;12:1186–92.
50. Hacker RI, Ritter G, Nelson C, Knobel D, Gupta R, Hopkins K, Marini CP, Barrera R. Subcutaneous heparin does not increase postoperative complications in neurosurgical patients: an institutional experience. J Crit Care. 2012;27:250–4.
51. Flemming KD, Brown Jr RD, Wiebers DO. Subarachnoid hemorrhage. Curr Treat Options Neurol. 1999;1:97–112.
52. Messori A, Trippoli S, Vaiani M, Gorini M, Corrado A. Bleeding and pneumonia in intensive care patients given ranitidine and sucralfate for prevention of stress ulcer: meta-analysis of randomised controlled trials. BMJ. 2000;321:1103–6.
53. O'Keefe GE, Gentilello LM, Maier RV. Incidence of infectious complications associated with the use of histamine2-receptor antagonists in critically ill trauma patients. Ann Surg. 1998;227:120–5.
54. Cook D, Guyatt G, Marshall J, Leasa D, Fuller H, Hall R, Peters S, Rutledge F, Griffith L, McLellan A, Wood G, Kirby A, for the Cana-dian Critical Care Trials Group. A comparison of sucralfate and ranitidine for the prevention of upper gastrointestinal bleeding in patients requiring mechanical ventilation. N Engl J Med. 1998;338:791–7.
55. Fletcher JJ, Brown DL, Rajajee V, Jacobs TL, Rochlen L, Meurer W. The association between proton pump inhibitor use and outcome after aneurysmal subarachnoid hemorrhage. Neurocrit Care. 2011;15(3):393–9.

56. MacLaren R, Reynolds PM, Allen RR. Histamine-2 receptor antagonists vs proton pump inhibitors on gastrointestinal tract hemorrhage and infectious complications in the intensive care unit. JAMA Intern Med. 2014;174:564–74.
57. Barletta JF, Erstad BL, Fortune JB. Stress ulcer prophylaxis in trauma patients. Crit Care. 2002;6:526–30.
58. Lu WY, Rhoney DH, Boling WB, et al. A review of stress ulcer prophylaxis in the neurosurgical intensive care unit. Neurosurgery. 1997;41(2):416–26.
59. Friedman D, Claassen J, Hirsch LJ. Continuous electroencephalogram monitoring in the intensive care unit. Anesth Analg. 2009;109:506–23.
60. Naidech AM, Kreiter KT, Janjua N, Ostapkovich N, Parra A, Com- michau C, Connolly ES, Mayer SA, Fitzsimmons BF. Phenytoin exposure is associated with functional and cognitive disability after subarachnoid hemorrhage. Stroke. 2005;36:583–7.
61. Zubkov AY, Wijdicks EF. Antiepileptic drugs in aneurysmal subarachnoid hemorrhage. Rev Neurol Dis. 2008;5:178–81.
62. Kirkpatrick PJ, Turner CL, Smith C, Hutchinson PJ, Murray GD, STASH Collaborators. Simvastatin in aneurysmal subarachnoid haemorrhage (STASH): a multicentre randomised phase 3 trial. Lancet Neurol. 2014;13(7):666–7.
63. Chiconie MR, Dacey RG. Clinical aspects of subarachnoid hemorrhage. In: Welch KMA, Caplan LR, Reis DJ, Siesjö BK, Weir B, editors. Primer on cerebrovascular disease. San Diego: Academic; 1997.
64. Dorai Z, Hynan LS, Kopitnik TA, Samson D. Factors related to hydrocephalus after aneurysmal subarachnoid hemorrhage. Neurosurgery. 2003;52:763–9.
65. Gigante P, Hwang BY, Appelboom G, Kellner CP, Kellner MA, Connolly ES. External ventricular drainage following aneurysmal subarachnoid haemorrhage. Br J Neurosurg. 2010;24:625–32.
66. Ramakrishna R, Sekhar LN, Ramanathan D, Temkin N, Hallam D, Ghodke BV, Kim LJ. Intraventricular tissue plasminogen activator for the prevention of vasospasm and hydrocephalus after aneurysmal subarachnoid hemorrhage. Neurosurgery. 2010;67(1):110–7; discussion 117.
67. Hoekema D, Schmidt RH, Ross I. Lumbar drainage for subarachnoid hemorrhage: technical considerations and safety analysis. Neurocrit Care. 2007;7:3–9.
68. Komotar RJ, Hahn DK, Kim GH, Khandji J, Mocco J, Mayer SA, Connolly Jr ES. The impact of microsurgical fenestration of the lamina terminalis on shunt-dependent hydrocephalus and vasospasm after aneurysmal subarachnoid hemorrhage. Neurosurgery. 2008;62(1):123–32; discussion 132–34.
69. Beydon L, Audibert G, Berré J, Boulard G, Gabrillargues J, Bruder N, Hans P, Puybasset L, Ravussin P, de Kersaint-Gilly A, Ter Minassian A, Dufour H, Lejeune JP, Proust F, Bonafé A. Pain management in severe subarachnoid haemorrhage. Ann Fr Anesth Reanim. 2005;24:782.
70. Binhas M, Walleck P, El Bitar N, Melon E, Palfi S, Albaladejo P, Marty J. Pain management in subarachnoid haemorrhage: a survey of French analgesic practices. Ann Fr Anesth Reanim. 2006;25:935–9.
71. Parkhutik V, Lago A, Tembl JI, Rubio C, Fuset MP, Vallés J, Santos MT, Moscardo A. Influence of COX-inhibiting analgesics on the platelet function of patients with subarachnoid hemorrhage. J Stroke Cerebrovasc Dis. 2012;21:755–9.
72. Rosen DS, Macdonald RL. Subarachnoid hemorrhage grading scales: a systematic review. Neurocrit Care. 2005;2:110–8.
73. Ryttlefors M, Howells T, Nilsson P, Ronne-Engström E, Enblad P. Secondary insults in subarachnoid hemorrhage: occurrence and impact on outcome and clinical deterioration. Neurosurgery. 2007;61:704–14.
74. Wartenberg KE. Update on the management of subarachnoid hemorrhage. Future Neurol. 2013;8:205–24.

75. Sendelbach S, Funk M. Alarm fatigue: a patient safety concern. AACN Adv Crit Care. 2013;24:378–86.
76. Roederer A, Holmes JH, Smith MJ, Lee I, Park S. Prediction of significant vasospasm in aneurysmal subarachnoid hemorrhage using automated data. Neurocrit Care. 2014;21: 444–50.
77. Boers AM, Zijlstra IA, Gathier CS, van den Berg R, Slump CH, Marquering HA, Majoie CB. Automatic quantification of subarachnoid hemorrhage on noncontrast CT. AJNR Am J Neuroradiol. 2014;35(12):2279–86.

Chapter 9
Intracerebral Hemorrhage

Moon Ku Han

Introduction

Spontaneous or nontraumatic intracerebral hemorrhage (ICH) is associated with poor outcome, a higher case fatality than ischemic stroke, and is one of the leading causes of death. Patients with ICH are among the highest number of admissions to the neurocritical intensive care unit (NICU) [1].

ICH represents 10–15 % of all strokes, but the median 1 month case fatality is 40–50 % with only 38 % surviving the first year [2]. The Oxfordshire Community Stroke Project estimated that about 60 % of the patients with ICH do not survive beyond one year [3]. Outcome is determined by the initial severity of the bleeding, and treatment regimens are limited [4].

The most common etiology of ICH is microangiopathy caused by arterial hypertension, which is estimated to constitute around 80 % of all causes. Since high blood pressure (BP) by itself often causes no symptoms, many people with ICH are not aware that they have high BP, or that their BP needs to be treated. Less common causes of ICH include amyloid angiopathy, trauma, infections, intracranial neoplasm, coagulopathy (either inherent or drug induced, such as chronic vitamin K antagonist therapy and thrombolytic therapy), cerebral venous thrombosis, and abnormalities of blood vessels (such as arteriovenous malformations, cavernous angioma, venous angioma). Other risk factors for ICH appeared to be advanced age, male sex, and high alcohol intake. High cholesterol tends to be associated with a lower risk of ICH [5].

M.K. Han, MD, PhD
Department of Neurology, Seoul National University Bundang Hospital,
Seongnam, South Korea
e-mail: mkhan@snu.ac.kr

© Springer International Publishing Switzerland 2015
K.E. Wartenberg et al. (eds.), *Neurointensive Care: A Clinical Guide
to Patient Safety*, DOI 10.1007/978-3-319-17293-4_9

145

Case

A 63-year-old Korean man with a history of hypertension and alcohol abuse was admitted to the hospital with sudden onset of nausea, vomiting, speech disturbance, and right hemiparesis. He was on amlodipine 5 mg and irbesartan 150 mg every morning for hypertension. The time of onset of symptoms was approximately 50 min ago. On arrival at the emergency department, the patient was found to be somnolent and responsive to painful stimuli. His Glasgow Coma Scale (GCS) score was 8. Vital signs were taken: BP: 180/100 mmHg, heart rate (HR): 98 bpm, respiratory rate (RR): 26, blood sugar by fingerstick: 160 mg/dL (8.8 mmol/L). Initial computed tomography (CT) scan showed a left basal ganglia ICH with intraventricular hemorrhage (IVH) into the left lateral ventricle (Fig. 9.1). Early intensive BP lowering (systolic BP ≤ 140 mmHg) was achieved and intraventricular administration of 1 mg tissue plasminogen activator (tPA) every 8 h via external ventricular drainage (EVD) was applied to reduce IVH volume and ICP.

Risks of Patient Safety and Management

Outcomes with ICH are significantly worse than with ischemic stroke, with up to 50 % mortality at 30 days. Morbidity and mortality in spontaneous ICH are correlated with low GCS score (≤8), hematoma volume, the presence of IVH, advanced age (≥80 years), and infratentorial hematoma [6]. Almost 40 % of patients with brain imaging obtained in the first 3 h after onset of symptoms of ICH experience hematoma expansion and this is highly associated with the increase of ICP and neurological deterioration [7]. The sudden increase in pressure within the brain can cause damage to the brain cells surrounding the hemorrhage. If the amount of blood increases rapidly, the sudden buildup in ICP can lead to unconsciousness or death. Expanding hematoma results from persistent and/or secondary bleeding at the periphery of an existing clot. Recent studies showed a strong association between contrast extravasation ("spot sign") on computed tomography angiography (CTA) and hematoma expansion and worse outcome [8].

Initial goals of treatment include stabilization of airway, breathing, and circulation, followed by preventing hemorrhage extension, as well as the prevention and management of elevated intracranial pressure along with other neurologic and medical complications. The patients should be monitored and treated in an NICU.

Blood Pressure

In general, the American Heart Association guidelines indicate that systolic BP exceeding 180 mmHg or mean arterial pressure (MAP) exceeding 130 mmHg should be managed with continuous-infusion antihypertensive agents (Table 9.1) [9]. There was concern about a reduction of cerebral blood flow surrounding the

Fig. 9.1 CT scan showing left basal ganglia intracerebral hemorrhage with extravasation into the left lateral ventricle

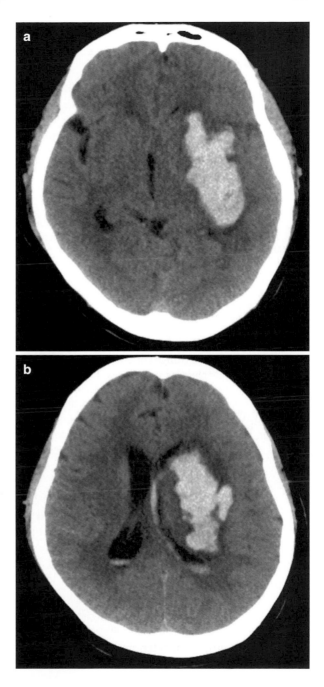

hemorrhage with aggressive BP reduction. However, despite a peri-hematomal reduction of cerebral metabolism, an ischemic zone was not found on several radiographic cerebral metabolism studies.

The use of nitroprusside has drawbacks since this agent may exacerbate cerebral edema and intracranial pressure, and sublingual agents are not preferred because of

Table 9.1 Intravenous anti-hypertensive agents for blood pressure reduction in ICH

Drug	Mechanism	Dose	Contraindications
Labetalol	α-1, β-1, β-2 receptor antagonist	10–80 mg bolus every 10 min, up to 300 mg; 0.5–2.0 mg/min infusion	Bradycardia, congestive heart failure, bronchospasm
Esmolol	β-1 receptor antagonist	0.5 mg/kg bolus; 50–300 μg/kg/min	Bradycardia, congestive heart failure, bronchospasm
Nicardipine	L-type calcium channel blocker (dihydropyridine)	5–15 mg/h infusion	Severe aortic stenosis, myocardial ischaemia
Enalapril	ACE inhibitor	0.625 mg bolus; 1.25–5 mg every 6 h	Variable response, sudden in BP with high-renin states
Fenoldopam	Dopamine-1 receptor agonist	0.1–0.3 μg/kg/min	Tachycardia, headache, nausea, flushing, glaucoma, portal hypertension
Nitroprusside	Nitrovasodilator (arterial and venous)	0.25–10 μg/kg/min	Increased ICP, variable response, myocardial ischemia, thiocyanate and cyanide toxicity

Abbreviations: *ACE* angiotension-converting enzyme, *BP* blood pressure

the need for precise BP control [10]. Therefore, nitroprusside should not be the first agent for BP reduction in patients with ICH. In general, no matter how high the BP is, the MAP should not be reduced beyond 15–30 % over the first 24 h [11].

Early elevation of BP is very common after ICH and is strongly associated with poor outcomes [12]. The adverse effects of high BP levels on outcomes in ICH are likely to involve a number of different mechanisms: elevated hydrostatic pressure in the region of the ICH is likely to result in a larger initial hemorrhage with more rapid increase of hematoma volume, whereas elevated BP may increase the likelihood of surrounding cerebral edema [13].

Current guidelines for the acute management of ICH provide an indication of perceived harm associated with "very high" BP levels. Early intensive BP lowering (systolic BP ≤ 140 mmHg) was feasible, well tolerated, and appeared to reduce hematoma growth over 72 h, which may translate into beneficial effects in patients treated within 6 h after acute ICH [14]. Early intensive lowering of BP (systolic BP ≤ 140 mmHg) with any agent did not result in a significant reduction in the rate of the death or major disability, but intensive treatment may improve functional outcomes and areas of perceived quality of life. The intensive treatment was not associated with an increase in the rates of death or serious adverse events [15]. Therefore, the guidelines for management of ICH by the European Stroke Organization recommend reduction of the systolic BP to less than 140 mmHg within 6 h of symptom onset which was shown to be safe [16].

Seizures

Clinical seizures should be treated with anti-epileptic drugs as recurrent seizures may increase mass effect and midline shift. Continuous EEG monitoring is indicated in ICH patients with depressed mental status out of proportion to the degree of brain injury. Patients with a change in mental status who are found to have electrographic seizures on EEG should be treated with anti-epileptic drugs. Prophylactic anticonvulsant medication should not be used [9, 16].

Treatment of Intraventricular Hemorrhage

Intraventricular extension of ICH that occurs in 45 % of cases is a known independent predictor of poor outcome. Several studies have demonstrated a direct relationship between IVH volume and poor outcome or mortality [17–19]. Another study showed that IVH volume predicts mortality independent of the GCS [20]. The mechanisms by which IVH volume affects outcome likely include increased intracranial pressure with reduced cerebral perfusion, mechanical disruption, ventricular wall distension, and possibly an inflammatory response [21–23]. Total volume of IVH in itself is associated with poor outcome and a "poor-outcome threshold" of 50 mL above which 100 % of patients had a poor outcome [18]. An IVH volume >60 mL was associated with a mortality rate of 60 %. Low-dose recombinant tissue plasminogen activator (r-tPA) administered via extraventricular drainage catheter in the treatment of ICH with IVH has an acceptable safety profile compared to placebo and historical controls of the natural history [24]. A dose of 1 mg of r-tPA every 8 h (followed by clamping of the EVD for 1 h) is reasonable until clearance of blood from the third or fourth ventricle has been achieved (*CLEAR INTRAVENTRICULAR HEMORRHAGE TRIAL* study protocol). However, prior to administration of r-tPA further hematoma expansion and the possible presence of EVD-associated hemorrhage should be excluded by repeat head CT. This treatment is currently under investigation in a phase III trial.

Intracranial Hypertension

Patients with a GCS score of 8 or less, or those with significant IVH or hydrocephalus, might be considered for ICP monitoring and treatment. Ventricular drainage as treatment for hydrocephalus is reasonable in patients with decreased level of consciousness [9].

The head of the bed should be elevated to 30°. Hyperosmolar therapy of mannitol or hypertonic saline is indicated in patients with intracranial hypertension and with impending herniation. Hypertonic saline was found to have a longer duration of effect. Safety concerns are renal failure with the use of mannitol and worsening of preexisting congestive heart failure with administration of hypertonic saline. In patients with renal failure, the osmolar gap should be followed instead of serum osmolarity to monitor the effect of mannitol.

Surgery has the greater potential to reduce the volume of ICH and there is clinical and experimental evidence that mass removal might reduce nervous tissue damage, possibly by relieving local ischemia or removal of noxious chemicals [25, 26]. Large, surgically accessible clots exerting a mass effect might benefit from early surgery, especially in younger patients; whereas, inaccessible clots with surgical approach paths that cross eloquent speech and motor regions probably do not. Most neurosurgeons would remove a large frontopolar or temporal ICH after recent deterioration of consciousness, an ICH of deeper location is not amendable to surgical removal. Minimally invasive techniques might be more beneficial for deeper clots and IVH.

In several prospective randomized controlled trials, the patient outcome early surgery for spontaneous supratentorial ICH was unchanged compared to controls. Some patients did worse with surgery (e.g., those with deep-seated bleeds or with IVH and hydrocephalus) and some had better results (e.g., patients with superficial lobar hematomas without IVH) [25]. The same effect was noted in a meta-analysis of other studies and in a large randomized trial: a benefit for mortality and functional from early surgery for ICH was not seen, there was a trend to better outcome with surgery of superficially located ICH [26, 27]. The results of STICH II showed no benefit for early surgery for patients with lobar ICH within 1 cm of the surface [28]. Therefore, the indication for surgical clot removal should be discussed individually and be based on the patient's age, the size and location of the hemorrhage, and the presence of mass effect.

For patient's safety, early aggressive BP lowering along with neuromonitoring, treatment of seizures, and early recognition of signs of intracranial hypertension followed by initiation of ICP reducing management are the most important steps.

Safety Barriers and Risk–Benefit Assessment

During all treatment steps discussed the patient must be monitored closely. The overall aim is to stop hemorrhage expansion and to limit the additional brain tissue reduction by mass effect and seizures. Intensive BP reduction is reasonable [15, 16]. The indication for craniotomy and clot removal needs to be carefully evaluated as hematoma evacuation may cause further tissue destruction and may be followed by rebleeding. In lobar ICH and younger patients, a CT angiogram upon presentation may help to exclude sources of bleeding which may be unmasked during hematoma evacuation and to identify patients at risk for hematoma expansion by demonstrating a "spot sign." Hemicraniectomy may be a reasonable alternative to hematoma evacuation, especially in younger patients.

All patients with ICH should be screened for coagulopathies, and anticoagulant medication effects antagonized emergently, especially before undergoing a neurosurgical procedure (see Table 9.2) [9].

Table 9.2 Emergency management of ICH due to coagulopathy

Scenario	Agent	Dose	Comments	Level of evidence[a]
Warfarin Target: INR < 1.4	Fresh frozen plasma (FFP) *or*	10–15 mL/kg	Usually 4–6 units (200 mL) each are given, risk of volume overload	Low
	Prothrombin complex concentrate (Factor II, IV, IX, X, protein C, S) *and*	10–50 U/kg	Works faster than FFP, but carries risk of DIC, thrombosis, infection, anaphylaxis	Low
	IV Vitamin K	10 mg	Can take up to 24 h to normalize INR	Low
Warfarin and emergency neurosurgical intervention	*Above plus consider* Recombinant factor VIIa	20–80 μg/kg	Contraindicated in acute thromboembolic disease, increased risk of ischemic stroke and myocardial infarction	Very low
Unfractionated or low-molecular-weight heparin Target PTT 25–35 s	Protamine sulfate	1–1.5/0.5–0.75/0.25–0.375 mg per 100 units of heparin (<30 min/ 30–120 min/ 2 h) 1 mg per 100 anti-Xa units LMWH if given within last 8 h	Slowly: less than 20 mg per min Maximum 50 mg Can cause flushing, bradycardia, or hypotension. More effective for tinzaparin than for dalteparin or enoxaparin Minimal efficacy against danaparoid or fondaparinux	Very low
Direct thrombin inhibitors (argatroban, hirudin, dabigatran) or **inhibitors of factor Xa** (apixaban, rivaroxaban, endoxaban)	Prothrombin complex concentrate 50 g charcoal if Xa inhibitor ingested within 2 h Hemodialysis for dabigatran overdose or renal insufficiency	30–60 U/kg	Carries risk of DIC, thrombosis, infection, anaphylaxis	Very low

(continued)

Table 9.2 (continued)

Scenario	Agent	Dose	Comments	Level of evidence[a]
Platelet dysfunction or thrombocytopenia	Platelet transfusion *and/or*	6 units or 1 single donor apheresis unit	Range 4–8 units based on size; within 12 h of symptom onset	Low
Target platelets > 100,000/μL If planned for neurosurgical procedure and documented platelet dysfunction	Desmopressin (DDAVP)	0.3 μg/kg	Single dose required	Low
Thrombolysis Complication	Cryoprecipitate	6–8 U	Mostly 4–6 units	Very low

Abbreviations: *DIC* disseminated intravascular coagulation, *INR* international normalized ratio, *LMWH* low molecular weight heparin, *PTT* prothrombin time

[a]According to the GRADE criteria: Low quality of evidence = The authors are not confident in the effect estimate and the true value may be substantially different; very low quality evidence = The authors do not have any confidence in the estimate and it is likely that the true value is substantially different from it

Summary

In management of ICH, acute severe hypertension should be aggressively, but carefully, controlled with IV medications to reduce systolic blood pressure to less than 140 mmHg. Coagulopathies need to be antagonized aggressively to prevent hematoma expansion. Suspected ICP elevation and symptomatic intracranial mass effect should be treated with head elevation, mannitol or hypertonic saline, surgical treatment should be considered for individual patients. Observation in a neurocritical care unit is strongly recommended for at least the first 24 h based on the risk of neurologic deterioration.

Dos and Don'ts

Dos

- Stabilize airway, breathing and circulation
- Observation in the NICU is strongly recommended for at least 24 h based on neurologic status and hemodynamics
- Prevention of extension of hemorrhage by BP control and antagonization of coagulopathy
- Patients with GCS of 8 or less with significant ICH or hydrocephalus should be considered for ICP monitoring
- Early intensive BP reduction of systolic BP to less than 140 mmHg within first 6 h
- Use continuous EEG monitoring with patients with depressed mental status out of proportion to brain injury
- Monitor for early signs and symptoms of intracranial hypertension
- Hypertonic saline is indicated for intracranial hypertension and impending herniation
- Indication for surgical clot removal depends on individual case
- In selected cases with right skills and resources, r-TPA administered via extraventricular drainage can be effective

Don'ts

- Reduction of the MAP beyond 15–30 % over the first 24 h
- Use nitroprusside IV as a first line agent to control BP in ICH
- Prophylactic anticonvulsant should not be used

References

1. Anderson RN, Smith BL. Deaths: leading causes for 2002. Natl Vital Stat Rep. 2005;53: 1–89.
2. Qureshi AI, Tuhrim S, Broderick JP, Batjer HH, Hondo H, Hanley DF. Spontaneous intracerebral hemorrhage. N Engl J Med. 2001;344:1450–60.
3. Dennis MS, Burn JP, Sandercock PA, Bamford JM, Wade DT, Warlow CP. Long-term survival after first-ever stroke: the Oxfordshire Community Stroke Project. Stroke. 1993;24:796–800.
4. Gebel JM, Broderick JP. Intracerebral hemorrhage. Neurol Clin. 2000;18:419–38.
5. Ariesen MJ, Claus SP, Rinkel GJ, Algra A. Risk factors for intracerebral hemorrhage in the general population: a systematic review. Stroke. 2003;34:2060–5.
6. Hemphill JC, Bonovich DC, Besmertis L, Manley GT, Johnston SC. The ICH score: a simple, reliable grading scale for intracerebral hemorrhage. Stroke. 2001;32:891–7.
7. Brott T, Broderick J, Kothari R, et al. Early hemorrhage growth in patients with intracerebral hemorrhage. Stroke. 1997;28:1–5.
8. Delgado Almandoz JE, Yoo AJ, Stone MJ, et al. The spot sign score in primary intracerebral hemorrhage identifies patients at highest risk of in-hospital mortality and poor outcome among survivors. Stroke. 2010;41:54–60.
9. Morgenstern LB, Hemphill 3rd JC, Anderson C, Becker K, Broderick JP, Connolly Jr ES, et al. Guidelines for the management of spontaneous intracerebral hemorrhage: a guideline for healthcare professionals from the American Heart Association/American Stroke Association. Stroke. 2010;41(9):2108–29.
10. Rose JC, Mayer SA. Optimizing blood pressure in neurological emergencies. Neurocrit Care. 2004;1:287–99.
11. Powers WJ, Asams RF, Yundt KD. Acute pharmacological hypotension after intracerebral hemorrhage does not change cerebral blood flow. Stroke. 1999;30:242.
12. Vemmos KN, Tsivgoulis G, Spengos K, Zakopoulos N, Synetos A, Manios E, Konstantopoulou P, Mavrikakis M. U-shaped relationship between mortality and admission blood pressure in patients with acute stroke. J Intern Med. 2004;255:257–65.
13. Kazui S, Minematsu K, Yamamoto H, Sawada T, Yamaguchi T. Predisposing factors to enlargement of spontaneous intracerebral hematoma. Stroke. 1997;28:2370–5.
14. Anderson CS, Huang Y, Arima H, et al. Effects of early intensive blood pressure lowering treatment on the growth of hematoma and perihematomal edema in acute intracerebral hemorrhage: the Intensive Blood Pressure Reduction in Acute Cerebral Haemorrhage Trial (INTERACT). Stroke. 2010;41:307–12.
15. Anderson CS, Heeley E, Huang Y, Wang J, Stapf C, Delcourt C, et al. INTERACT2 Investigators. Rapid blood-pressure lowering in patients with acute intracerebral hemorrhage. N Engl J Med. 2013;368:2355–65.
16. Steiner T, Al-Shahi Salman R, Beer R, Christensen H, Cordonnier C, Csiba L, Forsting M, Harnof S, Klijn CJ, Krieger D, Mendelow AD, Molina C, Montaner J, Overgaard K, Petersson J, Roine RO, Schmutzhard E, Schwerdtfeger K, Stapf C, Tatlisumak T, Thomas BM, Toni D, Unterberg A, Wagner M. European Stroke Organisation (ESO) guidelines for the management of spontaneous intracerebral hemorrhage. Int J Stroke. 2014;9(7):840–55.
17. Hallevi H, Albright K, Aronowski J, et al. Intraventricular hemorrhage: anatomic relationships and clinical implications. Neurology. 2008;70:848–52.
18. Young WB, Lee KP, Pessin MS, et al. Prognostic significance of ventricular blood in supratentorial hemorrhage: a volumetric study. Neurology. 1990;40:616–9.
19. Steiner T, Diringer MN, Schneider D, et al. Dynamics of intraventricular hemorrhage in patients with spontaneous intracerebral hemorrhage: risk factors, clinical impact, and effect of hemostatic therapy with recombinant activated factor VII. Neurosurgery. 2006;59:767–73.
20. Tuhrim S, Horowitz DR, Sacher M, et al. Volume of ventricular blood is an important determinant of outcome in supratentorial intracerebral hemorrhage. Crit Care Med. 1999;27: 617–21.

21. Mayer SA, Thomas CE, Diamond BE. Asymmetry of intracranial hemodynamics as an indicator of mass effect in acute intracerebral hemorrhage. A transcranial Doppler study. Stroke. 1996;27:1788–92.
22. Mayfrank L, Kissler J, Raoofi R, et al. Ventricular dilatation in experimental intraventricular hemorrhage in pigs characterization of cerebrospinal fluid dynamics and the effects of fibrinolytic treatment. Stroke. 1997;28:141–8.
23. Wasserman JK, Zhu X, Schlichter LC. Evolution of the inflammatory response in the brain following intracerebral hemorrhage and effects of delayed minocycline treatment. Brain Res. 2007;1180:140–54.
24. Naff N, Williams MA, Keyl PM, et al. Low-dose recombinant tissue-type plasminogen activator enhances clot resolution in brain hemorrhage: the intraventricular hemorrhage thrombolysis trial. Stroke. 2011;42:3009–16.
25. Xi G, Keep RF, Hoff JT. Mechanisms of brain injury after intracerebral haemorrhage. Lancet Neurol. 2006;5:53–63.
26. Keep RF, Xi G, Hua Y, Hoff JT. The deleterious or beneficial effects of different agents in intracerebral hemorrhage: think big, think small, or is hematoma size important? Stroke. 2005;36:1594–6.
27. Bhattathiri PS, Gregson B, Prasad KS, Mendelow AD, STICH Investigators. Intraventricular hemorrhage and hydrocephalus after spontaneous intracerebral hemorrhage: results from the STICH trial. Acta Neurochir Suppl. 2006;96:65–8.
28. Mendelow AD, Gregson BA, Rowan EN, Murray GD, Gholkar A, Mitchell PM, STICH II Investigators. Early surgery versus initial conservative treatment in patients with spontaneous supratentorial lobar intracerebral haematomas (STICH II): a randomised trial. Lancet. 2013;382:397–408.

Chapter 10
Patient Safety in Acute Ischemic Stroke

Ivan Rocha Ferreira da Silva and Bernardo Liberato

Introduction

Patient safety has been an increasing concern in modern medicine worldwide, and recent discussions about quality of care, safety precautions and performance measures of stroke care have gained growing interest. Healthcare systems throughout the world face the vexing problem of improving healthcare quality while at the same time confronted with ever-increasing costs and greater demands for accountability [1].

Stroke is a common and serious disorder. Each year, approximately 750,000 individuals have a new or recurrent stroke in the United States [2]. Also, stroke patients occupy 20 % of acute medical beds in the British National Health System [3]. Safety is a major issue in this population, as medical complications are frequent among individuals who have had a stroke, increasing the length of hospitalization as well as the costs of care [4]. Moreover, many of the complications described are potentially preventable or treatable if promptly recognized [5], and patients at risk for or who have had a stroke often do not receive medical care consistent with current evidence-based standards [6].

The aim of this chapter is to introduce the importance of structured stroke care, minimizing complications and risks, as well as promoting safe, effective, and durable care interventions.

I.R.F. da Silva, MD
Department of Neurocritical Care, Hospital Copa D'Or, Rio de Janeiro, Brazil

B. Liberato, MD (✉)
Department of Neurology, Hospital Copa D'Or, Rio de Janeiro, Brazil
e-mail: bbliberato@yahoo.com

© Springer International Publishing Switzerland 2015
K.E. Wartenberg et al. (eds.), *Neurointensive Care: A Clinical Guide to Patient Safety*, DOI 10.1007/978-3-319-17293-4_10

Case Scenario

A 75 year-old lady, with history of diabetes mellitus and hypertension, is brought to the emergency department by her son after a sudden onset of weakness on her right side and difficulty speaking. He mentioned that she was last seen normal approximately 45 min ago, and an immediate neurological exam discloses dense paresis of her right side, with severe aphasia and a left gaze deviation, with a National Institute of Health Stroke Scale (NIHSS) score of 18. An emergency computed tomography (CT) scan of the head was unremarkable, and so the decision was to proceed with intravenous thrombolysis with recombinant tissue plasminogen activator (r-tPA). The per-protocol bolus of the medication was uneventful, but during the first half of the infusion, the bedside nurse noticed a blood pressure of 200/115 mmHg and a finger test showed a capillary glucose of 210 mg/dL (11.6 mmol/L). Soon after, her level of consciousness declined suddenly, and a repeat CT disclosed a 35 mL intraparenchymal hemorrhage in the area of the left basal ganglia, with a 5 mm midline shift and intraventricular blood (Fig. 10.1). The r-tPA infusion was held, fresh-frozen plasma and cryoprecipitate were given and she was admitted to the neurocritical care unit (NICU). No surgical intervention was indicated at that point. During the first week in the NICU she was treated for aspiration pneumonia, not

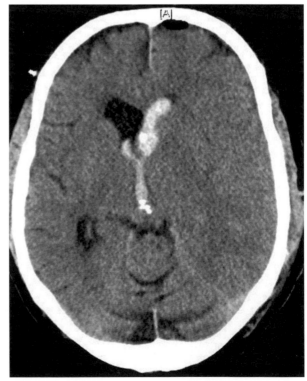

Fig. 10.1 CT scan of the 75-year-old patient with acute right sided hemiparesis and aphasia receiving intravenous thrombolysis showing the intraventricular hemorrhage originating from a left basal ganglia intracerebral hemorrhage and a 5 mm midline shift

requiring mechanical ventilation. Two weeks later the patient was moved to the neurology ward with some improvement of the right-sided weakness, but still with severe aphasia. During the following night, the patient was found on the ground by the on-call nurse, likely a consequence of the bed side-rail being down. She suffered no neurological insults, but a wrist fracture was noticed, prolonging her hospital stay and transfer to a rehabilitation facility.

Risks of Patient Safety

Stroke patients are exposed to several possible complications, which can occur at any time during the disease process, as early as a hemorrhagic transformation or intracerebral hemorrhage in the first few hours after thrombolysis, or later in the shape of aspiration pneumonia secondary to some degree of dysphagia, fall risk, deep venous thrombosis (DVT), and pressure ulcers during rehabilitation. Previous studies have shown that complications are common, with estimates of frequencies ranging from 40 to 96 % of patients [7–11]. As is true for long-term neurological recovery and overall mortality, age and stroke severity are associated with the development of complications, which most commonly occur in the first 4 days [12].

Several studies retrospectively analyzed the incidence and timing of medical complications in stroke patients. Davenport et al. [7] found that seizures and chest infections occurred early, whereas depression and painful shoulder were later problems. Dromerick et al. [8] noticed that the mean number of medical and neurological complications per patient were 3.6 and 0.6, respectively, and complications were independently related to both the severity of functional disability as judged by Barthel score and length of rehabilitation hospital stay. Finally, Johnston et al. [9] reported a 3-month mortality of 14 % in stroke patients, with 51 % of these deaths were attributed primarily to medical complications. Outcome was significantly worse in patients with serious medical complications [9].

A prospective cohort Scottish study [5] found that the most frequent complications during hospital stay were confusion (56 %), pain (34 %), falls (25 %), infections (24 %, mostly respiratory and urinary tract infections), depression (16 %,) and recurrent stroke (9 %), but during follow-up as outpatient, infections, falls, "blackouts," pain, and symptoms of depression and anxiety remained common.

Pneumonia, which is usually associated with immobility, ineffective cough and difficulty of airway protection, is an important cause of death after stroke [13–15]. Moreover, stroke-associated pneumonia increases length of stay, mortality, and hospital costs [16]. Early mobility and good pulmonary care can help to prevent pneumonia [16], as well as preventive measures in intubated patients, including ventilation in a semi-recumbent position, frequent suctioning, mouth hygiene, and early extubation. A retrospective study disclosed that patients with brain-stem stroke were more likely to develop early pneumonia. The incidence was higher in patients who failed swallowing evaluation and in those who were intubated [17].

Urinary tract infections are quite common, occurring in 15–60 % of stroke patients, independently predicting worse outcomes [5, 13, 18, 19]. Patients with major impairments as well as use of indwelling catheters are associated with urinary tract infections [20]. Early removal of indwelling catheters, bladder training and use of intermittent catheterization are strategies to lessen the risk of such infections [21].

Pulmonary embolism accounts for 10 % of deaths after stroke, and the complication may be detected in 1 % of stroke patients [22]. The risk of DVT is highest amongst immobilized and older patients with severe stroke [23–25], and is more frequent in the first 3 months after the stroke [12]. Besides being associated with a pulmonary embolism, symptomatic DVT also delays recovery and rehabilitation after stroke [21]. The alternatives for mitigating the risk of DVT include early mobilization, administration of antithrombotic agents, and the use of external compression devices. In patients with acute ischemic stroke, there is strong evidence that the use of low-molecular weight heparin is the therapy of choice to prevent DVT [26]. The late introduction of DVT prophylaxis with low-molecular weight heparin in hospitalized stroke patients, based on the unfounded concern for hemorrhagic transformation, adds to this problem, especially in patients with large hemispheric strokes who happen to be the most susceptible to thrombotic complications. The misconception that patients with a large hemispheric ischemic stroke should have the low-molecular weight heparin withheld for a few days only adds to the medical morbidity in such patients and is not supported by either anecdotal or evidence-based experience. Early introduction of DVT prophylaxis, even in the presence of small petechial bleeds should be the rule in all stroke patients.

Swallowing impairments are associated with an increased risk of death and pneumonia [14, 27]. Mann et al. [27] have shown that at presentation, a swallowing abnormality was detected clinically in 51 % of acute stroke patients and videofluoroscopically in 64 %, with 20 % having developed respiratory infections. An abnormal gag reflex, impaired voluntary cough, dysphonia, incomplete oral-labial closure, a high NIHSS score, or cranial nerve palsies should alert the care team to the risk of dysphagia [21]. A formal speech and swallow evaluation should be obtained early on in all stroke patients for detection of subtle signs of microaspiration. When such evaluation is not readily available, a water swallow test performed at the bedside is a useful screening tool [21], and dysphagia screening protocols have shown to lessen the risk of pneumonia in different settings [28, 29]. Although caution should be exerted to orally feed stroke patients, nutrition should be started as soon as possible, usually through nasogastric tubes, as it is associated with improved outcomes [30].

Stroke, as many neurological disorders, is associated with a high risk of falls [31]. It has been shown that up to 21 % of patients after an acute stroke might experience falls within the first 6 weeks [11], and studies investigating falls in the later phase report an incidence of up to 73 % in the first year post-stroke [32]. Falls can lead to a variety of consequences, such as traumatic brain injuries, fractures, fear of falling, reduced activity and death, and involve both personal suffering and economic costs for the community [33–35]. Exercises and physical therapy are recommended to improve gait stability, and assessment tools of fall risk on admission, both in the acute and subacute settings, seem to decrease the incidence of this complication [36, 37]. Professional advice with prescription of orthotic devices when appropriate and counseling regarding improvement in home safety measures might mitigate this problem.

Decubitus ulcers are an often neglected problem in hospitalized patients with stroke, and are considered a quality metric for many hospitals. Decubiti were reported in up to 21 % of acute stroke patients in a prospective study [5], and the Center for Medicare Services (CMS) does not reimburse wound care if the patient develops decubiti while hospitalized due to the potentially preventable nature of this complication [38]. This and other reinforcement tools might decrease its occurrence. Well known risk factors include immobility, lack of turning by nursing personnel, poor nutrition, and urinary incontinence.

Safety Barriers and Structured Stroke Care

Safety in healthcare is an essential part of modern medicine, and vast evidence has been produced recently on the matter. It is well known that protocol bundles might improve outcomes in critical care, such as decreasing mortality in severe sepsis [39], mitigating the incidence of central line associated infections [40, 41] and ventilator-associated pneumonia [42]. Furthermore, protocol bundles also optimize cost-effectiveness of care [43, 44]. A "bundle" is a group of evidence-based care components for a given disease that, when executed together, may result in better outcomes than when implemented individually, according to the Institute for Healthcare Improvement [45].

Unfortunately, no studies so far have assessed the implementation of safety bundles in patients with stroke. Important strategies such as DVT prophylaxis, dysphagia screening, fall prevention, blood pressure and serum glucose management are intuitive measures and are cited in guidelines [21, 46], but the impact of those actions taken together is unknown. At least in theory, all the benefits of the bundled care for the stroke patients can be found when they are admitted to a separate physical unit where attention is given to the specific needs of this patient population, e.g. the Stroke Unit. Also the presence of a team, experienced in the care of stroke patients offers a greater chance of protocol compliance, increased surveillance for potential medical complications and expedited discharge to an acute or subacute rehabilitation unit. Even more evident is the level of care for the severe stroke patients in a dedicated neurological ICU, where close attention and familiarity with the unstable neurological patient often make a difference in the outcome.

Recently, several attempts have been made to protocolize stroke care, with the aim of improving outcomes and minimizing complications. The Get With The Guidelines–Stroke is an ongoing voluntary, continuous quality-improvement initiative involving hospitals mainly in the United States and Canada that collects patient level data on characteristics, treatments, in-hospital outcomes, and adherence to quality measures in stroke, including ischemic stroke and hemorrhagic stroke. The initiative has been successful so far, with studies showing significant improvement of quality of care [47, 48]. Performance measures of quality of care in stroke are essential tools to assess what is offered to stroke patients, and several studies have been conducted in Germany [49, 50], Denmark [51], the United States [52–55], Chile [56], the Netherlands [57], and Austria [58] to better understand the gaps between the guidelines and bedside care. Recently, a study compared the performance measures used in several centers in Europe, and found significant differences in benchmarks, quality indicators and data documentation, suggesting that an equalization of such measurements should be done urgently [59].

The implementation of safety barriers is an important part of organized stroke care. Safe care can be promoted with patient and family's education, strict observance of established protocols, continuous feedback on performance measures and frequent training of healthcare personnel. Structured care, through establishment of neurocritical care and stroke units, can definitely change the outcomes in critically ill neurological patients [60–63]. The American Heart Association/American Stroke Association and the Joint Commission on Accreditation of Healthcare Organizations have merged efforts to create standards on stroke care, and recently started accrediting hospitals in the United States as Primary Stroke Centers or Comprehensive Stroke Centers, if strict criteria are fulfilled. A comparable accreditation process is available for regional, hyperregional, and comprehensive stroke centers in Germany and other countries in Europe through regional stroke societies and associations.

Some actions to prevent complications in stroke patients are well recognized, and will be discussed later in this chapter. The daily assessment of patient's needs, including measures to avoid complications, structured plan of care and fluid communication through all levels of the care team are essential to promote safety. The implementation of multidisciplinary rounds and the use of "check lists" to remind of important preventive measures are well established in critical care units [64, 65], and this successful model should be thoroughly used in the stroke population as well.

Risks and Benefits of Systemic Thrombolysis in Acute Ischemic Stroke

To this date, systemic thrombolysis with r-tPA is the only evidence-based treatment able to improve outcomes in patients with acute ischemic stroke. The landmark NINDS trial in 1995 randomized 624 patients, and produced clinical and statistical benefit over placebo for patients treated within 3 h of evaluation [66]. It showed that patients treated with r-tPA were at least 30 % more likely to have minimal or no disability at 3 months, with a 6.4 % risk of intracerebral hemorrhage [66]. Based on these results, r-tPA was approved for treatment of acute ischemic stroke in the United States in 1996 [67] for use within 3 h of onset of symptoms, but not without controversy. At that time, some authors [68–70], as well as associations of emergency medicine physicians [71, 72], criticized the study's methodology, and did not endorse its use by emergency specialists, as previous trials on thrombolysis in acute stroke were negative, such as the ECASS [73], ECASS II [74], and ATLANTIS

[75]. Worth mentioning, these studies used longer time windows (>3 h) and in ECASS a different dose of r-tPA was used. However, a Cochrane review using meta-analysis of various types of thrombolysis, including r-tPA, urokinase and streptokinase, concluded that this therapy was effective [76]. In a response to the emergency physicians, a re-analysis of the NINDS trial, now dividing into subgroups regarding the NIH stroke scale upon arrival and time of onset, was published in the Annals of Emergency Medicine, showing that the results were still similar after balancing again both groups [77].

The controversy finally settled almost a decade later. In order to have alteplase (r-tPA) approved under European Union regulations, the SITS-MOST study was conducted to assess the safety profile of alteplase in clinical practice by comparison with results in randomized controlled trials [78]. A total of 6,483 patients were recruited from 285 centers (50 % with little previous experience in stroke thrombolysis) in 14 countries between 2002 and 2006 for this prospective, open, monitored, observational study. Results showed that intravenous alteplase is safe and effective in routine clinical use when used within 3 h of stroke onset, even by centers with little previous experience in thrombolytic therapy for acute stroke. Two years later, the ECASS III trial found similarly positive results, now with patients with acute stroke within a time window within 3–4.5 h, leaving no doubt about the effectiveness and safety of this therapy [79].

A more elegant way of understanding the risk versus benefit in patients receiving r-tPA, and hence its safety implications, is to use the number needed to treat (NNT) and the number needed to harm (NNTH). The number needed to treat for benefit (NNT) is an effect measure that indicates how many patients need to be treated with an intervention for one patient to experience a benefit, with the opposite being the NNTH. The post-hoc analysis of the NINDS trial showed that for different dichotomized global functional end-points, the number needed to harm as a result of r-tPA-related cerebral hemorrhages ranges widely, from 36.5 to 707 [80]. To better refine, a reasonable key dichotomization for NNTH estimation is the number needed to treat for one additional patient to end up severely disabled or dead, with a calculated NNTH of 126 in the NINDS trial [80]. Finally, for every 100 patients treated with rtPA, across all levels of final global disability, approximately 32 will benefit and approximately three will be harmed, with odds of better results ten times higher than for harm [80]. Two years later another post-hoc analysis was conducted, now including the pooled data set of the first six major randomized acute stroke trials of intravenous r-tPA [81]. The results found that the NNT for benefit was 3.6 for patients treated between 0 to 90 min, 4.3 for 91 to 180 min, 5.9 for 181 to 270 min, and 19.3 with treatment between 271 and 360 min. This underscores not only the effectiveness of the therapy but also its strong time-dependency.

Some studies have shown that most complications related to r-tPA in acute ischemic stroke are derived from protocol violations (e.g., blood pressure control, patient selection, etc.) [82–84], and from a medico-legal standpoint, physicians have a much higher chance of being sued for not offering r-tPA for eligible candidates than for drug-related complications [85, 86]. Alteplase is the only Class I, Level of Evidence A treatment for acute ischemic stroke accordingly to the current American Heart Association and European Stroke Organization Guidelines

[21, 46]. It is recommended that institutions adhere to strict protocols in order to ensure minimal safety requirements. Continuous auditing and case-by-case discussion should be encouraged and regarded as basic safety measures, especially in centers with little experience (less than 5 cases/year). As is true in medical complications after an acute stroke the presence of checklists pre and post intravenous thrombolysis should be the rule with special emphasis on blood pressure monitoring per protocol, adequate glucose control, and frequent neurological assessments.

Finally, some case series and observational studies have shown that r-tPA can be probably safely administered in off label situations, such as in very elderly patients [87], patients with prior stroke and diabetes mellitus [88], stroke mimics [89], presence of unruptured aneurysm or arteriovenous malformation [90] and in pregnant patients [91–93].

Solutions to Potential Risks

Table 10.1 summarizes the most important and thoroughly studied actions to prevent and/or minimize the most frequent medical complications encountered in stroke patients.

Table 10.1 Solutions to potential risks

Risks	Possible solutions/prevention
Aspiration	Early screening for dysphagia per protocol, elevate head –of-bed 30°
Falls	Education of patients and family, elevate bed rails, assisted walking, early physical therapy, encourage use of corrective lenses, use of walking devices (e.g. cane, walker), assessment of fall risk on admission with clear identification of patients at risk
Urinary infections	Early removal of urinary catheters, bladder training, use of intermittent catheterization instead of indwelling catheters if needed later in the hospital stay
Pressure ulcers	Avoid immobility, aggressive skin care, frequent turning per protocol, adequate nutritional support, and control of urinary incontinence
Deep venous thrombosis	Avoid immobility, early use of low-molecular weight heparin (preferred) or unfractionated heparin, use of sequential compression devices in the first 24 h after systemic thrombolysis
Delirium	Support family at the bedside, early move to wards with windows and sunlight, encourage use of corrective lenses and hearing devices, mitigate the use of benzodiazepines and physical restraints, minimize metabolic derangements, use of orienting techniques, day-night structure
Secondary stroke prevention	Education of patients and family (blood pressure control, diabetes, stroke prevention, smoking cessation, nutrition), assure use of anti-platelet aggregation agents and statins upon discharge, referral for follow up soon after discharge

Summary

Patient safety has been an increasing worldwide concern in modern medicine, and recent discussions about quality of care, safety precautions and performance measures of stroke care have gained growing interest. Stroke patients are exposed to several possible complications, which can occur at any time during the disease process, and can potentially worsen their prognosis.

Unfortunately, no studies so far have studied the implementation of safety bundles in patients with stroke. Important strategies such as DVT prophylaxis, dysphagia screening, fall prevention, blood pressure and serum glucose management are cited in guidelines, but the impact of those actions taken together is unknown. The auditing for implementation of secondary prevention measures upon discharge, as suggested by the accrediting agencies and the American Heart Association – Get with the Guidelines, are also instrumental in maximizing the benefit and reducing the harm associated with early and late stroke recurrence.

The implementation of safety barriers is an important part of organized stroke care. Safe care can be promoted with patient and family's education, strict observance of established protocols, continuous feedback on performance measures and frequent training of healthcare personnel.

Dos and Don'ts

Dos

- Stroke patients should preferably be admitted to specialized units, e.g. stroke units
- Early physical/occupational therapy and speech/swallow evaluation
- Multidisciplinary teams are essential for adequate stroke care
- Check-lists should be used to remind of important preventive actions
- Clear identification (wrist band) of anticoagulated or recently thrombolized stroke patients
- Considered stroke a priority in your ER, with the same classification of urgency as trauma or acute myocardial infarction
- Education and training of healthcare personnel, as well as patients and their relatives is important.
- Adhere to approved guidelines for IV thrombolysis, especially in centers with little experience

Don'ts

- Do not underestimate medical complications in stroke patients
- Do not leave stroke patients with severe disabilities unattended

- Do not underestimate the aid of family members in stroke care
- Avoid protocol deviations in stroke care, especially utilizing systemic thrombolysis
- Do not admit stroke patients to your facility if stroke is not considered to be a priority in your ER, and receive the classification of urgency as trauma or acute myocardial infarction
- Do not admit stroke patients to your facility if it's unsure that quality care can be provided

References

1. Reeves MJ, Parker C, Fonarow GC, Smith EE, Schwamm LH. Development of stroke performance measures: definitions, methods, and current measures. Stroke. 2010;41(7):1573–8.
2. Alberts MJ, Latchaw RE, Selman WR, et al. Recommendations for comprehensive stroke centers: a consensus statement from the Brain Attack Coalition. Stroke. 2005;36(7): 1597–616.
3. Walsh K, Gompertz PH, Rudd AG. Stroke care: how do we measure quality? Postgrad Med J. 2002;78(920):322–6.
4. Kumar S, Selim MH, Caplan LR. Medical complications after stroke. Lancet Neurol. 2010;9(1):105–18.
5. Langhorne P, Stott DJ, Robertson L, et al. Medical complications after stroke: a multicenter study. Stroke. 2000;31(6):1223–9.
6. Holloway RG, Benesch C, Rush SR. Stroke prevention: narrowing the evidence-practice gap. Neurology. 2000;54(10):1899–906.
7. Davenport RJ, Dennis MS, Wellwood I, Warlow CP. Complications after acute stroke. Stroke. 1996;27(3):415–20.
8. Dromerick A, Reding M. Medical and neurological complications during inpatient stroke rehabilitation. Stroke. 1994;25(2):358–61.
9. Johnston KC, Li JY, Lyden PD, et al. Medical and neurological complications of ischemic stroke: experience from the RANTTAS trial. RANTTAS Investigators. Stroke. 1998;29(2):447–53.
10. Kalra L, Yu G, Wilson K, Roots P. Medical complications during stroke rehabilitation. Stroke. 1995;26(6):990–4.
11. McClatchie G. Survey of the rehabilitation outcome of strokes. Med J Aust. 1980;1(13): 649–51.
12. Indredavik B, Rohweder G, Naalsund E, Lydersen S. Medical complications in a comprehensive stroke unit and an early supported discharge service. Stroke. 2008;39(2):414–20.
13. Aslanyan S, Weir CJ, Diener HC, Kaste M, Lees KR. Pneumonia and urinary tract infection after acute ischaemic stroke: a tertiary analysis of the GAIN International trial. Eur J Neurol. 2004;11(1):49–53.
14. Martino R, Foley N, Bhogal S, Diamant N, Speechley M, Teasell R. Dysphagia after stroke: incidence, diagnosis, and pulmonary complications. Stroke. 2005;36(12):2756–63.
15. van der Worp HB, Kappelle LJ. Complications of acute ischaemic stroke. Cerebrovasc Dis (Basel, Switzerland). 1998;8(2):124–32.
16. Hilker R, Poetter C, Findeisen N, et al. Nosocomial pneumonia after acute stroke: implications for neurological intensive care medicine. Stroke. 2003;34(4):975–81.
17. Upadya A, Thorevska N, Sena KN, Manthous C, Amoateng-Adjepong Y. Predictors and consequences of pneumonia in critically ill patients with stroke. J Crit Care. 2004;19(1):16–22.
18. Kong KH, Young S. Incidence and outcome of poststroke urinary retention: a prospective study. Arch Phys Med Rehabil. 2000;81(11):1464–7.

19. Roth EJ, Lovell L, Harvey RL, Heinemann AW, Semik P, Diaz S. Incidence of and risk factors for medical complications during stroke rehabilitation. Stroke. 2001;32(2):523–9.
20. Ween JE, Alexander MP, D'Esposito M, Roberts M. Incontinence after stroke in a rehabilitation setting: outcome associations and predictive factors. Neurology. 1996;47(3):659–63.
21. Jauch EC, Saver JL, Adams Jr HP, et al. Guidelines for the early management of patients with acute ischemic stroke: a guideline for healthcare professionals from the American Heart Association/American Stroke Association. Stroke. 2013;44(3):870–947.
22. Wijdicks EF, Scott JP. Pulmonary embolism associated with acute stroke. Mayo Clin Proc. 1997;72(4):297–300.
23. Desmukh M, Bisignani M, Landau P, Orchard TJ. Deep vein thrombosis in rehabilitating stroke patients. Incidence, risk factors and prophylaxis. Am J Phys Med Rehabil. 1991;70(6): 313–6.
24. Kelly J, Rudd A, Lewis RR, Coshall C, Moody A, Hunt BJ. Venous thromboembolism after acute ischemic stroke: a prospective study using magnetic resonance direct thrombus imaging. Stroke. 2004;35(10):2320–5.
25. Warlow C, Ogston D, Douglas AS. Deep venous thrombosis of the legs after strokes. Part I–incidence and predisposing factors. Br Med J. 1976;1(6019):1178–81.
26. Sherman DG, Albers GW, Bladin C, et al. The efficacy and safety of enoxaparin versus unfractionated heparin for the prevention of venous thromboembolism after acute ischaemic stroke (PREVAIL Study): an open-label randomised comparison. Lancet. 2007;369(9570):1347–55.
27. Mann G, Hankey GJ, Cameron D. Swallowing function after stroke: prognosis and prognostic factors at 6 months. Stroke. 1999;30(4):744–8.
28. Hinchey JA, Shephard T, Furie K, Smith D, Wang D, Tonn S. Formal dysphagia screening protocols prevent pneumonia. Stroke. 2005;36(9):1972–6.
29. Martino R, Silver F, Teasell R, et al. The Toronto Bedside Swallowing Screening Test (TOR-BSST): development and validation of a dysphagia screening tool for patients with stroke. Stroke. 2009;40(2):555–61.
30. Dennis MS, Lewis SC, Warlow C. Effect of timing and method of enteral tube feeding for dysphagic stroke patients (FOOD): a multicentre randomised controlled trial. Lancet. 2005;365(9461):764–72.
31. Homann B, Plaschg A, Grundner M, et al. The impact of neurological disorders on the risk for falls in the community dwelling elderly: a case-controlled study. BMJ Open. 2013;3(11): e003367.
32. Verheyden GS, Weerdesteyn V, Pickering RM, et al. Interventions for preventing falls in people after stroke. Cochrane Database Syst Rev. 2013;(5):CD008728.
33. Batchelor FA, Mackintosh SF, Said CM, Hill KD. Falls after stroke. Int J Stroke. 2012;7(6):482–90.
34. Friedman SM, Munoz B, West SK, Rubin GS, Fried LP. Falls and fear of falling: which comes first? A longitudinal prediction model suggests strategies for primary and secondary prevention. J Am Geriatr Soc. 2002;50(8):1329–35.
35. Nystrom A, Hellstrom K. Fall risk six weeks from onset of stroke and the ability of the Prediction of Falls in Rehabilitation Settings Tool and motor function to predict falls. Clin Rehabil. 2013;27(5):473–9.
36. Rosario ER, Kaplan SE, Khonsari S, Patterson D. Predicting and assessing fall risk in an acute inpatient rehabilitation facility. Rehabil Nurs. 2014;39:86–93.
37. Smith J, Forster A, Young J. Use of the 'STRATIFY' falls risk assessment in patients recovering from acute stroke. Age Ageing. 2006;35(2):138–43.
38. Freeman WD, Dawson SB, Flemming KD. The ABC's of stroke complications. Semin Neurol. 2010;30(5):501–10.
39. Marwick C, Davey P. Care bundles: the holy grail of infectious risk management in hospital? Curr Opin Infect Dis. 2009;22(4):364–9.
40. Berenholtz SM, Lubomski LH, Weeks K, et al. Eliminating central line-associated bloodstream infections: a national patient safety imperative. Infect Control Hosp Epidemiol. 2014;35(1):56–62.

41. Hsu E, Lin D, Evans SJ, et al. Doing well by doing good: assessing the cost savings of an intervention to reduce central line-associated bloodstream infections in a Hawaii hospital. Am J Med Qual. 2014;29(1):13–9.
42. Morris AC, Hay AW, Swann DG, et al. Reducing ventilator-associated pneumonia in intensive care: impact of implementing a care bundle. Crit Care Med. 2011;39(10):2218–24.
43. Moller AH, Hansen L, Jensen MS, Ehlers LH. A cost-effectiveness analysis of reducing ventilator-associated pneumonia at a Danish ICU with ventilator bundle. J Med Econ. 2012;15(2):285–92.
44. Muscedere JG, Martin CM, Heyland DK. The impact of ventilator-associated pneumonia on the Canadian health care system. J Crit Care. 2008;23(1):5–10.
45. Institute for Healthcare Improvement. 2014. http://www.ihi.org/. Accessed 6 Feb 2014.
46. European Stroke Organisation (ESO) Executive Committee; ESO Writing Committee. Guidelines for management of ischaemic stroke and transient ischaemic attack 2008. Cerebrovasc Dis (Basel, Switzerland). 2008;25(5):457–507.
47. Fonarow GC, Reeves MJ, Smith EE, et al. Characteristics, performance measures, and in-hospital outcomes of the first one million stroke and transient ischemic attack admissions in get with the guidelines-stroke. Circ Cardiovasc Qual Outcomes. 2010;3(3):291–302.
48. Schwamm LH, Fonarow GC, Reeves MJ, et al. Get With The Guidelines-Stroke is associated with sustained improvement in care for patients hospitalized with acute stroke or transient ischemic attack. Circulation. 2009;119(1):107–15.
49. Heuschmann PU, Biegler MK, Busse O, et al. Development and implementation of evidence-based indicators for measuring quality of acute stroke care: the Quality Indicator Board of the German Stroke Registers Study Group (ADSR). Stroke. 2006;37(10):2573–8.
50. Nimptsch U, Mansky T. Quality measurement combined with peer review improved German in-hospital mortality rates for four diseases. Health Aff (Project Hope). 2013;32(9):1616–23.
51. Ingeman A, Andersen G, Hundborg HH, Svendsen ML, Johnsen SP. Processes of care and medical complications in patients with stroke. Stroke. 2011;42(1):167–72.
52. Jacobs BS, Baker PL, Roychoudhury C, Mehta RH, Levine SR. Improved quality of stroke care for hospitalized Medicare beneficiaries in Michigan. Stroke. 2005;36(6):1227–31.
53. Lakshminarayan K, Borbas C, McLaughlin B, et al. A cluster-randomized trial to improve stroke care in hospitals. Neurology. 2010;74(20):1634–42.
54. Pandey DK, Cursio JF. Data feedback for quality improvement of stroke care: CAPTURE Stroke experience. Am J Prev Med. 2006;31(6 Suppl 2):S224–9.
55. Roychoudhury C, Jacobs BS, Baker PL, Schultz D, Mehta RH, Levine SR. Acute ischemic stroke in hospitalized medicare patients: evaluation and treatment. Stroke. 2004;35(1):e22–3.
56. Hoffmeister L, Lavados PM, Comas M, Vidal C, Cabello R, Castells X. Performance measures for in-hospital care of acute ischemic stroke in public hospitals in Chile. BMC Neurol. 2013;13:23.
57. Lingsma HF, Dippel DW, Hoeks SE, et al. Variation between hospitals in patient outcome after stroke is only partly explained by differences in quality of care: results from the Netherlands Stroke Survey. J Neurol Neurosurg Psychiatry. 2008;79(8):888–94.
58. Steiner MM, Brainin M. The quality of acute stroke units on a nation-wide level: the Austrian Stroke Registry for acute stroke units. Eur J Neurol. 2003;10(4):353–60.
59. Wiedmann S, Norrving B, Nowe T, et al. Variations in quality indicators of acute stroke care in 6 European countries: the European Implementation Score (EIS) Collaboration. Stroke. 2012;43(2):458–63.
60. Josephson SA, Douglas VC, Lawton MT, English JD, Smith WS, Ko NU. Improvement in intensive care unit outcomes in patients with subarachnoid hemorrhage after initiation of neu-rointensivist co-management. J Neurosurg. 2010;112(3):626–30.
61. Knopf L, Staff I, Gomes J, McCullough L. Impact of a neurointensivist on outcomes in criti-cally ill stroke patients. Neurocrit Care. 2012;16(1):63–71.
62. Suarez JI, Zaidat OO, Suri MF, et al. Length of stay and mortality in neurocritically ill patients: impact of a specialized neurocritical care team. Crit Care Med. 2004;32(11):2311–7.

63. Varelas PN, Eastwood D, Yun HJ, et al. Impact of a neurointensivist on outcomes in patients with head trauma treated in a neurosciences intensive care unit. J Neurosurg. 2006;104(5): 713–9.
64. Irwin RS, Flaherty HM, French CT, et al. Interdisciplinary collaboration: the slogan that must be achieved for models of delivering critical care to be successful. Chest. 2012;142(6): 1611–9.
65. Vincent JL. Give your patient a fast hug (at least) once a day. Crit Care Med. 2005;33(6): 1225–9.
66. Tissue plasminogen activator for acute ischemic stroke. The National Institute of Neurological Disorders and Stroke rt-PA Stroke Study Group. N Engl J Med. 1995;333(24):1581–7.
67. Nightingale SL. From the food and drug administration. JAMA. 1996;276(6):443.
68. Lenzer J. Alteplase for stroke: money and optimistic claims buttress the "brain attack" campaign. BMJ (Clinical research ed). 2002;324(7339):723–9.
69. Lenzer J. Controversial stroke trial is under review following BMJ report. BMJ (Clinical research ed). 2002;325(7373):1131.
70. Li J. Questioning thrombolytic use for cerebrovascular accidents. J Emerg Med. 1998;16(5): 757–8.
71. Adams JG, Chisholm CD. The Society for Academic Emergency Medicine position on optimizing care of the stroke patient. Acad Emerg Med. 2003;10(7):805.
72. Brown DL, Barsan WG, Lisabeth LD, Gallery ME, Morgenstern LB. Survey of emergency physicians about recombinant tissue plasminogen activator for acute ischemic stroke. Ann Emerg Med. 2005;46(1):56–60.
73. Hacke W, Kaste M, Fieschi C, et al. Intravenous thrombolysis with recombinant tissue plasminogen activator for acute hemispheric stroke. The European Cooperative Acute Stroke Study (ECASS). JAMA. 1995;274(13):1017–25.
74. Hacke W, Kaste M, Fieschi C, et al. Randomised double-blind placebo-controlled trial of thrombolytic therapy with intravenous alteplase in acute ischaemic stroke (ECASS II). Second European-Australasian Acute Stroke Study Investigators. Lancet. 1998;352(9136): 1245–51.
75. Clark WM, Wissman S, Albers GW, Jhamandas JH, Madden KP, Hamilton S. Recombinant tissue-type plasminogen activator (Alteplase) for ischemic stroke 3 to 5 hours after symptom onset. The ATLANTIS Study: a randomized controlled trial. Alteplase Thrombolysis for Acute Noninterventional Therapy in Ischemic Stroke. JAMA. 1999;282(21):2019–26.
76. Wardlaw JM, Zoppo G, Yamaguchi T, Berge E. Thrombolysis for acute ischaemic stroke. Cochrane Database Syst Rev. 2003;(3):CD000213.
77. Kwiatkowski T, Libman R, Tilley BC, et al. The impact of imbalances in baseline stroke severity on outcome in the National Institute of Neurological Disorders and Stroke Recombinant Tissue Plasminogen Activator Stroke Study. Ann Emerg Med. 2005;45(4):377–84.
78. Wahlgren N, Ahmed N, Davalos A, et al. Thrombolysis with alteplase for acute ischaemic stroke in the Safe Implementation of Thrombolysis in Stroke-Monitoring Study (SITS-MOST): an observational study. Lancet. 2007;369(9558):275–82.
79. Hacke W, Kaste M, Bluhmki E, et al. Thrombolysis with alteplase 3 to 4.5 hours after acute ischemic stroke. N Engl J Med. 2008;359(13):1317–29.
80. Saver JL. Hemorrhage after thrombolytic therapy for stroke: the clinically relevant number needed to harm. Stroke. 2007;38(8):2279–83.
81. Lansberg MG, Schrooten M, Bluhmki E, Thijs VN, Saver JL. Treatment time-specific number needed to treat estimates for tissue plasminogen activator therapy in acute stroke based on shifts over the entire range of the modified Rankin Scale. Stroke. 2009;40(6):2079–84.
82. Katzan IL, Furlan AJ, Lloyd LE, et al. Use of tissue-type plasminogen activator for acute ischemic stroke: the Cleveland area experience. JAMA. 2000;283(9):1151–8.
83. Lopez-Yunez AM, Bruno A, Williams LS, Yilmaz E, Zurru C, Biller J. Protocol violations in community-based rTPA stroke treatment are associated with symptomatic intracerebral hemorrhage. Stroke. 2001;32(1):12–6.

84. Tsivgoulis G, Frey JL, Flaster M, et al. Pre-tissue plasminogen activator blood pressure levels and risk of symptomatic intracerebral hemorrhage. Stroke. 2009;40(11):3631–4.
85. Bambauer KZ, Johnston SC, Bambauer DE, Zivin JA. Reasons why few patients with acute stroke receive tissue plasminogen activator. Arch Neurol. 2006;63(5):661–4.
86. Weintraub MI. Thrombolysis (tissue plasminogen activator) in stroke: a medicolegal quagmire. Stroke. 2006;37(7):1917–22.
87. Mishra NK, Ahmed N, Andersen G, et al. Thrombolysis in very elderly people: controlled comparison of SITS International Stroke Thrombolysis Registry and Virtual International Stroke Trials Archive. BMJ (Clinical research ed). 2010;341:c6046.
88. Mishra NK, Ahmed N, Davalos A, et al. Thrombolysis outcomes in acute ischemic stroke patients with prior stroke and diabetes mellitus. Neurology. 2011;77(21):1866–72.
89. Scott PA, Silbergleit R. Misdiagnosis of stroke in tissue plasminogen activator-treated patients: characteristics and outcomes. Ann Emerg Med. 2003;42(5):611–8.
90. Aleu A, Mellado P, Lichy C, Kohrmann M, Schellinger PD. Hemorrhagic complications after off-label thrombolysis for ischemic stroke. Stroke. 2007;38(2):417–22.
91. Del Zotto E, Giossi A, Volonghi I, Costa P, Padovani A, Pezzini A. Ischemic stroke during pregnancy and puerperium. Stroke Res Treat. 2011;2011:606780.
92. Selim MH, Molina CA. The use of tissue plasminogen-activator in pregnancy: a taboo treatment or a time to think out of the box. Stroke. 2013;44(3):868–9.
93. Tassi R, Acampa M, Marotta G, et al. Systemic thrombolysis for stroke in pregnancy. Am J Emerg Med. 2013;31(2):448.e1–3.

Chapter 11
Cerebral Venous Thrombosis

Liping Liu and Ruijun Ji

Introduction

History and Definition

In the 1820s, occlusions of the cerebral veins that drain the brain were first reported. In 1825, Ribes [1–3] demonstrated the first case of dural sinus thrombosis. And then, in 1828, John Abercrombie [4] published the first case of venous thrombosis in the puerperal state. From now on, the prologue to the studies of cerebral venous thrombosis was opened.

Cerebral venous thrombosis, CVT, is a group of vascular diseases caused by backflow obstructions of the cerebral veins caused by thrombosis of intracranial venous sinus and veins. The characteristics of this group of diseases are complex etiology, diverse forms of pathogenesis, and a lack of specific clinical manifestations.

CVT accounts for 0.5–1 % of all cases of stroke and affects approximately five people per million annually. The age of onset is less than 61 years, and 78 % of patients are under 50 years. CVT occurs mainly in women and relatively young individuals. In Western countries, the incidence of CVT is about 1–4 per million during pregnancy and the postpartum period. The risk is highest during the last trimester and the first 4 weeks after delivery. This disease is also common in children, especially in those with fever and infection [5–11].

L. Liu, MD, PhD (✉) • R. Ji, MD, PhD
Neurology and Stroke Center, Beijing Tiantan Hospital, Beijing, China
e-mail: lipingsister@gmail.com

© Springer International Publishing Switzerland 2015
K.E. Wartenberg et al. (eds.), *Neurointensive Care: A Clinical Guide to Patient Safety*, DOI 10.1007/978-3-319-17293-4_11

Etiology

Underlying risk factors for the development of CVT include:

1. *Oral contraceptives;*
2. *Coagulopathy*: deficiency of antithrombin III, protein S and protein C, Leiden mutation of V factor, mutation of prothrombin G20210A, hyperhomocysteinemia, antiphospholipid antibody syndrome; [12–17]

    The largest study, International Study on Cerebral Vein and Dural Sinus Thrombosis (ISCVT) [5], a multinational, multicenter, prospective observational study with 624 patients demonstrated an inherited or acquired pro-thrombotic condition as the cause of CVT in 34 %.
3. *Pregnancy and Puerperium;*
4. *Infection*: aural region, mastoiditis, sinusitis, meningoencephalitis, brain abscess, and systemic infection.

    CVT caused by infection is more common in children. In a recent series of 70 children with CVT in the United States, 40 % had infection-related CVT. In ISCVT, 77 patients (12.3 %) over 15 years had CVT caused by infection, in 51 patients of those the infection source was found in the ear, face, mouth, and neck region, in 13 cases in the central nervous system [5].
5. *Other hematologic abnormalities*: iron-deficiency anemia, polycythemia, nephrotic syndrome etc.;
6. *Other drugs*: androgens, immunoglobulins, vitamin A.
7. *Tumor associated coagulopathy;*
8. *Systemic disease*: systemic lupus erythematosus, Wegener's granuloma, Behcet's disease, thyroid disease;
9. *Cryptogenic.*

General Clinical Characteristics and Diagnosis

At the end of the nineteenth century, Quinke described patients with headache, visual symptoms, papilledema, and evidence of raised intracranial pressure who always recovered and did not have brain tumors. He found an occlusion of both transverse sinuses and the vein of Galen in an autopsy of one of his patients.

1. *The symptoms of the whole brain*

    Headache: progressing, involving the entire head
    Papillary edema
    Disorders of consciousness
    Seizures

2. *Focal neurological deficits* depending on the location of thrombosis, scope, rate of progress, collateral circulation of veins, and the scope and extent of secondary brain injury

3. *Uncommon or rare*: cavernous sinus syndrome with cranial nerve deficits, subarachnoid hemorrhage, migraine with aura, circumscribed headache, transient ischemic attacks, tinnitus, cognitive disturbances, single or multiple cranial nerve damage.

Depending on the mechanism of neurological dysfunction, clinical findings are related to (1) increased intracranial pressure attributable to impaired venous drainage and (2) focal brain injury from venous ischemia/infarction or hemorrhage. CVT should be considered in new onset seizures, focal or generalized; subacute onset of symptoms, lobar hemorrhage with unclear etiology, signs of increased intracranial pressure.

The Imaging Examination of CVT

Neuroimaging is essential to the diagnosis of CVT [2, 18–24].

1. Computed tomography (CT) with contrast demonstrates the asa-dense triangle and the dense or empty delta sign in patients with thrombosis of the posterior portion of the superior sagittal sinus. An ischemic lesion with a hemorrhagic component is suggestive of CVT when an ischemic lesion crosses usual arterial boundaries or is located in a region close to a venous sinus. CVT may be seen on CT only during the subacute or chronic stage. And compared with the density of adjacent brain tissue, thrombus may be iso-dense, hypo-dense, or of mixed density.
   The magnetic resonance imaging (MRI) signal intensity of the venous thrombus varies according to the point of time of imaging from the onset of thrombus formation. The acute thrombus has a low intensity signal. In the first week, the venous thrombus frequently appears iso-intense to brain tissue on T1-weighted images and hypo-intense on T2-weighted images due to increased deoxyhemoglobin. By the second week, the thrombus contains methemoglobin, which results in a hyperintense signal on T1- and T2-weighted images. The early sign of CVT on non-contrast-enhanced MRI is absence of a flow void with alteration of signal intensity in the dural sinuses. The secondary signs include brain tissue damage including cerebral swelling, edema, and/or hemorrhage.
2. CT venogram is a rapid and reliable modality for detecting CVT. Because of the dense cortical bone adjacent to dural sinus, bone artifacts may interfere with the visualization of enhanced dural sinuses. To a certain extent, CTV is equivalent to magnetic resonance venogram (MRV) in the diagnosis of CVT, or may be more sensitive (less flow artifacts, shorter time, better depiction of smaller veins). This is contrasted with concerns about radiation exposure, the potential for iodine contrast material allergy, and contrast-induced nephropathy. Time-of-flight (TOF) MRV and contrast-enhanced MRI are the most commonly used MRV techniques. Phase-contrast MRI is used less frequently for the difficulty of defining the velocity of the encoding parameter which is operator-dependent. Nonthrombosed hypoplastic sinuses will not appear as abnormal low signal on

gradient echo or susceptibility-weighted images. Chronic thrombosis of the hypoplastic sinus appears as contrast-enhanced sinus with no flow on 2-dimensional TOF venography. Contrast-enhanced MRI offers improved visualization of cerebral venous structures.

In patients with persistent or progressive symptoms despite medical treatment, repeated neuroimaging (including a CTV or MRV) may help detect the development of a new ischemic lesion, intracerebral hemorrhage, edema, propagation of the thrombus, or other brain parenchymal lesions.

Invasive digital subtraction cerebral angiography (DSA) is less commonly needed to establish the diagnosis of CVT given the availability of MRV and CTV. A DSA should be performed if MRV or CTV results are inconclusive or if an endovascular procedure is being considered in propagation of the thrombus despite full therapeutic anticoagulation. CTV is diagnosed by failure of sinus appearance due to the occlusion; venous congestion with dilated cortical, scalp, or facial veins; enlargement of typically diminutive veins from collateral drainage; and reversal of venous flow.

3. A D-dimer of >500 ng/mL (0.5 mcg/mL) has been shown in 96 % of all patients with acute CVT [25].

Case Scenario

Case Report: CVT with Intracranial Infection and Secondary Cerebral Hemorrhage

We would like to present a young patient with CVT published by Te-Gyu Lee [26] in 1995. A 32 year old man was admitted to the emergency room with a generalized tonic seizure and otherwise good health until 6 months prior to admission. At that time, he suffered from purulent nasal discharge with foul odor and intermittent nasal stuffiness in the left nose, an elevated leukocyte count and erythrocyte sedimentation rate (ESR) were found. He denied orogenital ulcers, skull fractures, otitis or dental infection. He had no history of alcohol abuse or diabetes mellitus. Out of the blue, he felt a persistent bilateral throbbing headache in the frontal area with copious purulent rhinorrhea 2 days prior to admission. He presented with a generalized tonic seizure lasting about 3 min in the morning while sleeping 2 days later. He was found with postictal confusion, severe headache, and irritability for about 2 h. The contrast-enhanced MRI demonstrated severe inflammation in the left maxillary sinus and mild enhancement in the left anterior ethmoid sinus, a hyperintense lesion in the right frontal cortical area on T2-weighted images.

The routine examination of the cerebrospinal fluid (CSF) was normal except for the elevated opening pressure of 26 cmH_2O. After the young man regained consciousness, he complained of persistent global headache which was described as throbbing. Unfortunately, he had a second generalized tonic seizure in the evening of the admission day. The headache increased in intensity in the frontal area aggravated by sitting and standing. Neurological examination did not reveal any focal signs. Opioids and nonsteroidal anti-inflammatory drugs only had a modest effect on the headache.

After several routine examinations, the 6th day, the patient deteriorated in consciousness with stupor and recurrent generalized tonic clonic seizures along with fever. Seizure control was achieved with intravenous diazepam and phenytoin. The follow up MRI demonstrated high signal intensities in the superior sagittal sinus (SSS) and nonvisualization of the SSS and bilateral transverse venous sinuses. Intravenous heparinization was administered without any effect. Thereafter, on the 7th day, a CT scan showed intracalvarium hemorrhage and an empty delta sign of the superior sagittal sinus. The patient never regained consciousness. On the 8th day, a right parietotemporal lobectomy was done to prevent herniation due to the large intracerebral hemorrhage and surrounding edema. However, his neurological condition did not improve. He expired due to cardiopulmonary failure on the 11th day after admission.

Case Analysis: Gaps in Patient Safety of Wrong Diagnosis

The patient had rapidly progressive CVT with intracranial infection and intracerebral hemorrhage. Prior to developing seizures, he had exacerbated purulent nasal discharge and headache which was highly suggestive of acute sinusitis. The diagnosis of CVT was certain in this patient based on the clinical manifestation, MRI, and CT scan. Persistent leukocytosis, elevated sedimentation rates during the early phase, and high fever in the later phase pointed to the infectious origin of CVT. Initially, the clinical manifestations of the patient were bilateral frontal headache with copious purulent nasal discharge. This indicated that the headache was secondary to acute sinusitis, supported by persistent leukocytosis and elevated sedimentation rates. The seizures developed 2 days after the headache and rhinorrhea strongly suggested cerebral cortical involvement.

Because of the close proximity, the infection from the sphenoid sinus may spread to the intracranial venous system. In addition, the sphenoid wall can be extremely thin, and sometimes the sinus cavity is separated by just a thin mucosal barrier system from the adjacent structures. In cases of ethmoid or maxillary sinusitis sphenoid sinusitis may be missed [26]. This might have been the case in our patient, and the diagnosis of cerebral venous thrombosis was delayed.

Risks of Patient Safety

Clinical Diagnosis

All patients with intracranial hypertension and atypical headache should be considered for the diagnosis of CVT and undergo neuroimaging based on potential risk factors. Blood examinations should include biochemistry, prothrombin time (PT), activated partial thromboplastin time (aPTT), and D-Dimer. If the D-Dimer is low, the likelihood of diagnosing a CVT is low. However, if the clinical suspicion is high, further evaluation is warranted. The patient should be inquired about oral contraceptives, inflammatory diseases, infections, and previous thrombotic disease. A spinal tap may be helpful to exclude intracranial infections [27–31].

Misdiagnosis

Approximately 30–40 % of patients with CVT present with ICH. Typical clinical characteristics need to be inquired:

- Prodromal headache;
- Bilateral parenchymal abnormalities;
- Hypercoagulable states.

An isolated subarachnoid hemorrhage should also raise suspicion for CVT.

Isolated headache/idiopathic intracranial hypertension, cross-regional cerebral infarction of unclear etiology as well as isolated mental status changes may also be caused by CVT. CVT can only by excluded by CVT or MRV [27–31].

Follow Up Imaging

If the symptoms are persistent or progressive consistent with an extension of thrombus in patients undergoing anticoagulation for CVT, neuroimaging should be repeated early. For patients with a past history of CVT and new symptoms, repeat neuroimaging should be obtained. If CTV or MRV are inconclusive and the clinical suspicion of CVT is high, a cerebral angiogram is required. For the patients with stable CVT, CTV or MRV should be repeated 3–6 months after the diagnosis, in order to evaluate for recanalization of the occluded cortical veins or sinuses.

General Management of CVT

Complications of CVT encompass infection, intracranial hypertension, decreased visual acuity, epilepsy, hemorrhage, among others. The patients with CVT should be admitted to a monitoring unit or ICU initially [32].

Management for Intracranial Hypertension

Patients with neurological deterioration due to the serious mass effect or refractory intracranial hypertension caused by the intracranial hemorrhage should be evaluated for decompressive craniectomy. Tissue resection is not indicated.

If there is a decreased visual acuity, existing intracranial hypertension should be controlled. Longterm, acetazolamide can be applied. If there is a progressive decline in vision, other treatments such as lumbar puncture, optic nerve decompression or peritoneal shunt are effective as well.

Structural Epilepsy

The patients with CVT accompanied by seizures require antiepileptic drugs (AED). An AED should be maintained for 3–6 months and discontinued thereafter in patients without parenchymal lesions. However, routine use of antiepileptic drugs is not recommended.

Anticoagulation

Regardless of the presence of hemorrhage, anticoagulation should start immediately after the diagnosis of CVT. Unfractionated heparin (UFH) IV (dose titration) or low molecular weight heparin (LMWH, weight-based nadroparine) should be given initially, vitamin K antagonists constitute the long term therapy. If neurological condition is deteriorating despite full anticoagulation, endovascular treatment is the rescue therapy.

In provoked CVT (associated with a transient risk factor), vitamin K antagonists are continued for 3–6 months with a target INR of 2.0–3.0. In unprovoked CVT, vitamin K antagonists should be administered for 6–12 months with the same target INR. New oral anticoagulants are not approved for CVT.

Other Treatment

In case of bacterial infection, antimicrobial therapy is indicated. Brain abscess requires surgical drainage. Steroid use is not recommended.

Special Situations

If the cause of CVT is not obvious, an evaluation for coagulopathy is required. Testing for protein C, protein S, and antithrombin III is generally not meaningful until 2–4 weeks after discontinuation of anticoagulation.

The women with acute CVT during pregnancy should be treated with full-dose LMWH instead of UFH. The past history of CVT is not a contraindication for pregnancy. However, for the prothrombotic effect of pregnancy, frequent examination and consultations of experts are required for the affected women. In women with history of CVT, preventive application of low molecular weight heparin (LMWH) before pregnancy and postpartum may be considered. Figure 11.1 shows the clinical pathway of the management of CVT.

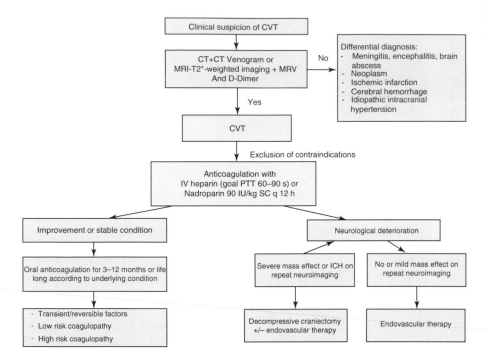

Fig. 11.1 Clinical pathway on diagnosis, treatment and prevention of CVT

Risk-Benefit Ratios of Management of the Disease

Anticoagulation

For patients with CVT, initial anticoagulation with adjusted unfractionated heparin (UFH, goal PTT 60–90 s) or weight-based low-molecular-weight heparin (LMWH) in full anticoagulant doses is reasonable, followed by vitamin K antagonists, regardless of the presence of ICH [30]. There are several rationales for anticoagulation therapy in CVT: to prevent thrombus growth, to facilitate recanalization, and to prevent DVT or PE. Controversy has ensued because cerebral venous infarction with hemorrhagic transformation or ICH is commonly present at the time of diagnosis of CVT.

There are two randomized controlled trials comparing anticoagulant therapy with placebo or open control in patients with CVT confirmed by contrast imaging [33, 34]. Taken together, these trials included only 79 patients. A meta-analysis of these two trials revealed a non-statistically significant relative risk of death or dependency with anticoagulation (relative risk 0.46, 95 % CI 0.16–1.31), with a difference in favor of anticoagulation of −13 % (95 % CI: −30 to 3 %). The relative risk of death was 0.33 (95 % CI: 0.08–1.21), with a risk difference of −13 % (95 % CI −27 to 1 %) in favor of anticoagulation [35].

In the special situation of CVT with intracerebral hemorrhage upon presentation or a patient with a major contraindication for anticoagulation (such as recent major hemorrhage), the clinician must balance the risks and benefits of anticoagulation, depending on the clinical situation [30]. In these settings, consultation with an expert in anticoagulation management may be appropriate, and low-intensity anticoagulation may be considered in favor of no anticoagulation until it might be safe to use full-intensity anticoagulation [36–40].

Chemical and Mechanical Thrombolysis

Although patients with CVT may recover with anticoagulation therapy, 9–13 % have poor outcomes despite anticoagulation [36]. Anticoagulation alone may not dissolve a large and extensive thrombus, and the clinical condition may worsen despite heparin treatment [36]. Incomplete recanalization or persistent thrombosis may explain this phenomenon. Recanalization rates may be higher for patients who receive thrombolytic therapy. In general, thrombolytic therapy is used if clinical deterioration continues despite anticoagulation or if a patient has elevated intracranial pressure that evolves despite other management approaches [30]. Many interventional approaches have been reported. These include direct intravenous thrombolysis via catheter and direct mechanical thrombectomy with or without thrombolysis. In direct intravenous thrombolysis, a standard microcatheter and microguidewire are delivered to the thrombosed dural sinus through a sheath or guiding catheter from the jugular bulb. Mechanical manipulation of the thrombus with the guidewire increases the amount of clot that might be impacted by the thrombolytic agent, potentially reducing the amount of fibrinolytic agent used. There are no randomized controlled trials to support these interventions. Most evidence is based on small case series or anecdotal reports.

Antiplatelets

There are no controlled trials or observational studies that directly assess the role of aspirin in management of CVT [30].

Outlook of Management of CVT: Improving Clinical Pathways for Management of CVT

The evaluation of patients presenting with CVT must begin with a thorough assessment of all potentially acquired risk factors. The identification of these risk factors will not only help to establish a causal mechanism but also help to define the prognosis and the appropriate duration of anticoagulant therapy. If an acquired causal mechanism can be firmly established, an assessment of coagulopathy is not warranted. Patients identified with a coagulopathy such as antiphospholipid antibody syndrome, protein C, protein S or antithrombin III deficiency, homozygous mutations of factor V Leiden or prothrombin G20210A mutation, or double heterozygous mutations for these variables ought to be considered for prolonged or lifelong anticoagulation. In other patients without active malignancy or other indications for prolonged anticoagulation therapy, a duration of anticoagulation of 3–6 months duration is likely sufficient. Though not formally tested in a randomized clinical trial, these recommendations stem from observations that the risk of recurrent CVT is reasonably low. For the rare case of cryptogenic CVT, treatment duration must be individualized as the risk of recurrence is not well defined. All treatment duration decisions must be weighed against the anticipated risk of major hemorrhage on vitamin K antagonist therapy based on the experience of the local medical institution where anticoagulation management will occur. If available, anticoagulation management should include specialized anticoagulation clinics [30].

Despite major progress in the evaluation and management of this rare condition in recent years, much of the literature remains descriptive. In some areas, evidence is lacking to guide decision making. Compared to arterial thrombosis, less attention has been paid to CVT. Continued research is essential to better understand issues related to the diagnosis, treatment and prediction of CVT. Identification of subgroups at higher risk would allow a more careful selection of patients who may benefit from selective interventions or therapies.

Summary

Cerebral venous thrombosis is an uncommon form of stroke, usually affecting young individuals. Despite advances in the recognition of CVT in recent years, diagnosis may be difficult because of the diversity of underlying risk factors and presenting symptoms. For patients with CVT, initial anticoagulation with adjusted-dose unfractionated heparin (UFH) or weight-based low-molecular-weight heparin (LMWH) in full anticoagulant doses is necessary. There are no randomized controlled trials for other treatment modalities in CVT, such as intravenous thrombolysis and antiplatelet therapy. Currently, there are no available risk stratification schemes for CVT, but patients with certain thrombophilic conditions or medical conditions, such as cancer, are considered high risk patients.

Dos and Don'ts

Dos

- Do screen for hypercoagulable states in high risk patients
- Do remember that a normal CT scan and MRI doesn't rule out CVT

- Do remember that signs of increased intracranial pressure require emergent diagnosis and treatment
- Initial anticoagulation with LMWH or UFH is the first treatment of choice
- Do consider direct thrombolysis and direct mechanical thrombectomy with or without thrombolysis for patients who are clinically deteriorating and have increased ICP
- Obtain a CTV or MRV in any patient with suspicion of CVT

Don'ts

- Don't rule out CVT without obtaining a CVT or MRV in idiopathic intracranial hypertension
- Don't rule out a high clinical suspicion of CVT because the D-Dimer is normal
- Don't use anti-epileptic drugs as routine practice in CVT
- Don't use steroids in CVT
- Don't forget to screen for infections as a cause for CVT which may require antibiotics

References

1. Kalbag RM, Woolf AL. Cerebral venous thrombosis. London: Oxford University Press; 1967.
2. Caplan LR. Posterior circulation disease: clinical findings, diagnosis, and management. Boston: Blackwell Science; 1996.
3. Ribes MF. Des recherches faites sur la phlebite. Revue Medicale Francaise et etrangere et Jornal de clinique de l'Hotal-Dieu et de la Charite de Paris. 1825;3:5–41.
4. Abercrombie J. Pathological and practical researches on diseases of the brain and spinal cord. Edinburgh: Waugh and Innes; 1828. p. 83–5.
5. Ferro JM, Canhao P, Stam J, et al. Prognosis of cerebral vein and dural sinus thrombosis. Stroke. 2004;35:664–70.
6. Cantu C, Barinagarrementeria F. Cerebral venous thrombosis associated with pregnancy and puerperium. Review of 67 cases. Stroke. 1993;24:1880–4.
7. Daif A, Awada A, Al-Rajeh S, et al. Cerebral venous thrombosis in adults. A study of 40 cases from Saudi Arabia. Stroke. 1995;26:1193–5.
8. Ameri A, Bousser M-G. Cerebral venous thrombosis. Neurol Clin. 1992;10:87–111.
9. Einhaupl K, Villringer A, Haberl RL, et al. Clinical spectrum of sinus venous thrombosis. In: Einhaupl K, Kemski O, Baethmann A, editors. Cerebral sinus thrombosis, experimental and clinical aspects. New York: Plenum; 1990. p. 149–55.
10. Tsai F, Wang A-M, Matovich VB, et al. MR staging of acute dural sinus thrombosis: correlation with venous pressure measurements and implications for treatment and prognosis. AJNR Am J Neuroradiol. 1995;16:1021–9.
11. Bousser M-G, Chiras J, Bories J, Castaigne P. Cerebral venous thrombosis—a review of 38 cases. Stroke. 1985;16:199–213.
12. Legnani C, Cosmi B, Valdre L, Boggian O, Bernardi F, Coccheri S, et al. Venous thromboembolism, oral contraceptives and high prothrombin levels. J Thromb Haemost. 2003;1:112–7.
13. Bertina RM, Koeleman BP, Koster T, Rosendaal FR, Dirven RJ, de Ronde H, et al. Mutation in blood coagulation factor v associated with resistance to activated protein c. Nature. 1994;369:64–7.

14. Martinelli I, Sacchi E, Landi G, Taioli E, Duca F, Mannucci PM. High risk of cerebral-vein thrombosis in carriers of a prothrombin-gene mutation and in users of oral contraceptives. N Engl J Med. 1998;338:1793–7.
15. Keijzer MB, den Heijer M, Blom HJ, Bos GM, Willems HP, Gerrits WB, et al. Interaction between hyperhomocysteinemia, mutated methylenetetrahydrofolatereductase (MTHFR) and inherited thrombophilic factors in recurrent venous thrombosis. Thromb Haemost. 2002;88:723–8.
16. den Heijer M, Koster T, Blom HJ, Bos GM, Briet E, Reitsma PH, et al. Hyperhomocysteinemia as a risk factor for deep-vein thrombosis. N Engl J Med. 1996;334:759–62.
17. Dentali F, Crowther M, Ageno W. Thrombophilic abnormalities, oral contraceptives, and risk of cerebral vein thrombosis: a meta-analysis. Blood. 2006;107:2766–73.
18. Bousser M-G, Ross Russell R. Cerebral venous thrombosis. London: Saunders; 1997.
19. Selim M, Caplan LR. Radiological diagnosis of cerebral venous thrombosis. Front Neurol Neurosci. 2008;23:96–111.
20. Singh V, Gress DR. Cerebral venous thrombosis. In: Babikian VL, Wechsler LR, Higashida RT, editors. Imaging cerebrovascular disease. Philadelphia: Butterworth-Heinemann; 2003. p. 209–21.
21. Rao CV, Knipp HC, Wagner EJ. Computed tomographic findings in cerebral sinus and venous thrombosis. Radiology. 1981;140:391–8.
22. Tovi F, Hirsch M. Computed tomographic diagnosis of septic lateral sinus thrombosis. Ann Otol Rhinol Laryngol. 1991;100:79–81.
23. De Slegte RGM, Kaiser MC, van der Baan S, Smit L. Computed tomographic diagnosis of septic sinus thromboses and their complications. Neuroradiology. 1988;30:160–5.
24. Bousser M-G, Goujon C, Ribeiro V, Chiras J. Diagnostic strategies in cerebral sinus vein thrombosis. In: Einhaupl K, Kempski O, Baethmann O, editors. Cerebral sinus thrombosis, experimental and clinical aspects. New York: Plenum; 1990. p. 187–97.
25. Crassard I, Soria C, Tzourio C, Woimant F, Drouet L, Ducros A, Bousser MG. A negative D-dimer assay does not rule out cerebral venous thrombosis: a series of seventy-three patients. Stroke. 2005;36(8):1716–9.
26. Lee TG. Cerebral venous thrombosis associated with maxillary and ethmoid sinusitis. J Korean Med Sci. 1995;10(5):388–92.
27. Bousser MG, Ferro JM. Cerebral venous thrombosis: an update. Lancet Neurol. 2007;6: 162–70.
28. Stam J. Thrombosis of the cerebral veins and sinuses. N Engl J Med. 2005;352:1791–8.
29. Stam J. Cerebral venous and sinus thrombosis: incidence and causes. Adv Neurol. 2003;92: 225–32.
30. Saposnik G, Barinagarrementeria F, Brown Jr RD, Bushnell CD, Cucchiara B, Cushman M, et al. Diagnosis and management of cerebral venous thrombosis: a statement for healthcare professionals from the American Heart Association/American Stroke Association. Stroke. 2011;42:1158–92.
31. McBane 2nd RD, Tafur A, Wysokinski WE. Acquired and congenital risk factors associated with cerebral venous sinus thrombosis. Thromb Res. 2010;126:81–7.
32. Younis RT, Lazar RH, Anand VK. Intracranial complications of sinusitis: a 15-year review of 39 cases. Ear Nose Throat J. 2002;81:636–8. 640–2, 644.
33. de Bruijn SF, Starn J. Randomized, placebo-controlled trial of anticoagulant treatment with low-molecular-weight heparin for cerebral sinus thrombosis. Stroke. 1999;30(3):484–8.
34. Einhaupl KM, Villringer A, Meister W, Mehraein S, Garner C, Pellhofer M, Haberl RL, Pfister HW, Schmiedek P. Heparin treatment in sinus venous thrombosis. Lancet. 1991;338(8767): 597–600.
35. Canhao P, Ferro JM, Lindgren AG, Bousser MG, Stam J, Barinagarrementeria F, et al. Causes and predictors of death in cerebral venous thrombosis. Stroke. 2005;36:1720–5.
36. Stam J, de Bruijn S, de Veber G. Anticoagulation for cerebral sinus thrombosis. Stroke. 2003;34:1054–5.

37. Gosk-Bierska I, Wysokinski W, Brown Jr RD, Karnicki K, Grill D, Wiste H, et al. Cerebral venous sinus thrombosis: incidence of venous thrombosis recurrence and survival. Neurology. 2006;67:814–9.
38. Shrivastava S, Ridker PM, Glynn RJ, Goldhaber SZ, Moll S, Bounameaux H, et al. D-dimer, factor viii coagulant activity, low-intensity warfarin and the risk of recurrent venous thromboembolism. J Thromb Haemost. 2006;4:1208–14.
39. Palareti G, Legnani C, Cosmi B, Valdre L, Lunghi B, Bernardi F, et al. Predictive value of d-dimer test for recurrent venous thromboembolism after anticoagulation withdrawal in subjects with a previous idiopathic event and in carriers of congenital thrombophilia. Circulation. 2003;108:313–8.
40. Palareti G, Cosmi B, Legnani C, Tosetto A, Brusi C, Iorio A, et al. D-dimer testing to determine the duration of anticoagulation therapy. N Engl J Med. 2006;355:1780–9.

Chapter 12
Bacterial Meningitis

Yasser B. Abulhasan and Pravin Amin$

Introduction

Bacterial meningitis is defined as inflammation of the leptomeninges. About 1.2 million cases of bacterial meningitis are estimated to occur annually worldwide with 135,000 deaths [1, 2]. Bacterial meningitis is coupled with high mortality and morbidity rates. Death rates are 20 % in high and 50 % in low-income countries [3]. Neurological deficits, such as hearing loss and neuropsychological impairment, occur in about 50 % of survivors [4]. Bacterial meningitis can be community-acquired or healthcare-associated. *Haemophilus influenzae*, *Streptococcus pneumoniae* and *Neisseria meningitidis*, are the three most common pathogens causing community-acquired bacterial meningitis globally. The major causes of healthcare-associated bacterial meningitis are staphylococci and aerobic gram-negative bacilli. Nosocomial bacterial meningitis may occur in patients following neurosurgery, with internal or external ventricular or lumbar drains and following trauma with skull base fracture and cerebrospinal fluid (CSF) leak.

$Author contributed equally with all other contributors.

Y.B. Abulhasan, MBChB, FRCPC (✉)
Faculty of Medicine, Health Sciences Center, Kuwait University, Kuwait, Kuwait

Department of Anesthesiology and Critical Care, Ibn Sina Hospital, Kuwait, Kuwait
e-mail: yasser.abulhasan@hsc.edu.kw

P. Amin, MD, FCCM
Department of Critical Care Medicine, Bombay Hospital Institute
of Medical Sciences, Mumbai, Maharashtra, India

© Springer International Publishing Switzerland 2015
K.E. Wartenberg et al. (eds.), *Neurointensive Care: A Clinical Guide
to Patient Safety*, DOI 10.1007/978-3-319-17293-4_12

Case Report

An 83-year-old gentleman presented with diminished hearing on the left side of 6 months duration. Over the last 3 weeks before admission to the hospital he presented with imbalance while walking and shooting pain in his left cheek. He had undergone coronary balloon angioplasty and stenting (PTCA) with stent placed in his left anterior descending (LAD) artery for angina pectoris and was currently on aspirin 150 mg daily. His magnetic resonance imaging (MRI) revealed a left acoustic schwannoma. He was operated a week later, after stopping aspirin. His postoperative course was uneventful and was transferred out of the neurocritical care unit on the second post-operative day. He was eating orally and was mobilized.

On the 5th postoperative day he developed high-grade fever, headache, vomiting and over the day became drowsy but arousable. He had neck rigidity and enhancement of the meninges was seen on contrast-enhanced CT scan. His lumbar puncture revealed the following: opening pressure of 20 cmH$_2$O, CSF protein 549 mg/dL. CSF glucose 5 mg/dL, with a simultaneous blood sugar of 133 mg/dL, WBC 5760 with 85 % polymorphonucleocytes. CSF lactate was 17.7 mmol/L.

He was empirically started on intravenous meropenem 2 g 8 hourly and intravenous vancomycin 1 g 12 hourly following a diagnosis of nosocomial meningitis.

Subsequently 2 days later, his blood culture and CSF grew *Acinetobacter baumannii*. The meropenem minimal inhibitory concentration (MIC) was 8 µg/mL and the MIC of colistin was ≤1 µg/mL. Vancomycin was stopped and colistin was started at a bolus dose of 9 million units followed subsequently by 3 million units 8 hourly and 1 million units intrathecally. The clinical and CSF reports improved gradually over a 4 week period.

A 16-year-old boy presented to the hospital with fever of 2 days duration. On arrival, the patient's blood pressure was 103/50 mmHg, pulse rate was 125/min and oral temperature was 38.9 °C. He was drowsy but arousable, while otherwise clinically stable. The patient also complained of headache, two episodes of vomiting, and severe dizziness. Physical examination showed generalized maculopapular rash. There was terminal neck rigidity. Kernig's and Brudzinski's signs were negative. There were no papilledema or any focal neurological signs, chest, cardiac and abdominal examination did not reveal any abnormality. A lumbar puncture was performed, which revealed an opening pressure of 22 cmH$_2$O, and the CSF was turbid. He was given dexamethasone 10 mg and ceftriaxone 2 g along with vancomycin 1 g intravenously.

Investigations showed white cell count of 21,300 cells per cubic meter with 87 % neutrophils; raised CSF protein of 807 mg/dL, CSF glucose was 20 mg/dL, with a simultaneous blood sugar of 185 mg/dL, CSF lactate was 12.6 mmol/L. Gram stain revealed gram negative diplococci. Subsequently, both blood culture and CSF culture grew *Neisseria meningitidis*. Ceftriaxone and dexamethasone were continued and vancomycin was stopped.

Clinical Features

Early clinical recognition of bacterial meningitis is of paramount importance so as to initiate immediate appropriate therapy. Early features associated with acute bacterial meningitis have a well-recognized pattern which include fever, vomiting, and headache described as bursting and splitting. Altered level of consciousness is considered characteristic and may range from irritability and confusion to stupor. Despite this altered mental status, most patients can be roused with forcible command or painful stimuli.

Nuchal rigidity, a common and important sign, tends to be difficult to elicit especially in the comatose patients. Classic diagnostic tests including neck stiffness, Kernig's sign and Brudzinski's sign still remain with questionable sensitivity and specificity, and their absence should not be used to rule out meningitis [5]. Rashes, in general, are not specific for any bacterial infections. The usual rashes associated with meningitis include petechiae, erythematous and maculopapular of different distribution. Petechiae rash, classically associated with *Neisseria meningitidis*, has also been described in viral meningitis. Meningococcal meningitis can result in purpura fulminans in severe cases [6]. Cranial nerves are initially spared. At extremity of age, acute confusional states and fever should raise the possibility of acute bacterial meningitis and thus investigated accordingly. Other signs including sluggish dilated pupils and papilledema [7], indicate progressive brain edema and high ICP and are signs of an advanced stage of the infection. Focal or generalized tonic-clonic seizures indicate extensive disease affecting the parenchyma. Meningitis caused by listeria has an increased propensity to develop seizures [8].

Potential sources for infection such as paranasal sinusitis, dental infections, middle ear infections and pneumonia should be investigated, these tend to be prevalent in the immunocompromised patients. A history of ear pain, sore throat, myalgias and fatigability occurring few days prior to clinical deteriorations and emergency room consultation is common.

In the post neurosurgical patient population, to differentiate chemical meningitis from bacterial meningitis using CSF and clinical data tends to be difficult which leads to a debatable antibiotics therapy situation [9].

Bacteria usually gain entry into the central nervous system (CNS) either by hematogenous spread via arterial blood, or direct extension from infected sinuses or bones. Once the organism has invaded the CNS, the local host defense mechanisms may invoke local and systemic responses [10]. Although these are defensive responses, often their effects are deleterious to the CNS tissue and lead to the clinical signs and symptoms described above [9].

Diagnosis

Laboratory data usually reveal leukocytosis; occasionally there may be leukopenia and thrombocytopenia. In more severe disease states, there can be disseminated intravascular coagulation and metabolic acidosis due to lactic acidosis. Blood cultures may be positive in very high percentages of patients with bacterial meningitis [7].

Table 12.1 The CSF findings in different types of meningitis

	Viral Meningitis	Bacterial meningitis	Tubercular Meningitis
Opening Pressure	Usually normal	Elevated	Variable
Glucose (mg/dL/ mmol/L)	Normal (>40/2.2	Low – Very low (<40/2.2)	Low (<40/2.2)
Proteins (mg/dL/ g/L)	Moderate increase (<100/1,000)	(Marked increase)>250/2,500	(Moderate to marked increase) 50–500/500–5,000
WBC (cells/µL)	<100 cells/µL.	>500 (usually>1,000)	Variable (10–1,000 cells/µL) <500 cells/µL
Cell type	Early: neutrophils. Late: lymphocytes	Predominance of Neutrophils	Predominance of Lymphocytes
Culture	Negative	May be Positive	May be Positive

The question of cranial CT prior to LP has been a matter of controversy for the past decade in neurologic emergency settings [11, 12]. A literature review in 1993 found no evidence to recommend CT of the brain before lumbar puncture in acute meningitis unless the patient showed atypical features or focal findings on neurological exam [11]. This is of great significance especially in remote areas where the next CT scanner is hours away. More specifically, performing a cranial CT prior to LP is appropriate mainly in the following circumstances: patients with focal neurological signs, patients with papilledema on fundoscopy, patients with known mass lesions and immunocompromised patients. On the other hand, a LP post a normal cranial CT does not preclude the development of a herniation syndrome especially if the patient has rapidly progressing cerebral edema. In these cases, the progression of the disease is thought to be the cause of herniation not the LP procedure itself [12].

When performing the LP, which is essential in establishing the diagnosis and later on tailoring the antibiotics therapy in bacterial meningitis, the patient should be in the left lateral decubitus position. An opening pressure should always be measured with a manometer before the collection of CSF. Opening pressure above 20 cm H_2O in this position is considered high warranting closer neurological observation and management of high intracranial pressure (ICP) (described below).

The CSF findings in different types of meningitis are elicited in Table 12.1. In bacterial meningitis, the WBC count amounts to 1,000–5,000/µL (range of 100 to >10,000) with neutrophils usually greater than 80 %, protein of 100–500 mg/dL, and glucose <40 mg/dL (with a CSF/serum glucose ratio of ≤0.4) [13]. The CSF picture in fungal meningitis may typically resemble tubercular meningitis. Every attempt should be made to do a gram stain in all suspected cases of bacterial meningitis [14]. CSF lactate concentration is useful to differentiate bacterial from aseptic meningitis [15]. Additional tests would include rapid diagnostic tests (Latex agglutination [16], and polymerase chain reaction [PCR] [17]) to determine antigens of organisms that cause bacterial meningitis.

Management of Bacterial Meningitis

Early Treatment

Although challenging, early recognition and initiation of specific treatment for bacterial meningitis is associated with improved patient outcome (see Fig. 12.1). Despite best efforts, certain clinical factors can be associated with delayed recognition of bacterial meningitis. For example, immunocompromised patients do not exhibit the classical signs of acute meningitis therefore clinicians should lower their pre-test probability for performing a complete work-up of these patients when indicated.

Delayed initiation of appropriate antibiotic therapy is not justified. In patients with moderate to high suspicion of bacterial meningitis, appropriate parenteral antibiotics (Tables 12.2, 12.3, and 12.4) should be initiated prior to LP or CT. Even with the most sensitive organisms, CSF sterilization only occurs after 4–6 h following antibiotic administration [18]. Still it is recommended that the CSF sample is obtained within 2 h post antibiotic administration.

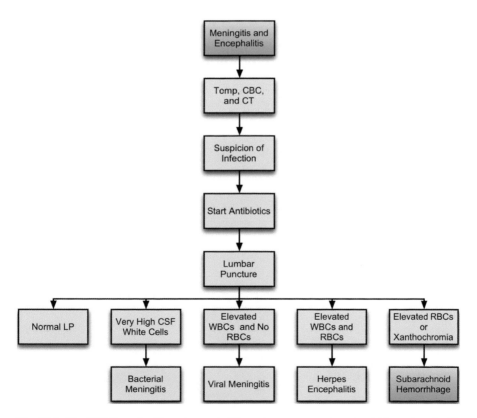

Fig. 12.1 The ENLS meningitis and encephalitis early management protocol (Reproduced with permission from the Neurocritical Care Society)

Results from the grams stain may facilitate the choice of antibiotics. The choice of antibiotics would vary considerably in nosocomial meningitis. The antibiotics should be revised following the availability of CSF culture sensitivity reports.

Duration of targeted antibiotic therapy should be based on culture sensitivity, immunocompetence, pharmacokinetics, clinical and laboratory response. The antibiotic choices based on organism [19] are listed in Tables 12.2, 12.3, and 12.4.

Intrathecal and/or intraventricular colistin represents the last resort treatment of multidrug-resistant (MDR) and extensively drug-resistant (XDR) *Acinetobacter baumannii* meningitis, presents a safe and effective form of therapy. The median dose of local colistin was 125,000 IU (10 mg) varying between 20,000 IU (1.6 mg) to 500,000 IU (40 mg) in adults, while a dose of 2,000 IU/kg (0.16 mg/kg) up to 125,000 IU (10 mg) was used in children [20]. Intrathecal and intraventricular application of antibiotics should be executed with caution in patients with high ICP.

The extensive achievement of advocating conjugate vaccines has had a vital effect on the incidence of bacterial meningitis in the affluent countries. How this has an impact on developing countries will depend on widespread availability of these vaccines at an affordable price.

Steroid Therapy in Bacterial Meningitis

Despite conflicting trial results, adjuvant corticosteroids (dexamethasone 0.15 mg/kg IV every 6 h) in acute bacterial meningitis are now considered standard of therapy in high income countries.

Table 12.2 Antibiotic therapy of meningitis based on microorganism

Microorganism	Recommended therapy	Alternative therapies
Streptococcus pneumoniae	Vancomycin + a third-generation cephalosporin	Meropenem, fluoroquinolone
Neisseria meningitidis	Third-generation cephalosporin	Penicillin G, ampicillin, chloramphenicol, fluoroquinolone, aztreonam
Listeria monocytogenes	Ampicillin or penicillin G	Trimethoprim-sulfamethoxazole, meropenem
Streptococcus agalactiae	Ampicillin or penicillin G	Third-generation cephalosporin
Haemophilus influenzae	Third-generation cephalosporin	Chloramphenicol, cefepime, meropenem, fluoroquinolone
Escherichia coli	Third-generation cephalosporin	Cefepime, meropenem, aztreonam, fluoroquinolone, trimethoprim-sulfamethoxazole
Pseudomonas aeruginosa, Acinetobacter baumannii	Meropenem	Meropenem + Colistin + Intrathecal and/or intraventricular Colistin

Modified from: Tunkel et al. [19] with permission

Table 12.3 Recommendations for empirical antimicrobial therapy for purulent meningitis based on patient age and specific predisposing condition

Predisposing factor	Common bacterial pathogens	Antimicrobial therapy
Age		
<1 month	*Streptococcus agalactiae, Escherichia coli, Listeria monocytogenes, Klebsiella* species	Ampicillin plus cefotaxime or ampicillin plus an aminoglycoside
1–23 months	*Streptococcus pneumoniae, Neisseria meningitidis, S. agalactiae, Haemophilus influenzae, E. coli*	Vancomycin plus a third-generation cephalosporin[a,b]
2–50 years	*N. meningitidis, S. pneumoniae*	Vancomycin plus a third-generation cephalosporin[a,b]
>50 years	*S. Pneumoniae, N. meningitidis, L. monocytogenes,* aerobic gram-negative bacilli	Vancomycin plus ampicillin plus a third-generation cephalosporin[a,b]
Head trauma		
Basilar skull fracture	*S. Pneumoniae, H. influenzae, group A β-hemolytic streptococci*	Vancomycin plus a third-generation cephalosporin[a]
Penetrating trauma	*Staphylococcus aureus,* coagulase-negative staphylococci (especially *Staphylococcus epidermidis*), aerobic gram-negative bacilli (including *Pseudomonas aeruginosa*)	Vancomycin plus cefepime, vancomycin plus ceftazidime, or vancomycin plus meropenem
Post neurosurgery	Aerobic gram-negative bacilli (including *P. aeruginosa*), *S. aureus,* coagulase-negative staphylococci (especially *S. epidermidis*)	Vancomycin plus cefepime, vancomycin plus ceftazidime, or vancomycin plus meropenem
CSF shunt	Coagulase-negative staphylococci (especially *S. epidermidis*), *S. aureus,* aerobic gram-negative bacilli (including *P. aeruginosa*), *Propionibacterium acnes*	Vancomycin plus cefepime,[c] vancomycin plus ceftazidime,[c] or vancomycin plus meropenem[c]

Adapted from: Tunkel et al. [19] with permission
[a]Ceftriaxone or cefotaxime
[b]Some experts would add rifampin if dexamethasone is also given
[c]In infants and children, vancomycin alone is reasonable unless Gram stains reveal the presence of gram-negative bacilli

Table 12.4 Recommended dosages of antimicrobial agents administered by the intraventricular route

Antimicrobial agent	Daily intraventricular dose, mg
Vancomycin	5–20
Gentamicin	1–8
Tobramycin	5–20
Amikacin	5–50
Polymyxin B	5
Colistin	10
Quinupristin/dalfopristin	2–5
Teicoplanin	5–40

Adapted from: Tunkel et al. [19] with permission

The steroids should be administered before or along with antibiotics but not after the administration of antibiotics. Twenty-four studies involving 4,041 participants have been identified. There was a trend toward lower mortality in adults receiving corticosteroids. Corticosteroids were associated with lower rates of hearing loss and neurological sequelae [21]. These results were not reproduced in low income countries. Subgroup analyses for causative organisms showed that corticosteroids reduced severe hearing loss in *Haemophilus influenzae* meningitis and reduced mortality in *Streptococcus pneumoniae* meningitis [22]. Dexamethasone is administered 15–20 min before or simultaneously with antibiotics. Two dose regimens are recommended: 0.15 mg/kg every 6 h for 4 days in the developed world, based upon the IDSA guidelines [19], and 0.4 mg/kg every 12 h for 4 days in the developing world, based upon the Vietnamese trial [23]. Adjunctive dexamethasone should not be given to adults who have already received antimicrobial therapy because it has no impact on outcomes. Corticosteroids have been used as an adjunct to antituberculous drugs to improve the outcome, in tubercular meningitis. Seven trials involving 1,140 participants (with 411 deaths) were analyzed and they revealed corticosteroids reduce the risk of death or disabling residual neurological deficit. Adverse events included gastrointestinal bleeding, bacterial and fungal infections and hyperglycaemia, but they were mild and treatable [24].

On the cellular level, corticosteroids have been shown to reduce the alteration of the blood–brain barrier by reducing the metalloproteinases [25]. This has raised the concern of penetration of hydrophilic antibiotics (vancomycin) into the CSF. Studies assessing the CSF vancomycin level were conflicting [26, 27]. Most centers still recommend administering dexamethasone prior to the appropriate antibiotics to treat acute bacterial meningitis.

Medical Management and Complications

Initially patients may present with hyponatremia which tends to be mild and easily corrected with normal saline. Free water should be restricted in these patients to avoid worsening of the hyponatremic state which might lower the threshold for seizures.

Complications of bacterial meningitis which might be seen during admission may include subdural effusions, abscess formation or cerebritis, cerebral venous thrombosis, early hydrocephalus and cerebral infarcts [28, 29]. These complications are devastating in nature and better diagnosed with MRI. Generalized myoclonus may be witnessed a number of days post cephalosporins treatment. In patients with co-existing renal failure, this indicates toxic cephalosporins levels. Although uncommon, late complications of bacterial meningitis include hearing loss, seizure disorder and neurological sequelae.

High ICP Management

Mortality and disability in bacterial meningitis are mainly due to raised ICP and herniation. Traditional aggressive therapy, especially in patients with high ICP, has not translated into improved outcome. This might be due to concomitant systemic and local effects such as arteritis leading to cerebral ischemia or infarctions, cerebritis, abscess formation, and punctate hemorrhages that can lead to serious infections, ischemic or hemorrhagic complications [30, 31].

Established treatment includes the basic ABC (Airway, Breathing, Circulation) of resuscitation. An initial assessment includes the airway and endotracheal intubation if decline in mental status is present to maintain a patent airway and prevent aspiration. Proper documentation of the neurological exam should be carried out prior to endotracheal intubation. Some patients with bacterial meningitis, as with other bacterial infections, will be in a hypovolemic state. In addition, a percentage of patients will either be in severe sepsis or septic shock thereby goal driven fluid and vasopressor resuscitation in line with the Surviving Sepsis Campaign recommendation should be followed [32]. Care is advised when following these recommendations as the relationship between aggressive fluid resuscitation and worsening cerebral edema and maintenance of cerebral perfusion pressure should be monitored.

If further neurological deterioration is encountered despite initial resuscitation, urgent cranial CT scan should be performed to rule out worsening cerebral edema. The use of hyperosmolar therapy (mannitol and/or hypertonic saline) in this situation should be guided by clinical exam and possibly ICP monitoring. Subdural empyema should also be ruled out using MRI imaging [33].

In a recent retrospective cohort study [34], we showed improved outcome in patients with severe bacterial meningitis by utilizing continuous lumbar drainage aimed at decreasing the inflammatory load released in the infected CSF and controlling intracranial hypertension. Contraindications to lumbar drainage which necessitate careful cranial CT assessment prior to the introduction of the lumbar drain include subdural hematomas, space-occupying lesions with mass effect and obstructive hydrocephalus in addition to coagulopathy.

Osmotic therapy in bacterial meningitis has been studied with glycerol in four poor quality trials comprising 1,091 participants. It had no effect on mortality in people with bacterial meningitis, and on seizures, however glycerol reduced the risk of subsequent deafness [35]. At the 27th congress of the International Pediatric Association held in August 2013 in Melbourne, Kumar RR et al. from Chandigarh, India presented data on comparison of osmotherapy with 20 % mannitol vs 3 % hypertonic saline in 16 pediatric patients with bacterial meningitis. Hypertonic saline was superior to mannitol in controlling raised ICP in acute CNS infections. The same group analyzed ideal sodium level in 251 patients with raised ICP in bacterial meningitis (in press). They concluded that serum sodium between 146 and 150 mEq/L is ideal for management of raised ICP in children with acute CNS infections.

ICP monitoring is an integral part of all Neurocritical care units (NCCU). A question arises whether this modality of monitoring predisposes to CNS infections. In a study from Turkey, the investigators prospectively compared the complications associated with intraparenchymal ICP monitoring using the fiberoptic Camino ICP device versus external ventricular drainage set (EVDS). A Camino ICP monitoring transducer was implanted in 631 patients. About half of the patients ($n=303$) also received an EVDS. Infection occurred in 6 patients with only an ICP transducer (6/328, 1.8 %) and 24 patients with an EVDS also (24/303, 7.9 %). The duration of monitoring had no effect on infection with the Camino transducer, whereas the use of an EVDS for more than 9 days increased infection risk by 5.11 times [36]. A group in Mumbai reduced ICP catheter infections by introduction of a simple technique of ensheathing the entire length of the external segment of the catheter in a sterile plastic sheath. This resulted in a decreased infection rate. In the study year, 1 of 78 patients developed catheter induced meningitis, compared to 7 of 64 patients in the year prior to introduction of the protective plastic sheath [37].

Risks of Patient Safety and Poor Outcome

Early diagnosis and treatment of bacterial meningitis is of paramount importance in reducing mortality and adverse neurological outcomes. In adults, the time of onset of symptoms has not been studied, however in children and adolescents a retrospective study addressed this issue in all meningococcal disease states [38]. In this study classical symptom of rash, meningism and altered sensorium was late in onset in the pre-hospital admission. Early signs prior to admission in adolescents (15–16 years.) with meningococcal disease were leg pain (53 %) and cold hands and feet (44 %). Patients with symptoms such as headache, nausea, and vomiting for the diagnosis of meningitis demonstrated a poor sensitivity and specificity. Of 493 cases of bacterial meningitis in adults showed that the typical symptoms of fever, neck rigidity, and altered mental status were present in only two-thirds of adults [6]. In 95 % of patients with culture positive bacterial meningitis presented with a minimum of two signs or symptoms of headache, fever, neck stiffness, and altered mental status. At least one of these four factors was present in 99 % of patients [7]; hence a high degree of suspicion of meningitis should be considered when two of these parameters are present. Such patients should be investigated in detail to prove or disprove bacterial meningitis.

Performance of a lumbar puncture may cause mild discomfort to potentially lethal brain herniation, which may be encountered in patients with raised ICP. In the case of the 16-year-old boy, the question one needs to ask is if the CT scan of brain was essential before performing LP when suspecting bacterial meningitis. Before the availability of CT scan, lumbar puncture in 129 patients with elevated ICP, 1.2 % of patients with papilledema and 12 % of patients without papilledema had adverse consequences within 48 h of the procedure [39]. The Canadians in a review stated that there were no Canadian legal precedents suggesting liability if physicians failed to perform CT in cases of meningitis [11]. In 301 adults with bacterial meningitis, the clinical features at baseline that was associated with abnormal findings of a CT scan of the head. This study formed the basis for recommendations to perform CT scan prior to LP and encompasses the following situations [12]:

1. Age of ≥60 years
2. A history of CNS disease (e.g., mass lesion, stroke, and focal infection)
3. An immunocompromised state (e.g., that due to HIV infection or AIDS, immunosuppressive therapy, or transplantation)

4. A history of seizure ≤1 week before presentation
5. Focal neurologic deficit (e.g., dilated nonreactive pupil, abnormalities of ocular motility, abnormal visual fields, gaze palsy, arm or leg drift)
6. Papilledema
7. Abnormal level of consciousness

Three important risk factors – hypotension, seizures and altered mental status – were separately linked with an poor outcome (hospital death or neurologic deficit at discharge) and placed these patients into three risk groups [40]:

1. Low risk (no risk factors) — 9 % poor outcome
2. Intermediate risk (one risk factor) — 33 % poor outcome
3. High risk (two or three risk factors) — 56 % poor outcome

Patients with bacterial meningitis have a high mortality risk based on their geographic location more so, in countries of low socio-economic strata. This is possibly due to the availability of better neurocritical care services in the affluent countries. There is strong data suggesting that managing bacterial meningitis in a neurocritical care unit improves outcomes. Risk classification is necessary for ascertaining the level of care that a patient will require in the hospital, mostly to determine which patients must be managed in a neurocritical care unit. The Swedish national guidelines for bacterial infections in the nervous system from 2004 recommend that neurointensive care unit admission should be considered under one or more of the following conditions [41]:

1. Reaction Level Scale grade ≥3B (drowsy, confused, responds to strong stimulation), Reaction Level Scale grade ≤3A (drowsy, very delayed reaction) but gradually worsening
2. Repeated seizures
3. Severe agitation
4. Cranial nerve palsy
5. Hypertonia
6. Bradycardia
7. Papilledema
8. Computed tomography indications of increased ICP.

The neurointensive care protocol applied followed ordinary management principles including ICP monitoring, CSF drainage and thiopental coma treatment in an escalated manner. Twenty of the 36 patients showed favorable outcomes by being managed in a neurocritical care unit [41]. Eighteen patients with severe bacterial meningitis were admitted to a NCCU University Hospital in Sweden. In 15 patients, ICP was measured continuously through an ICP measuring device. Mean ICP was significantly higher and CPP was markedly decreased in nonsurvivors compared with survivors [42]. Furthermore, a recently published study from the Post Graduate Institute of Medical Education and Research (PGIMER), India consisting of 110 pediatric patients with bacterial meningitis managed with ICP vs CPP, suggested that CPP-targeted therapy improves long-term neurological outcomes [43].

Treating both the underlying cause and managing complications is critical for limiting neurological damage.

The patient with nosocomial meningitis underwent neurosurgery 4 days after admission to the hospital as he had not stopped aspirin 1 week prior to admission. His risk for nosocomial infection increased as he had plenty of time to colonize with the *Acinetobacter* which finally caused nosocomial meningitis.

Safety Barriers

Isolation Precautions and Chemoprophylaxis

Respiratory isolation precautions are only indicated for patients who are suspected of being infected with *Neisseria meningitidis*. Isolation should be continued for the first 24 h of treatment. For all other patients suspected of having bacterial meningitis, no specific isolation measures are warranted apart from hand-washing.

Healthcare workers and other patients exposed to patients with community-acquired meningitis should receive appropriate chemoprophylaxis. Antibiotic prophylaxis is considered for those in close contact with cases of meningococcal meningitis during the first 7 days of illness. At 1 week after treatment, effective antibiotics are ciprofloxacin, rifampicin, minocycline and ampicillin. Between the 1 and 2 weeks follow-up, only rifampicin and ciprofloxacin are proven to be effective [44].

Certain bacteria that cause meningitis are contagious. Some bacteria can spread through exchange secretions (e.g., kissing). Generally, most of the bacteria that cause meningitis are not as contagious as the common influenza. These bacteria are not spread by casual contact or by air transmission. However, it would seem reasonable to isolate these patients initially so as to protect healthcare workers and fellow patients.

Basilar skull fractures (BSF) predispose the meninges to be in close proximity to colonized nasopharynx, sinuses, and middle ear. The risk of meningitis increases remarkably when skull base fractures are associated with CSF leak. The Cochrane group reviewed five RCTs and 17 non-RCTs comparing different types of antibiotic prophylaxis with placebo or no intervention in patients with BSF. They did not show evidence to support prophylactic antibiotic use in patients with BSF, even in the presence or absence of CSF leakage or not [45].

The first meningococcal conjugate vaccines, monovalent products against serogroup C, were available since 1999. The first meningococcal conjugate vaccine, covering serogroups A, C, W, and Y, was licensed in 2005 [46]. In January 2013, the first vaccine against endemic MenB was licensed in Europe. Meningococcal conjugate vaccines have been used for over 12 years in all age groups and have an acceptable record of safety. A serogroup A tetanus toxoid conjugate vaccine, called MenAfriVac (PsA-TT) was developed for the Sub Saharan region. In the first year after PsA-TT vaccination in Burkina Faso, the incidence of meningitis fell by 99.8 % and there were no cases of serogroup A meningococcal disease among vaccinated individuals [47]. By the end of 2012, over 100 million individuals were vaccinated with PsA-TT in the meningitis belt, and plans are in place for mass vaccination campaigns to occur in other meningitis belt countries by 2016. Early data suggest that the vaccine has the potential to eliminate serogroup A epidemics in Africa.

Hemophilus Influenzae type b (Hib) is one of the three big causes of acute bacterial meningitis. Eight randomized trials were found that compared the efficacy of Hib conjugate vaccine to placebo or no vaccine. From eight trials, the protective efficacy of the Hib conjugate vaccine was 84 % against invasive Hib disease, 75 % against meningitis, and 69 % against pneumonia [48].

Vaccination of the population at risk or in endemic areas would contribute to a reduction of the prevalence and mortality of meningitis.

Other safety barriers while starting drug therapy in patients with bacterial meningitis consist of time in initiating therapy and the nature of antibiotic used. The extremely important primary matter is averting any delay in ordering therapy and the initial choice of antibiotic. The delay in antibiotic therapy correlated independently to unfavorable outcome. The odds for unfavorable outcome may increase by up to 30 % per hour of treatment delay [49]. Rather than empiric therapy, IV antibiotics should be aimed at the assumed organism if the gram stain is diagnostic.

The First Hours Management Protocol

Figure 12.1 is a treatment protocol recently published by the Emergency Neurological Life Support (ENLS) group aimed at executing treatment within the first hours of presentation into an emergency department with meningitis and encephalitis [18].

Summary

- *Streptococcus pneumoniae* and *Neisseria meningitidis* remain the commonest pathogens in community acquired bacterial meningitis while the incidence of *Haemophilus influenza* is decreasing with the widespread vaccination programs.
- In adult patients, early empirical antibiotics consisting of third generation cephalosporin and vancomycin are recommended while in the elderly or immunosuppressed, the addition of ampicillin is warranted.
- Safety precaution (isolation) should be initiated when *Neisseria meningitidis* is the suspected pathogen.

Dos and Don'ts

- Early clinical recognition and treatment initiation translates into good clinical outcome
- In immunocompromised patients, clinicians should lower their pre-test probability for performing a complete work-up of these patients when indicated
- Specific intravenous antibiotics therapy capable of penetrating the blood–brain barrier should follow recommended treatment protocols and administered upon clinical suspension
- Adjuvant dexamethasone prior to antibiotic is considered standard of therapy in many centers
- Addition of vancomycin to treatment protocols have emerged due to bacterial resistance
- Lumbar puncture should be carried out (when appropriate) in the decubitus position and an opening pressure measured before CSF collection
- Respiratory isolation precautions is only indicated in *Neisseria meningitidis*
- Treatment revision should be carried upon the identification of bacterial sensitivity

References

1. Epidemic meningococcal disease. World Health Organization fact sheet 105. Geneva: WHO; 1998.
2. Scheld WM, Koedel U, Nathan B, Pfister HW. Pathophysiology of bacterial meningitis: mechanism(s) of neuronal injury. J Infect Dis. 2002;186 Suppl 2:S225–33.
3. Brouwer MC, Tunkel AR, van de Beek D. Epidemiology, diagnosis, and antimicrobial treatment of acute bacterial meningitis. Clin Microbiol Rev. 2010;23:467–92.
4. Kasanmoentalib ES, Brouwer MC, van de Beek D. Update on bacterial meningitis: epidemiology, trials and genetic association studies. Curr Opin Neurol. 2013;26:282–8.
5. Thomas KE, Hasbun R, Jekel J, Quagliarello VJ. The diagnostic accuracy of Kernig's sign, Brudzinski's sign, and nuchal rigidity in adults with suspected meningitis. Clin Infect Dis. 2002;35:46–52.
6. Durand ML, Calderwood SB, Weber DJ, Miller SI, Southwick FS, Caviness Jr VS, Swartz MN. Acute bacterial meningitis in adults. A review of 493 episodes. N Engl J Med. 1993;328: 21–8.
7. van de Beek D, de Gans J, Spanjaard L, Weisfelt M, Reitsma JB, Vermeulen M. Clinical features and prognostic factors in adults with bacterial meningitis. N Engl J Med. 2004;351: 1849–59.
8. Mylonakis E, Hohmann EL, Calderwood SB. Central nervous system infection with Listeria monocytogenes. 33 years' experience at a general hospital and review of 776 episodes from the literature. Medicine. 1998;77:313–36.
9. Brown EM, de Louvois J, Bayston R, Lees PD, Pople IK, British Society for Antimicrobial Chemotherapy Working Party on Neurosurgical Infections. Distinguishing between chemical and bacterial meningitis in patients who have undergone neurosurgery. Clin Infect Dis. 2002;34:556–8.
10. Bleck TP. Bacterial meningitis and other nonviral infections of the nervous system. Crit Care Clin. 2013;29:975–87.

11. Archer BD. Computed tomography before lumbar puncture in acute meningitis: a review of the risks and benefits. CMAJ. 1993;148:961–5.
12. Hasbun R, Abrahams J, Jekel J, Quagliarello VJ. Computed tomography of the head before lumbar puncture in adults with suspected meningitis. N Engl J Med. 2001;345: 1727–33.
13. Spanos A, Harrell Jr FE, Durack DT. Differential diagnosis of acute meningitis. An analysis of the predictive value of initial observations. JAMA. 1989;262:2700–7.
14. Fitch MT, van de Beek D. Emergency diagnosis and treatment of adult meningitis. Lancet Infect Dis. 2007;7:191–200.
15. Sakushima K, Hayashino Y, Kawaguchi T, Jackson JL, Fukuhara S. Diagnostic accuracy of cerebrospinal fluid lactate for differentiating bacterial meningitis from aseptic meningitis: a meta-analysis. J Infect. 2011;62:255–62.
16. Shameem S, Vinod Kumar CS, Neelagund YF. Bacterial meningitis: rapid diagnosis and microbial profile: a multicentered study. J Commun Dis. 2008;40:111–20.
17. Wu HM, Cordeiro SM, Harcourt BH, Carvalho M, Azevedo J, Oliveira TQ, Leite MC, Salgado K, Reis MG, Plikaytis BD, Clark TA, Mayer LW, Ko AI, Martin SW, Reis JN. Accuracy of real-time PCR, Gram stain and culture for Streptococcus pneumoniae, Neisseria meningitidis and Haemophilus influenzae meningitis diagnosis. BMC Infect Dis. 2013;13:26.
18. Gaieski DF, Nathan BR, Weingart SD, Smith WS. Emergency neurologic life support: meningitis and encephalitis. Neurocrit Care. 2012;17 Suppl 1:S66–72.
19. Tunkel AR, Hartman BJ, Kaplan SL, Kaufman BA, Roos KL, Scheld WM, Whitley RJ. Practice guidelines for the management of bacterial meningitis. Clin Infect Dis. 2004;39: 1267–84.
20. Karaiskos I, Galani L, Baziaka F, Giamarellou H. Intraventricular and intrathecal colistin as the last therapeutic resort for the treatment of multidrug-resistant and extensively drug-resistant Acinetobacter baumannii ventriculitis and meningitis: a literature review. Int J Antimicrob Agents. 2013;41:499–508.
21. Brouwer MC, McIntyre P, Prasad K, van de Beek D. Corticosteroids for acute bacterial meningitis. Cochrane Database Syst Rev. 2013;(6):CD004405.
22. van de Beek D, de Gans J, McIntyre P, Prasad K. Corticosteroids for acute bacterial meningitis. Cochrane Database Syst Rev. 2007;(1):CD004405.
23. Nguyen TH, Tran TH, Thwaites G, Ly VC, Dinh XS, Ho Dang TN, Dang QT, Nguyen DP, Nguyen HP, To SD, Nguyen VV, Nguyen MD, Campbell J, Schultsz C, Parry C, Torok ME, White N, Nguyen TC, Tran TH, Stepniewska K, Farrar JJ. Dexamethasone in Vietnamese adolescents and adults with bacterial meningitis. N Engl J Med. 2007;357:2431–40.
24. Prasad K, Singh MB. Corticosteroids for managing tuberculous meningitis. Cochrane Database Syst Rev. 2008;(1):CD002244.
25. Paul R, Lorenzl S, Koedel U, Sporer B, Vogel U, Frosch M, Pfister HW. Matrix metalloproteinases contribute to the blood–brain barrier disruption during bacterial meningitis. Ann Neurol. 1998;44:592–600.
26. Cabellos C, Martinez-Lacasa J, Martos A, Tubau F, Fernandez A, Viladrich PF, Gudiol F. Influence of dexamethasone on efficacy of ceftriaxone and vancomycin therapy in experimental pneumococcal meningitis. Antimicrob Agents Chemother. 1995;39:2158–60.
27. Ricard JD, Wolff M, Lacherade JC, Mourvillier B, Hidri N, Barnaud G, Chevrel G, Bouadma L, Dreyfuss D. Levels of vancomycin in cerebrospinal fluid of adult patients receiving adjunctive corticosteroids to treat pneumococcal meningitis: a prospective multicenter observational study. Clin Infect Dis. 2007;44:250–5.
28. Schut ES, Brouwer MC, de Gans J, Florquin S, Troost D, van de Beek D. Delayed cerebral thrombosis after initial good recovery from pneumococcal meningitis. Neurology. 2009;73: 1988–95.
29. Schut ES, Lucas MJ, Brouwer MC, Vergouwen MD, van der Ende A, van de Beek D. Cerebral infarction in adults with bacterial meningitis. Neurocrit Care. 2012;16:421–7.
30. Breeze RE, McComb JG, Hyman S, Gilles FH. CSF production in acute ventriculitis. J Neurosurg. 1989;70:619–22.

31. Kim YS, Sheldon RA, Elliott BR, Liu Q, Ferriero DM, Tauber MG. Brain injury in experimental neonatal meningitis due to group B streptococci. J Neuropathol Exp Neurol. 1995;54: 531–9.
32. Dellinger RP, Levy MM, Rhodes A, Annane D, Gerlach H, Opal SM, Sevransky JE, Sprung CL, Douglas IS, Jaeschke R, Osborn TM, Nunnally ME, Townsend SR, Reinhart K, Kleinpell RM, Angus DC, Deutschman CS, Machado FR, Rubenfeld GD, Webb SA, Beale RJ, Vincent JL, Moreno R, Surviving Sepsis Campaign Guidelines Committee including the Pediatric Subgroup. Surviving sepsis campaign: international guidelines for management of severe sepsis and septic shock: 2012. Crit Care Med. 2013;41:580–637.
33. Wijdicks EFM. The practice of emergency and critical care neurology. New York: Oxford University Press; 2010.
34. Abulhasan YB, Al-Jehani H, Valiquette MA, McManus A, Dolan-Cake M, Ayoub O, Angle M, Teitelbaum J. Lumbar drainage for the treatment of severe bacterial meningitis. Neurocrit Care. 2013;19:199–205.
35. Wall EC, Ajdukiewicz KM, Heyderman RS, Garner P. Osmotic therapies added to antibiotics for acute bacterial meningitis. Cochrane Database Syst Rev. 2013;(3):CD008806.
36. Bekar A, Dogan S, Abas F, Caner B, Korfali G, Kocaeli H, Yilmazlar S, Korfali E. Risk factors and complications of intracranial pressure monitoring with a fiberoptic device. J Clin Neurosci. 2009;16:236–40.
37. Kapadia F, Rodrigues C, Jha AN. A simple technique to limit ICP catheter infection. Br J Neurosurg. 1997;11:335–6.
38. Thompson MJ, Ninis N, Perera R, Mayon-White R, Phillips C, Bailey L, Harnden A, Mant D, Levin M. Clinical recognition of meningococcal disease in children and adolescents. Lancet. 2006;367:397–403.
39. Korein J, Cravioto H, Leicach M. Reevaluation of lumbar puncture; a study of 129 patients with papilledema or intracranial hypertension. Neurology. 1959;9:290–7.
40. Aronin SI, Peduzzi P, Quagliarello VJ. Community-acquired bacterial meningitis: risk stratification for adverse clinical outcome and effect of antibiotic timing. Ann Intern Med. 1998;129:862–9.
41. Edberg M, Furebring M, Sjolin J, Enblad P. Neurointensive care of patients with severe community-acquired meningitis. Acta Anaesthesiol Scand. 2011;55:732–9.
42. Lindvall P, Ahlm C, Ericsson M, Gothefors L, Naredi S, Koskinen LO. Reducing intracranial pressure may increase survival among patients with bacterial meningitis. Clin Infect Dis. 2004;38:384–90.
43. Kumar R, Singhi S, Singhi P, Jayashree M, Bansal A, Bhatti A. Randomized controlled trial comparing cerebral perfusion pressure-targeted therapy versus intracranial pressure-targeted therapy for raised intracranial pressure due to acute CNS infections in children. Crit Care Med. 2014;42:1775–87.
44. Prasad K, Karlupia N. Prevention of bacterial meningitis: an overview of Cochrane systematic reviews. Respir Med. 2007;101:2037–43.
45. Ratilal BO, Costa J, Sampaio C, Pappamikail L. Antibiotic prophylaxis for preventing meningitis in patients with basilar skull fractures. Cochrane Database Syst Rev. 2011;(8):CD004884.
46. Bilukha OO, Rosenstein N, National Center for Infectious Diseases CfDC, Prevention. Prevention and control of meningococcal disease. Recommendations of the Advisory Committee on Immunization Practices (ACIP). MMWR Recomm Reports. 2005;54:1–21.
47. Novak RT, Kambou JL, Diomande FV, Tarbangdo TF, Ouedraogo-Traore R, Sangare L, Lingani C, Martin SW, Hatcher C, Mayer LW, Laforce FM, Avokey F, Djingarey MH, Messonnier NE, Tiendrebeogo SR, Clark TA. Serogroup A meningococcal conjugate vaccination in Burkina Faso: analysis of national surveillance data. Lancet Infect Dis. 2012;12:757–64.
48. Obonyo CO, Lau J. Efficacy of Haemophilus influenzae type b vaccination of children: a meta-analysis. Eur J Clin Microbiol Infect Dis. 2006;25:90–7.
49. Koster-Rasmussen R, Korshin A, Meyer CN. Antibiotic treatment delay and outcome in acute bacterial meningitis. J Infect. 2008;57:449–54.

Chapter 13
Brain Abscess

Bijen Nazliel

Introduction

Brain abscess is a focal collection within the brain parenchyma, which can arise as a complication of a variety of infections, trauma or surgery. Successful treatment of a brain abscess requires a high index of suspicion and a combination of surgical excision, drainage, and antimicrobial therapy [1].

The management of brain abscess aims to reduce the space-occupying activity, reduce the intracranial pressure, and eradicate the pathogenic microorganism. The anatomical location, number and size of abscess, stage of abscess formation, age and neurological status of the patient can influence the strategy for managing brain abscess [2].

Cerebellar abscesses compromise 6–35 % of all brain abscesses. They are often ominously silent and carry significant mortality [3]. Associated supra or infra tentorial abscess or empyema may be present [4]. The cerebellar abscess needs to be treated differently from supratentorial abscess because of their ability to cause sudden total occlusion of CSF pathways early in the course of disease [3].

B. Nazliel, MD
Neurology-Neurointensive Care Unit,
Gazi University Faculty of Medicine, Ankara, Turkey
e-mail: bijennazliel@yahoo.com

© Springer International Publishing Switzerland 2015
K.E. Wartenberg et al. (eds.), *Neurointensive Care: A Clinical Guide to Patient Safety*, DOI 10.1007/978-3-319-17293-4_13

Case

A Streptococcal Cerebellar Abscess

A 59-year-old male was admitted to the Emergency Department with a 2-day history of headache, vertigo, nausea, and vomiting. On examination, he was febrile, but his other vital signs were normal. The head and neck examination revealed intact, non-inflamed tympanic membranes and normal mastoid regions bilaterally. The cardiac examination revealed a normal S1 and S2; there were no murmurs or gallops.

The neurological examination revealed that the patient was awake, alert, and cooperative. He had ataxia, a wide-based gait, and left dysmetria. No cranial, motor, or sensory abnormalities were present. His medical history was unremarkable.

On admission, his blood urea nitrogen (12.3 mg/dL), creatinine (0.61 mg/dL), aspartate aminotransferase (AST; 22 IU/L), alanine aminotransferase (ALT; 17 IU/L), white cell count (9,600/µL), and other blood cell counts and routine biochemical analyses were normal. The patient was negative for human immunodeficiency virus (HIV) antibodies.

Computed tomography (CT) of the head revealed a 3-cm solitary ring-enhancing lesion in the left cerebellum compressing the forth ventricle with surrounding edema. Magnetic resonance imaging (MRI) with gadolinium confirmed the presence of a solitary cerebellar abscess.

He was transferred to the neurology intensive care unit for further evaluation and treatment. A provisional diagnosis of cerebellar abscess was made and antibiotic therapy that included cefotaxime 2 g q6h intravenously (IV), amikacin 750 mg o.d. IV, and metronidazole 100 mg q8h IV was started.

The following day, stereotactic aspiration of the abscess was performed under aseptic conditions and 8 mL of greenish yellow pus were sent for investigation. Gram staining showed Gram-positive cocci in chains and pairs. Antimicrobial susceptibility testing was performed and the isolate was identified as *Streptococcus pneumonia*, which was susceptible to penicillin and the first-line drugs. Therefore, ofloxacin 100 mg q12h was added to the treatment.

Three days postoperatively, he became drowsy and had a generalized tonic–clonic seizure. He did not regain consciousness following the seizure. CT revealed the presence of perilesional edema, blood in the abscess cavity, and a shift with a mass effect on the fourth ventricle. He was treated with a loading dose of phenytoin, dexamethasone 10 mg IV, and mannitol 150 mL. He was immediately transferred to the operating room and underwent a left suboccipital craniotomy. The cerebellar abscess was drained, without placing drains. He was in a deep coma following the procedure and died the next day due to cerebellar herniation.

Risks of Patients Safety

Mortality from brain abscess ranges from 8 to 25 % [5, 6]. However, mortality increases to 27–85 % when the abscess ruptures in to the ventricle [6]. Factors associated with increased risk of rupture include deep location, location close to the ventricle wall, and the presence of multiple abscesses [7]. Severe mental status changes on admission, stupor or coma (60–100 % mortality), rupture in to the ventricle (80–100 % mortality) are the determinants of prognosis. Neurologic sequelae develop in 20–70 % of survivors [5].

Safety Barriers

Successful management of a brain abscess usually requires a combination of antibiotics and surgical drainage for both diagnostic and therapeutic purposes [1].

The nature of the abscess, its anatomic location, the number, size, and the initial neurological status of the patient all influence the treatment strategy [7].

Antibiotics are the first-line treatment and should be started immediately unless the patient is to be taken to the operating room, in which case antibiotics are held until aspiration of the lesions contents yields a sample culture [8].

The goals of surgical management of brain abscess are to decompress the space occupying lesion, reduce intracranial pressure, and eradicate the infection as well as primary infection source if present. The surgical options include aspiration, craniotomy, and complete excision, or craniotomy and marsupialisation [9]; therefore surgical drainage provides the most optimal therapy.

Aspiration is generally preferable to surgical excision since the neurologic sequelae are reduced [1]. Aspiration results in rapid relief in intracranial pressure while confirming the diagnosis of abscess and obtaining a sample for identification of the causative organism [10]. It is relatively safe and therefore can be performed even in patients who are poor surgical candidates. Complications of aspiration include subarachnoid or subdural leakage of pus resulting in empyema or meningitis, or intraventricular rupture of abscess. The biggest drawback of stereotactic aspiration is that abscess capsule is left intact and removal of purulent material is frequently incomplete, as a result most patients require multiple aspiration procedures to achieve resolution of the abscess [10]. Also the risk of repeated aspiration is that the procedure may cause bleeding. Risk factors for failure of aspiration requiring repeat procedure include inadequate antibiotic coverage, incomplete aspiration, and lack of catheter placement when larger abscesses are drained [8]. Surgical excision, once the mainstay of therapy for brain abscess, has been overshadowed by the advent of stereotaxic aspiration which has become the treatment of choice in many institutions [10]. Surgical evacuation offers the advantages of decreasing the infectious burden, confirming the diagnosis by sampling the capsular tissue, and relieving the mass effect in the acutely deteriorating patient [8]. Surgical excision is a more radical approach that generally results in greater neurologic deficits and is now infrequently performed [1]. Surgery carries the risk of spread of the infectious agent to the ventricular system, resulting in ventriculitis. Contraindications to surgical excision include the presence of multiple lesions and a deep location of the lesion [8]. But failure to perform surgical drainage can lead to a higher mortality rate.

Discussion of Risk/Benefit Ratios in Management of Brain Abscess

Many modern series advocate aspiration above craniotomy except in certain circumstances such as multiloculated abscess, posterior fossa abscess, abscess associated with foreign body or open head injury that have failed aspiration procedures and fungal abscess [10].

Cerebellar abscess should be completely excised through suboccipital craniectomy or craniotomy. Excision of the abscess significantly helps to reduce the cerebellar edema and relieves brain stem compression. If treated within reasonable time period, the prognosis following evacuation of cerebellar abscess is excellent. The long term outcome of patients with cerebellar abscess is directly proportional to their preoperative consciousness level [4].

Most series of brain abscess including both patients treated with closed aspiration and those treated with excision report no significant difference in effectiveness of the two procedures [10].

In patients undergoing an open procedure the reoperation rate was 16 % whereas most patients required multiple aspiration procedures in order to achieve the resolution of the abscess [10]. In series by Cavusoglu et al. [2, 10] 90 % of patients treated with aspiration required repeated aspiration, usually two to three times but occasionally more. Mamelak et al. [10, 11] reported that 62 % of patients in their series required additional surgery for drainage after the initial aspiration. The need for serial follow-up imaging is reduced in abscess excision, because closed aspiration usually leaves a persistent ring-enhancing lesion that must be followed closely until resolution [10].

Open surgery approximately takes 90 min from start to end and closed aspiration is not of shorter duration [10]. The course of intravenous antibiotic therapy can be shortened to 4 weeks following excision compared with drainage. Excised lesions are less likely to relapse than lesions that have only been drained [1].

Solutions

Empiric antibiotic therapy should be broad, started promptly, and narrowed only when a specific microbial cause is known. Empiric therapy is based on the usual microbial causes associated with the patient's risk factors for brain abscess [5].

Once a causative microorganism is identified, antimicrobial therapy can be tailored [12]. Expert microbiological advice is invaluable when selecting antimicrobials.

Medical management alone is considered appropriate in certain cases of brain abscess, such as small lesions (2.5–3 cm in diameter) in which the causative organism is known and if there is no compromise in neurologic status or signs of increased intracranial pressure [10].

Abscesses <3 cm and >1.5 cm in diameter are considered for stereotactic aspiration [7]. Stereotactic aspiration has been shown particularly helpful in the aspiration of deep seated abscess and those in speech areas and regions of the sensory or motor cortex and in comatose patients [1, 10].

Excision is generally recommended for abscesses that are superficially located with thick membranes as well as posttraumatic, gas containing, encapsulated fungal, and multiloculated abscess [7]. Open surgery is especially recommended for large multiloculated cortical lesions and cerebellar lesion where obstruction of the cerebrospinal fluid (CSF) can lead to rapid decompensation of the patient [8].

Cerebellar abscess should be completely excised through suboccipital craniectomy or craniotomy. Excision of abscess significantly helps to reduce the cerebellar edema and relieves brain stem compression. If treated within reasonable time period, the prognosis following evacuation of cerebellar abscess is excellent. The long term outcome of patients with cerebellar abscess is directly proportional to their preoperative consciousness level [4].

In cases of intraventricular rupture in addition to combination of intrathecal and intravenous antimicrobial treatment, rapid evacuation and debridement of the abscess cavity via urgent craniotomy, lavage of the ventricles, intraventricular drainage, and intraventricular administration of gentamicin are recommended [7].

Seizures are an important complication of brain abscess and may be an early or late complication occurring in 13–25 % of cases [12–16]. Seizures can occur as one of the initial complications of brain abscess and the rates of subsequent attacks are high [7]. It is believed that posterior fossa lesions are less likely to cause seizures, although reports have failed to demonstrate a correlation between abscess location and the likelihood of seizures [8].

Even though seizures in bacterial brain abscess patients may have a delayed manifestation, most seizures occur during the acute phase [16]. The mean time intervals from bacterial brain abscesses to first seizure in early seizures group was 2.3 days [16]. Early seizures predispose to the development of late seizures [7].

Several pathophysiological mechanisms though requiring further elucidation are implicated in the occurrence of seizures after bacterial brain abscesses including a combination of sudden development of space occupying lesion with mass effect, striking edema, and a surrounding zone of prominent perivascular inflammatory response which might possibly account for seizures in the early phase of brain abscesses [16].

The use of prophylactic antiepileptic drugs (AED) in the prevention of seizures in abscess remains controversial although the possible benefit of AEDs is the reduction of functional morbidity after seizures following bacterial brain abscesses [16]. Even though seizures may not affect the overall mortality rate [12–15] an anticonvulsant should be prescribed to prevent seizure in the early course of therapy.

Seizure prophylaxis and continuation of anticonvulsive therapy for an extended period are recommended for patients with brain abscess [7, 17]. Some authors have proposed seizure prophylaxis for all patients; the patients should then be re-evaluated by neurological and EEG examinations several months after the treatment of the brain abscess. The duration of AED treatment is dependent on EEG results [16].

The use of corticosteroids in the management of brain abscess is controversial. Some believe that steroid therapy can reduce antibiotic penetration in to the abscess, slowing capsule formation or increasing the risk of ventricular rupture [10, 18]. Dexamethasone has been used for reducing intracranial pressure, especially in patients with impending brain herniation. Although the benefit of dexamethasone in treatment of brain abscess remains unclear [12, 15, 19–21], in some cases extensive edema may surround the abscess and contribute to raised intracranial pressure [9]. Local vasogenic edema is the predominant type of edema leading to increased intracranial pressure, causing significant mortality and morbidity in patients with brain abscesses. Although there is no-well controlled randomized clinical study examining the use of corticosteroids for controlling cerebral edema accompanying brain abscess, corticosteroids are recommended preoperatively for reducing intracranial pressure and avoiding brain herniation. It is important to remember that prolonged use of corticosteroids may decrease the penetration of antimicrobial agents or impair the clearance of some pathogens and may also decrease the enhancement of the abscess wall on radiological examinations, particularly in the cerebritis stage [7, 22]. In patients with severe cerebral edema a short course of steroids may be of benefit [10] Utilization of steroid therapy should be done on a case by case basis [10]. Unnecessary or prolonged use of corticosteroids should be avoided because of its numerous adverse effects [12].

Summary

Despite advances in diagnosis and treatment, brain abscess still remains as life-threatening disease [7]. Non-surgical management alone is not recommended for lesions >3 cm in diameter [8]. Aspiration is the gold standard for treatment of brain abscesses. Stereotactic or intraoperative ultrasound guidance may be very useful [7]. Surgical excision, once the mainstay of therapy for brain abscess, has been overshadowed by the advent of stereotaxic aspiration which has become the treatment of choice in many institutions [10]. Open surgery is reserved for large multi-loculated cortical lesions and cerebellar lesion where obstruction of the CSF can lead to rapid decompensation of the patient. Open surgery is also recommended for fungal lesions, because the penetration of antifungal agents across the blood-brain barrier is poor [8].

The choice of antibiotic agents should be based on culture results, and therapy with 3rd generation cephalosporins combined with metronidazole and vancomycin can be considered. In patients with severe cerebral edema a short course of steroids may be of benefit [10], and even though seizures may not affect the overall mortality rate [12–15] an anticonvulsant should be prescribed to prevent seizure in the early course of therapy

Dos and Don'ts

Dos (In Patients with Cerebral-Cerebellar Abscess)

- Patients should be immediately evaluated both clinically and radio logically.
- Make a contact with a neurosurgeon, neurologist, neuroradiologist & infectious disease specialist
- Infections (including otitis/mastoiditis and sinus, pulmonary and dental infections) that may lead to brain abscess should be identified
- Empiric antibiotic therapy should be broad, started promptly
- Once the etiological agent is identified, treatment is tailored to the sensitivity of the specific agent
- Continue antibiotics minimum of 4–6 weeks of therapy if the abscess has been excited or aspirated and 6–8 weeks if treated conservatively
- An anticonvulsant should be prescribed to prevent seizure in the early course of therapy.
- In patients with severe cerebral edema a short course of steroids may be of benefit
- Utilization of steroid therapy should be done on a case by case basis.
- Unnecessary or prolonged use of corticosteroids should be avoided
- Determine the best choice of surgical approach (stereotactic guided aspiration versus excision)
- In patients with multiple abscess, the largest lesion is usually aspirated and other lesions monitored with post-operating imaging
- Serial neuroimaging should be performed to follow the effect of treatment

Don'ts (In Patients with Cerebral-Cerebellar Abscess)

- Do not perform lumber puncture due to increased risk of herniation
- Do not medically treat patients if the causative organism is unknown
- Do not perform craniectomy if the abscess is on speech areas and regions of the sensory or motor cortex
- Do not perform drainage in the early cerebritis phase without evidence of cerebral necrosis

References

1. Treatment and prognosis of brain abscess. http://www.uptodate.com/contents/treatment-and-prognosis-of-brain-abscess. Accessed 20 Sept 2013.
2. Cavusoglu H, Kaya RA, Turkmenoglu ON, Colak IB, Aydın Y. Brain abscess: analysis of results in a series of 51 patients with a combined surgical and medical approach during an 11-year period. Neurosurg Focus. 2008;24(6):E9.
3. Sharma BS, Gupta SK, Khosla VK. Current concepts in the management of pyogenic brain abscess. Neurol India. 2000;48:105.
4. Muzumdar D, Jhawar S, Goel A. Brain abscess: an overview. Int J Surg. 2011;9:136–44.
5. Derber CJ, Troy SB. Head and neck emergencies. Bacterial meningitis, encephalitis, brain abscess, upper airway obstruction and jugular septic thrombophelebitis. Med Clin North Am. 2012;96:1107–26.
6. Tunkel A. Brain abscess. In: Mandel GL, Bennet JE, Dolin R, editors. Mandell, Douglas and Bennett's principles and practice of infectious diseases, vol. 1. 7th ed. Philadelphia: Churchill Livingstone Elsevier; 2009. p. 1265–78.
7. Hakan T. Management of bacterial brain abscess. Neurosurg Focus. 2008;24(6):E4,1–6.
8. Brain abscess. http://bestpractice.bmj.com/best-practice/monograph/925/treatment/step-by-step.html. Accessed 20 Sept 2013.
9. Whitfield P. The management of intracranial abscess. AJNR. 2005;1:13–5.
10. Gadgil N, Patel AJ, Gopinath SP. Open craniotomy for brain abscess: a forgotten experience. Surg Neurol Int. 2013;4:34.
11. Mamelak AN, Mampulum TJ, Obamu WG, Rosenbum ML. Improved management of multiple brain abscess. A combined medical and surgical approach. Neurosurgery. 1995;36:76–84.
12. Honda H, Warren DK. Central nervous system infections: meningitis and brain abscess. Infect Dis Clin North Am. 2009;23:609–23.
13. Xiao F, Tseng MY, Teng JL, Tseng HM, Tsai JC. Brain abscesses: clinical experience and analysis of prognostic factors. Surg Neurol. 2005;63(5):442–9.
14. Tseng JH, Tseng MY. Brain abscess in 142 patients: factors influencing outcome and mortality. Surg Neurol. 2006;65(6):557–62.
15. Hakan T, Ceran N, Erdem I, Berkman MZ, Goktas P. Bacterial brain abscesses: an evaluation of 96 cases. J Infect. 2006;52(5):359–66.
16. Chuang MJ, Chang WN, Chang HW, Lin WC, Tsai NW, Hsieh MJ, Wang HC, Lu CH. Predictors and long-term outcome of seizures after bacterial brain abscess. J Neurol Neurosurg Psychiatry. 2010;81:913–7.
17. Klipatrick C. Epilepsy and brain abscess. J Clin Neurosci. 1997;4(1):26–8.
18. Quartey GR, Johston JA, Rozdilsky B. Decadron in the treatment of cerebral abscess. An experimental study. J Neurosurg. 1976;45:301.
19. Seydoux C, Francioli P. Bacterial brain abscesses: factors influencing mortality and sequelae. Clin Infect Dis. 1992;15(3):394–401.
20. Tonon E, Scotton PG, Galluci M, Vaglia A. Brain abscess clinical aspects of 100 patients. Int J Infect Dis. 2006;10(2):103–9.
21. Kao PT, Tseng HK, Liu CP, Su SC, Lee CM. Brain abscesses: clinical analysis of 53 cases. J Microbiol Immunol Infect. 2003;36(2):129–36.
22. Kramer AH, Bleck TP. Neurocritical care of patients with central nervous system infections. Curr Infect Dis Rep. 2007;9:308–14.

Chapter 14
Seizures and Status Epilepticus in the Intensive Care Units

Johnny Lokin

Introduction

The risk of occurrence of seizures in the Intensive Care Unit (ICU) either triggered by a primary brain lesion or as a complication of another medical illness is around 3.3 % [1]. It ranks second to metabolic encephalopathy as a cause of neurologic complications admitted in the ICU [1]. Status epilepticus (SE), defined as continuous seizures of more than 5 minutes or intermittent seizures without regaining consciousness, is an admitting diagnosis in only 0.2 % of the time [2].

On the other hand, seizures and SE in the Neurologic Intensive Care Unit (NICU) are often due to a primary disease of the brain. Patients who are admitted to the NICU may suffer from various traumatic and nontraumatic cerebral illnesses that can predispose them to develop seizures. These conditions include brain tumors, central nervous system infections (meningitis or encephalitis), intracerebral hemorrhage, cerebral infarction, cerebral venous thrombosis, complications of neurosurgical interventions and traumatic brain injury [3, 4]. In patients with subarachnoid hemorrhage, SE has an occurrence rate of 8 % while for traumatic brain injury, it ranges between 1.9 and 8 % [3, 4]. Approximately 8–34 % of comatose patients in NICU's have been described as having nonconvulsive status epilepticus (NCSE) [3, 4]. The most frequent causes for SE in this setting are hypoxia (42 %) and stroke (22 %) [3], while in another study, antiepileptic drug withdrawal or noncompliance to such medications, as well as alcohol withdrawal were identified as causes for seizures in the ICU [5, 6].

Patient safety in the NICU in the light of seizure occurrence poses a challenge to critical care specialists and neurologists as difficulties may be encountered with

J. Lokin, MD
Neuro-Intensive Care Unit, Chinese General Hospital
and Medical Center/University of Santo Tomur Hospital, Manila, Philippines
e-mail: j_lokin@yahoo.com

© Springer International Publishing Switzerland 2015
K.E. Wartenberg et al. (eds.), *Neurointensive Care: A Clinical Guide to Patient Safety*, DOI 10.1007/978-3-319-17293-4_14

identifying the etiology of seizures, with treatment and prevention of complications. Therefore, errors may transpire in various forms: diagnostic (failure to order the appropriate test, delay in the diagnosis, failure to act on results or monitoring), treatment (error in the performance of an operation, procedure or test; error in administering treatment, drug administration mistakes), prevention of recurrence (failure to provide appropriate monitoring, failure to provide prophylaxis), and others (failure in communication, equipment failure, system failure) [7].

Case Scenario

A 36-year-old male was admitted to the NICU with SE. The patient had been maintained on valproic acid given as 2 mg/kg/day with a blood level of 30 µmL. The NICU staff was busy preparing unlabelled medications when the patient suddenly had recurrence of seizures. It was after the sixth minute that the nurse saw the patient. The patient fell from his bed and was found on the floor, cyanotic and with an upward gaze. The nurse got frantic and ran to the nursing station trying to call for assistance. It took a few minutes before she realized that the nurse aid was out on an errand while the neuro-intensivist was attending to another patient. She went back to the room to attend to the patient who was in a postictal state at the time, unarousable to verbal and tactile stimuli. The nurse reviewed the chart and saw that the physician only ordered for the continuation of valproic acid and requested a complete blood complete count. No precautions or emergency medications for seizure recurrence had been ordered [7].

Risks of Patient Safety

Patient's safety is put at risk at different levels once admitted to the NICU. This can be summarized as: (1) failure and delay in the recognition or diagnosis of seizures and SE, (2) failure to administer appropriate, adequate, and timely management for seizures and SE, and (3) prevention of complications/injuries as a consequence of seizures.

Failure and Delay in the Recognition or Diagnosis of Seizures and Status Epilepticus

In most cases, the witnessed seizure occurring in a critically ill patient is classified as generalized tonic-clonic or focal with secondary generalization as well as complex-partial. Sometimes this constitutes a diagnostic dilemma as these may be difficult to differentiate from posturing, myoclonic jerks, or syncopal episodes. Even more challenging are the nonconvulsive seizures that may be misinterpreted as encephalopathies, other neurological disorders or even a psychiatric condition [8]. Delay in the diagnosis puts a patient at risk since focal and nonconvulsive seizures, especially SE have different etiologies. Hence, a different and definite approach is required in their treatment. However, in times of an emergency, the diagnosis and treatment should be prioritized equally due to the dreadful consequences posed with delayed management [9].

NICUs should ideally have monitoring units such as continuous video electroencephalography (cEEG) as used in epilepsy monitoring units (EMUs) to document and recognize seizures. Despite these advances, there are still reported cases of missed seizures even in the EMUs and these are defined as the seizures that occur "during which there was lack of recognition or delayed recognition by the video-monitors and/or inadequate intervention when they were recognized (malfunctioning equipment, poor nurse response postictally or during postictal psychosis, and delayed antiepileptic drug administration)" [10].

Failure to Administer Appropriate, Adequate, and Timely Management for Seizures and Status Epilepticus

As for treatment, there are also various ways wherein errors may be committed: administration (53 %), prescription (17 %), preparation (14 %), and transcription (11 %) [11]. In a study by the group of Agalu, the prevalence of medical administration errors was 51.8 % in the ICU and these were comprised of wrong timing (30.3 %), omission due to unavailability of the drug (29 %), missed doses (18.3 %), wrong route (9.1 %), wrong dose (4.2 %), unauthorized drug administration (2.7 %), wrong rate of infusion (1.4 %), and wrong duration (0.9 %) [12]. Anticonvulsants rank third among the drugs associated with medication administration errors [12, 13].

The physician/specialist/intensivist must be knowledgeable in the different indications of each drug as well as the contraindications, side effects, and interactions. Prescribing an erroneous drug, an incorrect dose, inappropriate route, and unsuitable schedule to the patient may lead to irreversible adverse events. One of the causes of these errors is inadequate communication in the form of ambiguous orders, illegible writing, or misunderstanding in verbal communication. Calculations, especially of the dose of medications with a narrow therapeutic window can be detrimental to the safety of patients with seizures in the ICU.

Prevention of Complications/Injuries Secondary to Seizures

Preventive measures in the NICU or ICU should be implemented particularly in patients with seizures. Attacks may occur unexpectedly, in various forms, and may have grave complications or consequences. SE and postictal psychosis are common causes of patient's falls even in the epilepsy monitoring unit [10].

Safety Barriers for Patients with Seizures/Status Epilepticus in the ICU

Barriers in ensuring patient safety in the ICUs include factors that may be categorized into: (1) problems with the organization and structure of the unit and (2) problems with the process of care.

Problems with the Organization and Structure of the Unit

It is quite evident that the nurse-to-patient-ratio is an important factor that must be addressed because it reflects the amount of work that needs to be done, and quality of patient care is highly dependent on this factor [14]. Other contributors to this problem include: nurses working out of their scope of practice in the ICU, receiving inadequate orientation, deficiency in workplace training, shortage of adequate clinical and educational support systems, and poor training in general [15].

Problems with the Process of Care

On the other hand, process of care pertains to issues with teamwork, collaboration, and communication. Among those that need particular attention is the nurse–physician collaboration in the ICU and transmission of information [14]. Identified barriers to effective communication are hierarchical differences, inter-professional and intra-professional rivalries, health literacy of the patient, differences in language and use of jargons, cultural and generational differences [7].

Risk/Benefit Ratios in the Management of the Seizures/Status Epilepticus in the ICU

It is equally imperative to examine the management of seizures and SE in the ICUs including the ICU in terms of the risks and benefits in their diagnosis and treatment.

Risks and Benefits in the Diagnosis of Seizure in the ICU

The neurologist or critical care specialist must be keen in diagnosing patients with SE since there are cases of "pseudostatus" or nonepileptic spells simulating SE.

These occur even in patients with real seizure disorders and may prove to be challenging to differentiate from SE. Manifestations are volitional behavioural problems and nonvolitional somatization. While other indicators such as preserved consciousness, purposeful movements, poorly coordinated thrashing, back arching, eyes held shut, head rolling, and pelvic thrusting can be frequently encountered. In such cases, benzodiazepines are still the effective therapy [16].

A detailed neurologic assessment with characterization of seizures described as convulsions, automatisms, onset of focal deficits, pupillary changes, and level of consciousness are invaluable in the management of seizures in the ICUs is as well as in pre-hospital and emergency room settings. Determining the underlying etiology is vital especially in prolonged SE (i.e. seizures beyond 60 min). Prolonged SE may be caused by other medical or secondary neurologic problems like hyperthermia, hypoglycemia, hypotension, pulmonary edema, renal failure, or rhabdomyolysis [17]. Failure to recognize and provide adequate treatment may lead to cerebral ischemia from hypoperfusion of susceptible areas like the limbic system and cortical structures [18].

In the diagnosis of seizure etiology, blood and serum chemistries are useful. Complete blood count, metabolic panel, serum calcium and magnesium, toxicology screening, and antiepileptic drug level determination are just a few of the noteworthy tests that should be undertaken [16]. Prudent use of neuroimaging is advised in patients who do not return to a normal level of consciousness; have new focal neurologic findings; or new onset SE without an identifiable etiology [16]. cEEG is an invaluable tool in identifying nonconvulsive SE, especially in patients who do not regain full consciousness despite treatment. It will likewise provide other diagnostic information and guide practitioners in therapy [16].

Risks and Benefits in the Treatment of Seizures and Status Epilepticus in the ICU

Rapid and early initiation of seizure control is important in the treatment and prevention of SE [19]. This is supported by studies showing a reduction of neuronal injury, prevention of duration-dependent kindling and cytokine-mediated effects in experimental models with early termination of SE [20, 21]. In one study, therapy initiated within 30 min from the onset of seizures had 80 % response rate to first-line antiepileptic drugs while therapy given beyond a 2-h window period had a decreased response rate of 40 %. The use of benzodiazepines has been proven to be effective in such scenarios [5]. However, one must consider that benzodiazepines are most effective when given shortly after seizure onset and its effectiveness decreases with prolonged seizure duration [22].

Medical practitioners must also be knowledgeable in the alternative routes of administration of benzodiazepines: diazepam per rectum and intranasal; buccal, or intramuscular midazolam. All routes were shown to be effective alternatives to intravenous administration and must be utilized in times when there is lack of intravenous access to avoid delay in the administration [23].

Despite having protocols or guidelines regarding the pharmacologic therapy of seizures and SE, some physicians still prefer alternative approaches. Some studies report that although phenobarbital remains a reasonable option for control of SE by acting on the GABA receptor, it may be a less rational choice in those who have not responded to benzodiazepines [24]. The use of propofol in SE also poses certain threats of developing propofol-infusion syndrome. Its rather rare occurrence should not undermine its potentially fatal outcome. This is characterized by refractory cardiac arrhythmia with hepatomegaly, hyperlipidemia, metabolic acidosis, or rhabdomyolysis [25, 26].

Solutions for the Patients at Risk

The management of patients with seizures should focus on the identified barriers as previously discussed: (1) problems with the organization and structure of the unit, (2) problems with the process of care, and (3) problems with the provision of resources.

A competent protocol that serves as a guide to the personnel should be in place, it must consist of customized orders, treatment parameters, safety limits such as when and how to call the physician, 24 h limit on intravenous benzodiazepines, and ward capabilities and limitations. Practice guidelines on the management of SE should be clear and implemented judiciously [27].

Implementation of such protocols may be ensured through proper communication among the health care team especially during shift changes. Written sign outs should be comprised of diagnosis, clinical status of the patient, pending results, allergies, what to watch out for, and actions to be taken when seizures and complications occur. Physicians may personally notify and demonstrate the different findings and specific details of monitoring. Important matters and standardized protocols should always be reiterated. It is detrimental to the practitioner and the patient to make assumptions [7].

The ICU's should be adequately staffed with a patient-to-nurse-ratio higher than regular wards according to ICU guidelines. The presence of family members who are knowledgeable of seizure episodes is valuable during monitoring and detection of seizures. A seizure button, apart from the call light, is a very useful apparatus inside the patient's room [28].

Staff education modules may be provided by the hospital administrators. Special topics such as seizure classification, clinical presentations, diagnostic tests, first aid and treatment, proper response and care for patients during seizures, role of seizure observation and reporting of observations during and after the seizure should also be discussed. On the other hand, physician education may prioritize discussions on identification and review of patients at high risk of adverse events, on safety reports and causes of any adverse events [10].

Preparation for responses to seizure episodes should be part of any ICU setting. A neurologist/specialist should be available at all times. Rescue medications should be easily accessed through the emergency kits. Protocols for seizure first aid should have visual aids. While regular skills training should keep the staff alerted and updated on how to manage seizures and SE. This entails (1) responding to changes in consciousness, mental status, or behavior; (2) monitoring vital signs during acute seizures, during and after administration of intravenous antiepileptic drugs; (3) turning of patients on lateral decubitus position and removal of hazards within the area; (4) availability of suctioning and oxygen supplementation equipment; (5) recording the duration of the event with documentation of observations; (6) having a set of criteria for informing the specialists about a seizure, when to give rescue medications, and prudent resumption of pre-admission anticonvulsants.

The physician's orders and instructions should be clear. Written orders account for a large percentage of inpatient errors such as drug dosing. Handwriting should be legible. Standardized orders could help to decrease orders of omission but may increase orders of commission due to duplication of requested ancillaries or medications. Electronic health record systems may be advantageous.

Pre-admission screening should be done to prepare the staff for seizure episodes [29]. Salient features that should be identified in the patient's history are: (1) seizure character, frequency, and triggers, (2) information on the patient's ictal and postictal behavior, (3) which factor among the ictal and postictal behavior and complications has the propensity to put the patient or the staff at risk, (4) risk for SE such as history of drug withdrawal or noncompliance, and SE as an admission diagnosis [30]. Checklists are vital instruments in ensuring patient safety. In a study by Spanaki et al., a checklist was developed to identify patients with increased risk for falls and injuries during seizures which includes those with generalized tonic-clonic seizures, previous injuries during seizure, elderly, developmentally challenged, demented, or with motor weakness [10].

Seizure precautions should include cardiac monitoring. Ictal asystole occurs in 0.27 % of epilepsy while late hypotension is seen more often in SE. Another reason why the patients' cardiac status should be monitored in seizure patients in the NICU is sudden unexpected death in epilepsy (SUDEP) [31]. It is also recommended that pulse oximeter and oxygen supplementation be made available at anytime. Intravenous access should be placed for ease of administration of parenteral anticonvulsant medications. Patients should be advised to limit off-ward trips and to alert staff in cases when aura is experienced.

Patient safety during postictal aggression begins with its recognition such as awareness of its occurrence after one episode or after a cluster of seizures, its tendency to cause harm, its natural course as it resolves spontaneously; as well as its conservative management of limiting patient contact. There is no need to restrain the patient unless his behavior becomes a grave threat to his safety and to the people around him [32].

Another complication that should be monitored is postictal psychosis with an onset of less than a week after seizures. The patient is described to be irritable with a labile mood and insomnia. The duration of the psychosis is estimated to be from 15 h to approximately 2 months. Delirium, paranoid delusions, auditory, and visual hallucinations are the common manifestations. Although it has a self-limiting course, the psychosis should be treated if it worsens. sedatives, benzodiazepines, and neuroleptics may be indicated [33].

The ICU must be well furnished and equipped before admitting patients, especially those with seizures. The patient's room should be limited to the essential tools for monitoring seizures and the fixtures should be kept simple and safe. Potentially dangerous objects should be removed. The heights of beds should be kept low with padded side rails [28]. Bathrooms are high risk areas for falls. Hence, some suggestions to keep patient safe include outswing design for the door, use of a curtain instead of a door, padded sink edges and toilet seats, and placement of assistive rails [28].

Summary/Key Points

Patient safety in the management of seizures in the intensive care units specially with NICU starts with the physician's keen clinical acumen in the detection and diagnosis of seizures. Timely, appropriate, and adequate management and control of seizures are expected. Anticipation and prevention of SE, as well as the complications such as falls and head trauma tend to move the patient out of harm's way. Proper communication, a good administrative plan and implementation help to administer and employ the different protocols for seizures in the ICU patients. Finally, proper communication and collaboration among professionals are the important factors in the prevention of errors committed in the management of patients with seizures in the intensive care units.

Dos and Don'ts

Dos

- ICU, particularly the NICU should have continuous video EEG
- Protocol and check list for management of seizures
- Ensure adequate nurse-to-patient ratio 1:1–1:2
- Neuroimaging is recommended for patients who do not regain consciousness or have new neurological deficits or new onset of seizures
- Install a seizure button inside patient's room
- Continuous ICU staff education on classification of seizures and management
- Electronic medical record system to avoid medication errors

Don'ts

- Don't delay the diagnosis and management of seizures
- Don't leave seizure patients at risk for injuries; falling without a risk of fall sign at the bedside
- Don't exclude cardiac monitoring as a seizure precaution
- Don't restrain the patient unless his behaviour becomes a grave threat to his safety and to the medical staff

References

1. Bleck TP, Smith MC, Pierre-Louis SJ, Jares JJ, Murray J, Hansen CA. Neurologic complications of critical medical illnesses. Crit Care Med. 1993;21(1):98–103.
2. Varelas PN, Mirski MA. Seizures in the adult intensive care unit. J Neurosurg Anesthesiol. 2001;13(2):163–75.
3. Towne AR, Waterhouse EJ, Boggs JG, et al. Prevalence of nonconvulsive status epilepticus in comatose patients. Neurology. 2000;54:340–5.
4. Jordan KG. Continuous EEG, and evoked potential monitoring in the neuroscience intensive care unit. J Clin Neurophysiol. 1993;10:445–75.
5. Lowenstein DH, Alldredge BK. Status epilepticus at an urban public hospital in the 1980s. Neurology. 1993;43:483–8.
6. Aminoff MJ, Simon RP. Status epilepticus: causes, clinical features and consequences in 98 patients. Am J Med. 1980;69:657–66.
7. Patient safety 101 for neurologists. American Academy of Neurology. 2012. https://www.aan.com/uploadedfiles/website_library_assets/documents/3.practice_management/2.quality_improvement/2.patient_safety/2.patient_safety_education/patient%20safety_abust%20and%20violence%20101%20power%20point.pdf
8. Ziai WC, Kaplan PW. Seizures and status epilepticus in the intensive care unit. Seminars in Neurology. Thieme Medical Publishers. 2008;28(5):668–81.
9. Varelas PN, Spanaki MV. Seizures in Critical Care: A guide to diagnosis and therapeutics 2nd edition. Totowa, New Jersey: Humana Press; 2010;14:305–64.
10. Spanaki MV, et al. Developing a culture of safety in the epilepsy monitoring unit: a retrospective study of safety outcomes. Epilepsy and Behavior. 2012;25(2):185–188.
11. Moyen E, et al. Clinical review: medication errors in critical care. Critical Care. BioMed Central. 2008;12(2):208.
12. Agalu A, et al. Medication administration errors in an intensive care unit in Ethiopia. International Archives in Medicine. BioMed Central. 2012;5(1):15.
13. Gordon PC, et al. Drug administration errors by South African anesthetists-a survey. South African Medical Journal. 2006:96(7):631–2.
14. Moreno RP, Rhodes A, Donchin Y. Patient safety in intensive care medicine: the Declaration of Vienna. Intensive Care Med. 2009;35:1667–72. Springer and ESICM.
15. Morrison A. The effects of nursing staff inexperience on the occurrence of adverse patient experiences in ICUs. Aust Crit Care. 2001;14:116–21.
16. Claasen J, Silbergleit R, Weingart S, Smith W. Emergency neurological life support: status epilepticus. Neurocritical Care. Neurocritical Care Society. Springer. 2012;17:S73–8.
17. Lothman E. The biochemical basis and pathophysiology of status epilepticus [review]. Neurology. 1990;40(5 Suppl 2):13–23.
18. Walton NY. Systemic effects of generalized convulsive status epilepticus [review]. Epilepsia. 1993;34 Suppl 1:S54–8.

19. Brophy GM, Bell R, Claassen J, et al. Neurocritical care society status epilepticus guideline writing committee. Guidelines for the evaluation and management of status epilepticus. Neurocrit Care. 2012;17(1):3–23.
20. Morimoto K, Fahnestock M, Racine RJ. Kindling and status epilepticus models of epilepsy: rewiring the brain. Prog Neurobiol. 2004;73:1–60.
21. Ravizza T, Vezzani A. Status epilepticus induces time-dependent neuronal and astrocytic expression of interleukin-1 receptor type I in the rat limbic system. Neuroscience. 2006;137: 301–8.
22. Kapur J, Macdonald RL. Rapid seizure-induced reduction of benzodiazepine and Zn2+ sensitivity of hippocampal dentate granule cell GABAA receptors. J Neurosci. 1997;17:7532–40.
23. Ortega-Gutierrez S, Desai N, Clansen J. The neuro ICU book. The McGraw-Hill Companies. 2012:3;52–76.
24. Berning S, Boesebeck F, van Baalen A, Kellinghaus C. Intravenous levetiracetam as treatment for status epilepticus. J Neurol. 2009;256:1634–42.
25. Vasile B, Rasulo F, Candiani A, Latronico N. The pathophysiology of propofol infusion syndrome: a simple name for a complex syndrome [review] [published online ahead of print August 6, 2003]. Intensive Care Med. 2003;29:1417–25.
26. Kam PC, Cardone D. Propofol infusion syndrome [review]. Anaesthesia. 2007;62:690–701.
27. Manford M. Practical guide to epilepsy. Burlington: Butterworth-Heinemann; 2003.
28. Sanders PT, Cysyk BJ, Bare MA. Safety in long-term EEG/video monitoring. J Neurosci Nurs. 1996;28(5):305–13.
29. Lee JW, Shah A. Safety in the EMU: reaching consensus. Epilepsy Currents. American Epilepsy Society. Open Access. 2013;13(2):107–9. .
30. Dewar A, Pack A. Preadmission screening, discharge planning, and safety with seizure provocation. In: Labiner D (Chair) 2008 American Epilepsy Society. Symposium conducted at the meeting of American Epilepsy Society, Seattle; 2008.
31. Schuele S, Bermeo A, Alexopoulos A, Locatelli E, Burgess R, Dinner D, Foldvary-Schaefer N. Video-electrographic and clinical features in patients with ictal asystole. Neurology. 2007;69(5):434–41.
32. Gerard EM, Spitz MC, Towbin JA, Shantz D. Subacute postictal aggression. Neurology. 2011;50:384–7.
33. Falip M, Carreño M, Donaire A, Maestro I, Pintor L, Bargalló N, Setoaín J. Postictal psychosis: a retrospective study in patients with refractory temporal lobe epilepsy. Seizure. 2009;18(2):145–9.

Chapter 15
Traumatic Brain Injury

Tamer Abdelhak and Guadalupe Castillo Abrego

Introduction

Individuals of all ages, background, and health status are susceptible to traumatic brain injury (TBI). Every year in the United States 1.7 million people suffer from TBI, and TBI is listed as a contributing cause in approximately one third of injury-related deaths [1]. Approximately 290,000 patients require hospitalization, and 51,000 die of their injuries [2].

Although most cases of TBI are mild, our focus in the intensive care environment has been the small percentage severe TBI which historically carried a poor prognosis regardless of the cause. While the numbers suggest a grim state concerning TBI treatment there have been improvements in its management. Over the past 30 years, deaths from severe TBI have reduced from 50 % to fewer than 25 % [3]. Evidence-based guidelines for TBI management were introduced in 1995 by the Brain Trauma Foundation (BTF) in the United States because of variable treatment approaches. In the years following there have still been lapses in consistent implementation [4, 5]. Mortality is not the only concern in TBI. It is estimated that 3.2 million people are living with long-term disability related to traumatic brain injury (TBI) [6]. In addition to the personal toll, the direct and indirect costs of these disabilities are estimated to exceed $60 billion annually [7].

T. Abdelhak, MD
Department of Neurology, Southern Illinois University School of Medicine,
Springfield, IL, USA

G. Castillo Abrego, MD (✉)
Critical Care Department, Caja de Seguro Social Hospital, Panama City, Panama
e-mail: Guadalupe.castilloabrego@neuroandcriticalcare.com,
guadalupecastilloabrego@hotmail.com

© Springer International Publishing Switzerland 2015   219
K.E. Wartenberg et al. (eds.), *Neurointensive Care: A Clinical Guide
to Patient Safety*, DOI 10.1007/978-3-319-17293-4_15

One important factor to emphasize is center referral and specialization. A very large prospective study of the cost and outcomes associated with trauma center designation found more than a 25 % reduction in in-hospital mortality for those with severe TBI who were initially treated at a level I trauma center compared to similarly injured patients treated at hospitals of similar size that were not designated trauma centers [8].

The true incidence of TBI is unknown because current surveillance methodologies do not capture those treated in nonhospital settings (e.g., primary care office) or those who do not seek treatment at all.

One problem in the development of reliable guidelines for treatment of TBI is the varied pathophysiology of injury. TBI may be penetrating or nonpenetrating, diffuse or focal, vary in severity, location, and patient characteristics. Additionally, since TBI is often accident-related, there are limited primary prophylactic measures.

For the purpose of this book this chapter will be focused on management of adult patients in civilian environment with nonpenetrating severe traumatic brain injury. The BTF guidelines for management of this population were last updated in 2007 [9]. These guidelines addressed 15 topics concerning the in-hospital management of severe traumatic brain injury.

    I. Blood Pressure and Oxygenation
   II. Hyperosmolar Therapy
  III. Prophylactic Hypothermia
  IV. Infection Prophylaxis
   V. Deep Vein Thrombosis Prophylaxis
  VI. Indications for Intracranial Pressure Monitoring
 VII. Intracranial Pressure Monitoring Technology
VIII. Intracranial Pressure Thresholds
  IX. Cerebral Perfusion Thresholds
   X. Brain Oxygen Monitoring and Thresholds
  XI. Anesthetics, Analgesics, and Sedatives
 XII. Nutrition
XIII. Antiseizure Prophylaxis
XIV. Hyperventilation
 XV. Steroids

These guidelines too are probably outdated after 7 years of continued research. A PubMed search of code words *Traumatic brain injury* revealed 74,062 citations. Of these 19,196 have been published over past 5 years only (25 %). Adding the word *Safety* to the whole search yielded only 1,128 citations (1.5 %). So there is a clear gap about our understanding of the safety of clinical management of traumatic brain injury based on evidence-based medicine.

In this chapter, we are going to follow the same template of the BTF guidelines in addressing each of the categories of treatment and its safety and updated literature review.

Case Scenario

A 22-year-old male was skate boarding holding on to a moving car. He tripped and fell. He was extracted by EMS and placed in neck collar and transported to the nearest trauma center which was a level II. He was comatose, Glasgow Coma Scale (GCS) was 6, and his systolic blood pressure (SBP) was 85/50 mmHg. Two large bore IV lines were placed and he was given 2 L Lactated Ringers solution. He was intubated with inline stabilization of the C spine. Trauma surveys revealed skin lacerations all over the head and body. X-rays demonstrated a broken left ankle and rib fractures. The CT scan of the head revealed multiple frontal parietal contusions with right-sided acute subdural hematoma with midline shift (Fig. 15.1). He was taken emergently to the operating room (OR) where he underwent right hemicraniectomy with evacuation of the hematoma. He was then transferred to the nearest level I trauma center. Upon arrival he was still comatose, intubated, GCS was 5. Repeat CT scan upon arrival showed a new left-sided subdural hematoma and increasing hemorrhagic components of the frontal and temporal parietal contusion and diffuse cerebral edema (Fig. 15.2). He was taken to the OR and a left-sided hemicraniectomy was performed with evacuation of the hematoma. He was then brought back to the NeuroICU. He was placed in a 30° sitting position. His blood

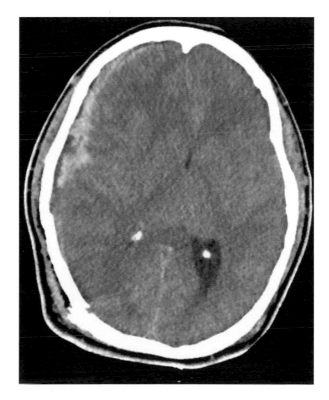

Fig. 15.1 Initial CT scan at outside hospital showing hyperacute right subdural hematoma and depressed skull fracture near the occipital region. Notice the complete effacement of the ventricular system

Fig. 15.2 CT scan few hours
post initial surgery showing
suboptimal right
hemicraniectomy with
subdural evacuation and
cortical hemorrhagic
contusion. Notice the
developing left subdural
hematoma as a result of
countercoup injury

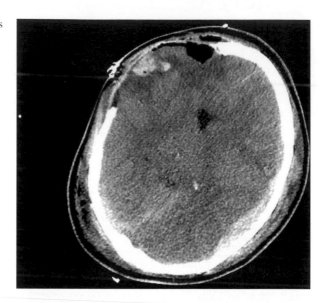

Fig. 15.3 CT scan as soon as
the patient transferred
showing worsening of left
subdural with loss of basal
cisterns and uncal herniation.
Notice the nasal bone fracture
with fluid in the ethmoid
sinuses

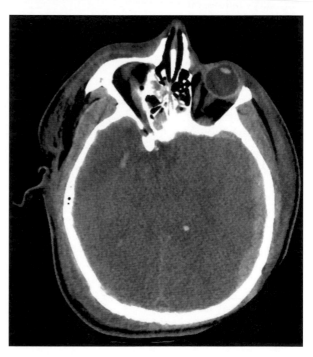

pressure was maintained with mean arterial pressure (MAP) >70 mmHg (assuming
the intracranial pressure (ICP) was <10 mmHg given bilateral hemicraniectomy to
maintain a presumptive cerebral perfusion pressure (CPP) >60 mmHg). Minimal
sedation with use of fentanyl and midazolam drips achieved to maintain synchrony

Fig. 15.4 CT scan following the second surgery showing bilateral hemicraniectomy that were connected anteriorly to decompress the frontal lobes. The anterior part of the superior sagittal sinus was ligated. Notice the bilateral hemorrhagic contusions and the opening of the lateral ventricular system following the decompression

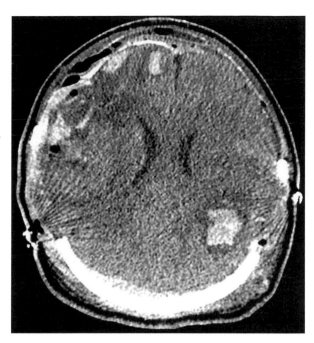

with ventilator. Ventilator settings were adjusted to target oxygen saturations >95 %, partial pressure of oxygen (PaO$_2$) >90 mmHg, partial pressure of carbon dioxide (pCO$_2$) 35–45 mmHg. Enteral nutrition was started through an orogastric tube. Phenytoin seizure prophylaxis was initiated upon arrival with a loading dose of 20 mg/kg, then maintenance of 100 mg every 8 h intravenously. Neck collar was loosened as the patient was bedbound and a CT of the cervical (C) spine did not show any fractures. Within 48 h the MRI of the C spine showed no evidence of ligamentous injury, so the neck collar was removed. As the CT head showed a significant degree of cerebral edema even with hemicraniectomy (Figs. 15.3 and 15.4), osmotic therapy using 3 % NaCl solution infusion was initiated upon arrival to NeuroICU and sodium goal was targeted to 10 mEq higher than patient's baseline sodium. Labs were checked initially every 6 h to monitor electrolytes, hemoglobin, INR, and arterial blood gas. The patient required a central line for osmotic therapy so a femoral line was placed initially to avoid putting the head down initially. This was changed 48 h later to a subclavian central line to avoid internal jugular vein thrombosis. Hemoglobin goal was directed to be >8 g/dL. Platelets goal was >70,000/dL, INR <1.5.

The patient stabilized over next few days, though he remained comatose with GCS 6–7. He received a tracheostomy and gastrostomy on day 7. He was transferred to a TBI long-term care facility on day 35 of admission following a long hospital stay complicated by persistent fever that required aggressive normothermia protocols, and recurrent pneumonia. Long-term follow-up showed him to be in a minimally conscious state without ventilator dependence but requiring tube feeding

Fig. 15.5 Follow-up CT
4 months post injury and
after cranioplasty. Notice the
bilateral hydrocephalus ex
vacuo secondary to
encephalomalacia. A trial of
cerebrospinal fluid drainage
did not result in improvement
in neurological status.
However, the patient had a
ventriculoperitoneal shunt
placed at outside facility to
improve the appearance of
the ventricles

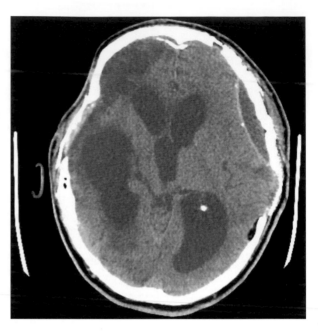

through gastrostomy tube. His bone flaps were placed back 10 weeks following the
injury. The follow-up CT showed areas of encephalomalacia with hydrocephalus ex
vacuo (Fig. 15.5).

Blood Pressure and Oxygenation

The recommendations from BTF were the following:

Level II – Blood pressure should be monitored and hypotension (systolic blood
pressure < 90 mm Hg) avoided [9].

Level III – Oxygenation should be monitored and hypoxia (PaO_2 < 60 mm Hg or O_2
saturation < 90 %) avoided [9].

It is imperative to avoid secondary brain injury after initial insult. Hypoxic ischemic brain injury is the most common secondary injury resulting from hypotension
or hypoxemia. Hypoxemia and hypotension occur commonly before the patient
reaches hospital and significantly increase the risk of secondary brain injury and the
likelihood of a poor outcome [10, 11].

Hypotension, defined as a SBP of less than 90 mmHg, should be treated aggressively. In two US studies, hypotensive episodes were observed in 16 % [10] and
32 % [11] of patients with severe traumatic brain injury at the time of hospital
arrival and during surgical procedures, respectively. A single episode of hypotension was associated with increased morbidity and doubling of mortality. An
Australian study reported similar findings [11]. Normovolemia should be restored

by infusing isotonic fluids as needed. Hypotonic intravenous solutions can exacerbate cerebral edema and should be avoided.

If the patient is anemic, packed red blood cells should be transfused to restore hemodynamic stability. The real value of adequate hemoglobin value in TBI is still unknown and could be anywhere between 8 and 10 g/dL. If hypotension is refractory to volume resuscitation, the patient should be given a continuous IV infusion of a vasopressor medication, with the dose titrated to raise the SBP > 90 mmHg. Norepinephrine has been shown to be most efficacious at maintaining MAP and CPP without deleteriously affecting ICP [12].

Hypoxemia defined as pulse oximetry saturation below 90 OR $PaO_2 < 60$ is best avoided with the use of tracheal intubation and mechanical ventilation if the patient is comatose, i.e., GCS <9 or not protecting airway or if in need for urgent surgery for other reasons.

The fraction of inspired oxygen should be titrated to provide an arterial PaO_2 around 100 mmHg which should provide a good margin above 60 mmHg as cutoff value. Normobaric hyperoxia might also be beneficial (see below). Traumatic or neurogenic acute respiratory distress syndrome (ARDS) can develop in patients with severe chest injuries or TBI. In such cases, adequate oxygenation requires the use of positive end-expiratory pressure (PEEP). Concern has been raised that the use of PEEP in patients with TBI may increase the ICP. However, clinical studies have shown that in the presence of ARDS, up to 14–15 cm H_2O of PEEP can be used without measurable changes in ICP, most likely because ARDS significantly reduces pulmonary compliance.

Maintaining an arterial pCO_2 of approximately 35–45 mmHg is advised to avoid cerebral vasoconstriction associated with aggressive hyperventilation and hypocapnia. Hypoventilation should also be avoided to prevent hypercapnia induced cerebral vasodilation and cerebral edema.

Hyperosmolar Therapy

The recommendations from BTF were the following:

Level II – Mannitol is effective for control of raised intracranial pressure (ICP) at doses of 0.25–1 g/kg body weight. Arterial hypotension (systolic blood pressure < 90 mm Hg) should be avoided [9].

Level III – Restrict Mannitol use prior to ICP monitoring to patients with signs of transtentorial herniation or progressive neurological deterioration not attributable to extracranial causes [9].

Mannitol is a sugar alcohol that is been long used in management of cerebral edema and intracranial hypertension since the early twentieth century. It is available as a 20 % solution (Osmolarity 1,100 mOsm/L) and used as intravenous bolus infusion of 0.5–1 g/kg. The bolus administration can be repeated at 0.25–1 g/kg every 4–6 h. The mechanism of action is not fully understood but mainly includes osmotic dehydration of the brain using blood–brain barrier (BBB) as a semi permeable dialysis membrane, minimal cerebral vasoconstriction (similar to hyperventilation) and reduction in production of cerebrospinal fluid (CSF).

Mannitol is an osmotic diuretic and will cause diuresis and hypotension in volume challenged patients. It is why it is contraindicated in hypotensive patients on vasopressor support and with anuria. It can also worsen or induce acute kidney injury via osmotic stress of the nephron. With repeated dosing renal parameters can be monitored via checking the osmotic gap (difference between calculated serum osmolality and measured one) and keeping it less than 20 prior to dose administration. A minimal amount of mannitol can cross the intact BBB (Reflection coefficient 0.9) which would explain its failure resulting in rebound cerebral edema with prolonged infusions in the past.

Hypertonic saline solution (HSS) is a different option that has been introduced over past four decades. HSS is available in different concentrations of sodium chloride in water, e.g., 2, 3, 7.5, 14.6, 20, and 23.4 % (highest possible concentration) or in a combination of sodium chloride and other sodium salts (acetate or lactate) to avoid hyperchloremia. In contrast to mannitol, HSS is a volume expander and is not associated with hypotension or kidney damage unless heart failure or hyperchloremic metabolic acidosis ensues. It also has a reflection coefficient of 1 which means that HSS-sodium does not pass freely through the intact BBB which would favor prolonged infusions. HSS is useful in cases of elevated ICP which does not respond to other therapies. For instance, repeated administration of 14.6 % HS in a cohort of patients with elevated ICP completely refractory to other therapies was shown successful in reducing ICP [13]. Other studies have confirmed this finding by directly comparing mannitol and HS in similar refractory cases of elevated ICP. One of the studies also revealed HS to significantly elevate brain oxygenation compared to mannitol [14]. By reducing ICP, hyperosmolar agents may elevate CPP which is beneficial when focal regions are hypoperfused after trauma; mannitol and HSS both have demonstrated this effect in an acute TBI cohort of 8 patients [15]. Yet, when compared with mannitol directly in a randomized trial, HSS increased cerebral blood flow (CBF) and CPP to higher values and for an increased duration [16]. Although the data for HSS is appealing, the BTF does not see enough evidence to support HSS over mannitol in 2007. Both agents should also be used as part of tiered approach to intracranial hypertension in conjunction with other methods or medications. (Suggested tiered management protocol of intracranial hypertension appears later in this chapter.)

Prophylactic Hypothermia

The recommendations from BTF were the following:

Level III – Pooled data indicate that prophylactic hypothermia is not significantly associated with decreased mortality when compared with normothermic controls. However, preliminary findings suggest that a greater decrease in mortality risk is observed when target temperatures are maintained for more than 48 h [9].

Prophylactic hypothermia is associated with significantly higher Glasgow Outcome Scale (GOS) scores when compared to scores for normothermic controls [9].

There are three types of hypothermia in TBI patients, spontaneous upon admission, prophylactic to be initiated as early as the patient is resuscitated, and therapeutic for ICP control during the ICU stay. Spontaneous hypothermia upon time of admission is associated with poorer prognosis [17–19] because it might be a sign of hypotension and global tissue hypoperfusion. Therapeutic hypothermia has been used successfully in refractory intracranial hypertension and cerebral edema. Prophylactic hypothermia is a controversial issue in the literature because multiple variables are involved in its successful implementation; these include temperature at time of injury, initial onset of cooling, rate of cooling, final temperature targeted, and mechanism of cooling as well as re-warming rate. Since brain temperature cannot be predicted from body temperatures with high confidence, separate monitoring is recommended [20]. The National Acute Brain Injury Study: Hypothermia II (NABISH trial) was a large-scale RCT which failed to confirm any benefit of prophylactic hypothermia [21]. However, recent retrospective analysis of pooled neurotrauma data revealed patients receiving hypothermia treatment had significantly more favorable outcomes compared to normothermic patients and those with no temperature management; it is important to note that hypothermic patients were, on average, significantly younger [22]. Another study demonstrated that hypothermia of 32.7 °C in severe TBI, maintained for 72 h produced favorable outcomes [23]. A meta-analysis by Fox et al. (2010) suggests a rationale for discrepancies among the study results. Hypothermia studies with long-term/goal-directed strategies in their design demonstrated patients to have lower mortality rates and more favorable outcome, whereas studies implementing short-term strategies were often inconclusive [24]. Besides strategic design, another key variable influencing prophylactic hypothermia studies is the re-warming strategy. For instance, the NABISH II trial re-warmed patients from 33 °C to 0.5 °C every 2 h, there was no difference in Glasgow outcome scale (GOS) scores or mortality between hypothermic and normothermic patients [21]. Another prospective study cooled patients to 32.7 °C and allowed them to spontaneously re-warm at room temperature. In that study, hypothermic patients had significantly improved GOS scores compared to the normothermic group [23]. Re-warming strategies are important during therapeutic temperature management for optimizing patient outcomes due to the rebound effect of releasing free radicals or cerebral metabolic demand–perfusion mismatch.

Infection Prophylaxis

The recommendations from BTF were the following:

Level II – Periprocedural antibiotics for intubation should be administered to reduce the incidence of pneumonia. However, it does not change length of stay or mortality [9].

Early tracheostomy should be performed to reduce mechanical ventilation days. However, it does not alter mortality or the rate of nosocomial pneumonia [9].
Level III – Routine ventricular catheter exchange or prophylactic antibiotic use for ventricular catheter placement is not recommended to reduce infection [9].
Early extubation in qualified patients can be done without increased risk of pneumonia [9].

TBI patients have an increased incidence of infections given aspiration of secretions and vomitus while unconscious, mechanical ventilation, and other invasive aspects of patient monitoring and treatment.

One possible source of infection is the insertion of ICP devices. The incidence of ICP device infection can range from less than 1–27 % [25]. Even with these striking infection rates, there are conflicting data concerning the appropriate prophylactic measures. Most studies cited by the 2007 guidelines have shown no difference in infection rates with or without prophylactic antibiotics in patients with external ventricular drainage (EVD) catheters. Additionally, one study showed that patients receiving bacitracin flushes experienced a significantly higher infection rate than those without prophylactic measures [24]. Routine change of ventriculostomy catheters has also been shown to increase rates of infection. Antibiotic impregnated catheters have been used over the past years with some evidence for a decreased incidence of gram-positive bacterial infections, but solid randomized trials have not been done. Pre insertion single dose antibiotics have been used in some hospital protocols to prevent catheter related infections. Good clinical practice protocols exist regarding ventriculostomy management to reduce rates of infection. These include early removal, sterile insertion technique, routine site cleaning and maintenance, and minimizing access to the CSF drainage system via elimination of surveillance cultures to avoid contaminating the system.

Prophylactic antibiotic use in patients with TBI has not resulted in a meaningful reduction of nosocomial infections [24]. In addition, an increase in serious gram-negative infections was noted in this population. The guidelines also cite data showing an increase in resistant or gram-negative bacterial nosocomial pneumonias, observed after the administration of prophylactic antibiotics for longer than 48 h in general trauma patients. In contrast, one study showed a decrease in the incidence of pneumonia when prophylactic antibiotics were given to patients with TBI. No difference in mortality was noted [24]. More evidence is expected regarding the benefit of early tracheostomy to decrease ventilator days. However, early tracheostomy did not reduce ventilator associated pneumonia or mortality. Currently, there is no evidence to support early tracheostomy in TBI patients.

Since the publication of the 2007 guidelines, one further study in patients with TBI has been completed [25]. This study retrospectively evaluated the use of antibiotic prophylaxis in patients with ICP monitors. Of the 155 patients included in the analysis, only two developed central nervous system (CNS) infections, both in the group that received prophylactic antibiotics. Additionally, complications from infections and multidrug resistant bacterial infections were significantly increased in the prophylactically treated group.

In summary, there are currently no convincing data to support infection prophylaxis with antibiotics in patients with TBI [24, 25].

Deep Vein Thrombosis Prophylaxis

The recommendations from BTF were the following:

Level III – Graduated compression stockings or intermittent pneumatic compression (IPC) stockings are recommended, unless lower extremity injuries prevent their use. Use should be continued until patients are ambulatory [9].
Low-molecular-weight heparin (LMWH) or low dose unfractionated heparin should be used in combination with mechanical prophylaxis. However, there is an increased risk for expansion of intracranial hemorrhage [9].
There is insufficient evidence to support recommendations regarding the preferred agent, dose, or timing of pharmacologic prophylaxis for deep vein thrombosis (DVT) [9].

Patients who are comatose, those being maintained on neuromuscular blocking agents, and those with pelvic or long-bone fractures are at high risk for deep venous thrombosis and pulmonary embolism. They should receive early prophylaxis, which typically includes the use of lower extremity sequential compression devices as well as subcutaneous heparin or LMWH. The early (2–3 days after injury) use of unfractionated heparin (5,000 units subcutaneous every 8 h) or low-molecular-weight heparin (enoxaparin 30 mg subcutaneous every 12 h or 40 mg subcutaneous once daily) is safe and has not been found to cause or worsen intracranial hemorrhage after TBI [26, 27]. However it is important to obtain a CT scan demonstrating stability prior to initiation of pharmacologic prophylaxis to avoid expansion of intracranial hemorrhages [28].

Indications for Intracranial Pressure Monitoring

The recommendations from BTF were the following:

Level II – Intracranial pressure (ICP) should be monitored in all salvageable patients with a severe traumatic brain injury (TBI; Glasgow Coma Scale [GCS] score of 3–8 after resuscitation) and an abnormal computed tomography (CT) scan. An abnormal CT scan of the head is one that reveals hematomas, contusions, swelling, herniation, or compressed basal cisterns [9].
Level III – ICP monitoring is indicated in patients with severe TBI with a normal CT scan if two or more of the following features are noted at admission: age over 40 years, unilateral or bilateral motor posturing, or systolic blood pressure (SBP)<90 mmHg [29].

Intracranial pressure (ICP) monitoring and management is one of the most controversial issues in TBI. Practice of TBI management worldwide has differed greatly between countries in that regard. In developed countries there is a trend toward routine placement of ICP monitors in severe TBI patients. In developing countries the trend is much less given the cost, lack of technology, and manpower.

It is well reported and documented that intracranial hypertension is strongly associated with high mortality and morbidity. According to BTF guidelines continuous ICP monitoring is considered essential for all patients who have severe TBI and abnormal CT findings, because intracranial hypertension develops in 53–63 % of such patients [30].

Controversies surrounding threshold of detrimental ICP, methods of measurement and methods of treatment do exist. However, the main controversy is that ICP guided treatment protocols trials have shown mixed results in outcomes of patients with TBI in various trials. A recent randomized trial, the BEST TRIP trial, showed no difference in outcomes between patient groups randomized to either ICP guided management protocols versus frequent radiological scanning and clinically guided protocols [31]. This trial was conducted in Bolivia and Ecuador, although funded by the USA NIH (NINDS). Therefore, the study had good internal validity, but not external validity. Concerns regarding prehospital care and posthospital care were raised [31, 32].

The controversies surrounding ICP measurement were addressed in the International Multidisciplinary Consensus Conference on Multimodality Monitoring in 2014 to create a consensus statement for healthcare professionals from the Neurocritical Care Society and the European Society of Intensive Care Medicine [33]. Measurement of ICP was considered as follows:

1. ICP and CPP monitoring are recommended as a part of protocol-driven care in patients who are at risk of elevated intracranial pressure based on clinical and/or imaging features. (Strong recommendation, moderate quality of evidence.)
2. We recommend that ICP and CPP monitoring be used to guide medical and surgical interventions and to detect life-threatening imminent herniation; however, the threshold value of ICP is uncertain on the basis of the literature. (Strong recommendation, high quality of evidence.)
3. We recommend that the indications and method for ICP monitoring should be tailored to the specific diagnosis (e.g., SAH, TBI, encephalitis). (Strong recommendation, low quality of evidence.)
4. While other intracranial monitors can provide useful information, we recommend that ICP monitoring be used as a prerequisite to allow interpretation of data provided by these other devices. (Strong recommendation, moderate quality of evidence.)
5. We recommend the use of standard insertion and maintenance protocols to ensure safety and reliability of the ICP monitoring procedure. (Strong recommendation, high quality of evidence.)
6. Both parenchymal ICP monitors and external ventricular catheters (EVD) catheters provide reliable and accurate data and are the recommended devices to measure ICP. In the presence of hydrocephalus, use of an EVD when safe and practical is preferred to parenchymal monitoring. (Strong recommendation, high quality of evidence.)

7. We recommend the continuous assessment and monitoring of ICP and CPP including waveform quality using a structured protocol to ensure accuracy and reliability. Instantaneous ICP values should be interpreted in the context of monitoring trends, CPP, and clinical evaluation. (Strong recommendation, high quality of evidence.)
8. While refractory ICP elevation is a strong predictor of mortality, ICP per se does not provide a useful prognostic marker of functional outcome; therefore, we recommend that ICP not be used in isolation as a prognostic marker. (Strong recommendation, high quality of evidence) [33].

In summary, it is the conclusion of this author based on all of the above guidelines and literature that ICP monitoring should still be used as a standard essential method of monitoring and management of patients with severe TBI requiring ICU care.

Intracranial Pressure Monitoring Technology

In the current state of technology, the ventricular catheter connected to an external strain gauge is the most accurate, low-cost, and reliable method of monitoring intracranial pressure (ICP). It also can be recalibrated in situ [34]. ICP transduction via fiberoptic or micro strain gauge devices placed in ventricular catheters provide similar benefits, but at a higher cost. Parenchymal ICP monitors cannot be recalibrated during monitoring. Parenchymal ICP monitors, using micro strain pressure transducers, have negligible drift. The measurement drift is independent of the duration of monitoring. Subarachnoid, subdural, and epidural monitors (fluid coupled or pneumatic) are less accurate.

The overall complication rate for ventricular ICP monitoring is 7.7 % (infection, 6.3 %; hemorrhage, 1.4 %), [63] and some studies indicate that the infection rate increases significantly when a catheter remains in place for more than 5 days [35].

Intracranial Pressure Thresholds

The recommendations from BTF were the following:

Level II – Treatment should be initiated with intracranial pressure (ICP) thresholds above 20 mmHg [9].
Level III – A combination of ICP values, and clinical and brain CT findings, should be used to determine the need for treatment [9].

Intracranial hypertension is defined as sustained ICP greater than 20 mmHg. Several clinical studies have found that mortality and morbidity increase significantly when the ICP persistently remains above this threshold [35].

Based on this association and the widely accepted premise that elevated ICP can compromise cerebral perfusion and cause ischemia, the aggressive treatment of intracranial hypertension is almost uniformly endorsed. Before beginning therapy for intracranial hypertension, however, medical or physiologic conditions that can increase

ICP should be considered and treated, if present. These include seizures, fever, jugular venous outflow obstruction (e.g., poorly fitting cervical collars), and agitation.

Several medical and surgical options are available to reduce ICP. Depending on the type of brain injury, some may be more effective than others, and each is associated with potential adverse effects. A stepwise approach is usually followed, with the least toxic therapies utilized first and more toxic therapies added only if the initial treatment is unsuccessful. Sedation and neuromuscular blockade are often an effective first treatment, particularly if the patient is agitated or posturing. Narcotics (e.g., morphine, fentanyl), short-acting benzodiazepines (e.g., midazolam), or hypnotic agents such as propofol can be used for sedation, and vecuronium bromide as the paralytic agent. Narcotic-induced hypotension can be averted by using relatively low doses and ensuring the patient is normovolemic before treatment. Because the ability to obtain an accurate GCS score is lost during this treatment, the pupillary reaction, ICP, and CT scans should be monitored closely.

If intracranial hypertension is refractory to sedation and neuromuscular blockade, ventricular CSF drainage is used via ventriculostomy.

If these measures fail to reduce the ICP, a bolus administration of mannitol is recommended (0.25–1 g/kg every 3–6 h as needed) [36]. Bolus or continuous infusions are utilized. Infusions of hypertonic saline for a target serum sodium 8–12 mEq above baseline or roughly serum sodium of 150–155 mEq/L are an effective alternative to mannitol [37].

If despite these measures the ICP remains above 20 mmHg, the ventilator rate can be adjusted to reduce the arterial pCO_2 to 30 mmHg. Hyperventilation should be used cautiously during the first 24–48 h after injury, it causes cerebral vasoconstriction at a time when CBF is already critically reduced. Evidence also suggests that even brief periods of hyperventilation can lead to secondary brain injury by causing an increase in extracellular lactate and glutamate levels [38]. Prophylactic hyperventilation is always contraindicated in the absence of elevated ICP [39].

If hyperventilation is used, the brain tissue oxygenation ($pbtO_2$) or jugular venous oxygen saturation should be monitored to detect cerebral hypoxia. The risk of tissue ischemia and poor outcome may increase if the brain tissue $PbtO_2$ falls below 10 mmHg [40].

If intracranial hypertension persists despite all these treatments, particularly if the ICP rises rapidly or if the patient's initial CT scan showed a small contusion or hematoma, another CT scan should be obtained immediately to determine whether there is a new mass lesion or a preexisting lesion has enlarged. Even if the lesion has enlarged only slightly, an emergent craniotomy and evacuation of the contusion or hematoma may be the most effective way to reduce the mass effect.

If the CT scan does not reveal an intracranial mass lesion requiring surgery, the next recommended treatment for intracranial hypertension is high-dose barbiturates. Barbiturates are thought to be effective by reducing cerebral metabolic demand and blood flow, and preclinical studies suggest significant cerebral protective effects [41]. Pentobarbital is the most commonly used drug for this purpose and is administered as an IV loading dose of 10–15 mg/kg over 1–2 h (thiopental 1.5–7 mg/kg), followed by a maintenance infusion of 1–2 mg/kg per hour. The dose can be increased until intracranial hypertension subsides or MAP begins to fall. Continuous electroencephalography (EEG) monitoring is recommended while increasing the dose until a burst suppression pattern is observed. Hypotension, the most common adverse effect of barbiturates, can usually be averted by ensuring a normal intravascular volume before administering the drug.

Only a few options remain when intracranial hypertension is recalcitrant to all these measures, and they are controversial and not uniformly embraced. Therapeutic moderate hypothermia has been used in several clinical trials over the past decade. They have consistently shown that hypothermia significantly reduces ICP and does not cause significant medical complications when used for no longer than 48 h [42, 43].

Some advocate the use of decompressive craniectomy, such as large lateral or bifrontal bone flaps, with or without a generous temporal or frontal lobectomy. In one study of patients with severe TBI, 6-month outcomes were similar for a group that had large decompressive craniectomy and a group that did not, even though the craniectomy group had lower initial GCS scores and more severe radiographic injuries [44]. Importantly, the craniectomy group did not have a higher incidence of persistent vegetative state. Two studies reported good outcomes in 56–58 % of patients whose refractory intracranial hypertension was treated with decompressive craniectomy as a last resort [45, 46]. Another study suggested that decompressive craniectomy with temporal lobectomy, when performed soon after injury, improves the outcome for young patients [47]. However, others found that decompressive craniectomy does not improve ICP, CPP, or mortality rates [48]. The most recent trial, the DECRA trial, concluded after studying 155 TBI patients that early bifrontotemporoparietal decompressive craniectomy decreased the ICP and length of stay in the ICU but was associated with more unfavorable outcomes. This trial was heavily criticized for its selection bias in the surgical group as well as its surgical technique choice [49]. The RescueICP trial from Cambridge group, UK, finished recruiting 400 patients in May 2014 and the analysis is still ongoing. Results are expected in early 2015.

Cerebral Perfusion Thresholds

The recommendations from BTF were the following:

Level II – Aggressive attempts to maintain cerebral perfusion pressure (CPP) above 70 mmHg with fluids and pressors should be avoided because of the risk of adult respiratory distress syndrome (ARDS) [9].
Level III – CPP less than 50 mmHg should be avoided [9].
The CPP value to target lies within the range of 50–70 mmHg. Patients with intact pressure autoregulation tolerate higher CPP values. Ancillary monitoring of cerebral parameters that include blood flow, oxygenation, or metabolism facilitates CPP management [9].

The cerebral perfusion pressure (CPP), defined as the difference between MAP and ICP, is a calculated physiologic measurement that is used to describe actual cerebral perfusion. It was suggested that maintaining the CPP above a certain threshold is more important than any particular MAP or ICP [50]. Most TBI center and Neurocritical care unit protocols target CPP >60 mmHg (median between 50 and 70 mmHg). Patients with CPP values <50 mmHg were shown to have poor outcomes with evidence of secondary hypoxic ischemic brain damage. There are some points of controversy. (1) It is unclear if the MAP measured at right atrial zero point is same as the MAP inside cerebral circulation. Gravitationally the intracranial MAP should be lower in the sitting position and the same in flat position. This would mean lower perfusion pressure if MAP is measured with the zero point at the level of the right atrium. To solve this conflict, some TBI centers zero the arterial line to the same zero point for ICP (tragus of the ear corresponding to foramen of Monro). There is no clinical evidence available to prove one point versus the other [51]. (2) Another point of controversy is whether delivering blood under perfusion pressure is the main factor in brain oxygen delivery. Other factors like presence or absence of cerebral autoregulation and oncotic pressure, hemoglobin content, oxygen saturation additionally control adequate cerebral oxygen delivery which is the ultimate goal in management of brain injury to meet cerebral metabolic demand and to prevent further cerebral tissue hypoxia, resulting in cortical laminar necrosis and long white matter tract demyelination. (3) The final and most sophisticated point is whether CPP should be kept at a static point of >60 mmHg or be regarded as a dynamic value. Lately, research mainly from Cambridge, UK, was directed to finding the optimum CPP value (CPP optimum) at certain points of time. This is based on gauging cerebral autoregulation through reactivity of ICP to changes in blood pressure. A software has been developed with retrospective analysis of CPP and cerebral reactivity. No major clinical trials have been conducted to prove the clinical value [52].

In summary, CPP can serve as one of the surrogate markers of cerebral perfusion and optimizing that to values >60 mmHg mm Hg might be reasonable in management of patients with TBI till more evidence is available.

Brain Oxygen Monitoring and Thresholds

The recommendations from BTF were the following:

Level III – Jugular venous saturation (>50 %) or brain tissue oxygen tension (>15 mmHg) are treatment thresholds. Jugular venous saturation or brain tissue oxygen monitoring measure cerebral oxygenation [9].

Several studies have found that direct brain tissue pbtO$_2$ monitoring may be an ideal complement to ICP monitoring in TBI treatment [53–59]. Brain partial pressure of O$_2$ values between 30 and 50 mmHg are regarded as normal, whereas reductions to less than 10 or 15 mmHg are associated with hypoxia. In particular, a significant relationship between poor outcome and cerebral hypoxia has been consistently observed: the number, duration, and intensity of cerebral hypoxia episodes (brain tissue $pbtO_2$, 15 mmHg) and any brain tissue $pbtO_2$ values less than 6 mmHg [60–63] are associated with worse patient outcome. Consistent with these results, prolonged systemic hypoxia following TBI is also associated with worse clinical outcomes [64]. There are many factors that influence brain tissue $pbtO_2$, some of which are not detected by an ICP monitor. Furthermore, a direct relationship between CPP and $pbtO_2$ is not observed in every patient, in large part because autoregulation frequently is disturbed (see above) [65]. Results from recent studies have also demonstrated that an increase in brain tissue $pbtO_2$ is associated with improved cerebral metabolism [66]. Therefore, it is reasonable to assume that the use of a brain tissue PO_2 monitor and efforts to increase brain O_2 delivery may improve TBI outcome.

There is mixed literature about the outcomes of brain tissue oxygen guided treatment protocols in patients with TBI. Most literature is retrospective, nonrandomized, or inadequately powered (<200 patients). However, a larger randomized prospective controlled phase III trial of protocolled utilization brain tissue oxygen monitoring in management of severe TBI is underway, named BOOST.

In summary, brain tissue oxygen monitoring might be a useful tool to guide therapy in the context of adjusting other cerebral variables within a management protocol.

Anesthetics, Analgesics, and Sedatives

The recommendations from BTF were the following:

Level II – Prophylactic administration of barbiturates to induce burst suppression EEG is not recommended [9].
High-dose barbiturate administration is recommended to control elevated ICP refractory to maximum standard medical and surgical treatment. Hemodynamic stability is essential before and during barbiturate therapy [9].
Propofol is recommended for the control of ICP, but not for improvement in mortality or 6 month outcome. High-dose propofol can produce significant morbidity [9].

Head-injured patients are severely stressed with a markedly raised concentration of plasma catecholamines. To avoid stress-induced increase in ICP and release of catecholamines, patients are sedated with various combinations of drugs.

Benzodiazepines are commonly used, e.g., midazolam, lorazepam as boluses or more commonly as infusions. They serve the purpose of sedation and seizure prophylaxis, anxiolysis, treatment of alcohol withdrawal symptoms. Midazolam is more commonly used as a shorter acting agent. Attention should be paid in patients with liver disease or injury as benzodiazepines can remain in the system for a longer duration of time and impair validity of neurological examination.

Narcotics are used as analgesic agents in patients with TBI. Short-acting agents like fentanyl and remifentanyl are used to interrupt sedation for neurological examination within a brief period of its discontinuation. There were few reports in the past of occasional increases in ICP with narcotics.

Propofol is one of the most commonly used agents for sedation in TBI patients. It has a very short half-life and is administered in a white lipid solution. It induces burst suppression thus reducing cerebral metabolic demand and intracranial pressure. It is a powerful vasodilator and can cause severe hypotension. Prolonged use >48 h, concomitant use with catecholamines and high doses >80 mcg/kg in small muscle mass patients can be associated with the propofol infusion syndrome. This syndrome is characterized by rhabdomyolysis, lactic acidosis, hypertriglyceridemia and cardiac arrhythmias including asystole. It has a high fatality rate and best treatment is prevention by stopping propofol infusions after a short period of time.

A new agent, dexmedetomidine is becoming popular for sedation in the ICU. It is an alpha 2 agonist leading to a central decrease in catecholamine release similar to clonidine. It is administered as an intravenous infusion. It is associated with bradycardia and hypotension, but does not cause respiratory depression.

Barbiturates were used in past for sedation and treatment of alcohol withdrawal, but they fell out of favor because of their potent cardiac suppressor effect and long duration of action in the face of newer drugs. This sedative is now mostly reserved for patients with refractory intracranial hypertension with or without the use of decompressive hemicraniectomy. Patients on barbiturates enter a phase of burst suppression and they usually loose all neurological reflexes including pupillary exam. Side effects include hypotension, ileus, and occasionally hypothermia [41, 67].

Nutrition

The recommendations from BTF were the following:

Level II – Patients should be fed to attain full caloric replacement by day 7 post-injury [9].

Malnutrition is common after severe TBI. The resting metabolic expenditure typically increases by 140 % in a nonparalyzed patient with severe TBI [68]. Branched-chain amino acids from muscle protein are used preferentially for energy metabolism, potentially compromising the effectiveness of physical therapy. Nitrogen wasting is also increased, with excretion of as much as 9–12 g/day. Thus, early enteral or parenteral feeding is advisable, with the aim of providing at least 140 % of the daily basal metabolic caloric requirements by the third or fourth day after injury [69].

A normal-sized adult patient usually needs 25–30 kcal/kg/day. Because parenteral feeding increases the risk of infection, continuous enteral administration is preferable. For a patient expected to be in a prolonged coma, a percutaneous gastrostomy or surgical jejunostomy provides a convenient and well-tolerated route to administer tube feeding. Hyperglycemia is associated with TBI, with prolonged hospital stay and with increased mortality [70, 71].

Aggressive management of hyperglycemia has been shown to decrease complications and improve long-term outcome, but the optimal blood glucose range in patients with severe TBI remains controversial. Tight glucose control may be problematic [72].

However, a recent paper analyzed all articles addressing nutrition in severe TBI. There is inconsistency within the nutrition intervention methods and outcome measures which means that the present evidence base is inadequate for the construction of best practice guidelines for nutrition in TBI [73].

Antiseizure Prophylaxis

The recommendations from BTF were the following:

Level II – Prophylactic use of phenytoin or valproate is not recommended for preventing late posttraumatic seizures (PTS). Anticonvulsants are indicated to decrease the incidence of early PTS (within 7 days of injury). However, early PTS is not associated with worse outcomes [9].

Seizures are common post-TBI occurring in approximately 50 % of patients 15 years after a penetrating injury. Post-traumatic seizures may be classified as early (<1 week post-injury) or late (>1 week post-injury), with an incidence of 4–25 % and 9–42 %, respectively, in untreated patients [74–76]. There are numerous factors which put patients at increased risk for post-traumatic seizures, including: GCS < 9, cortical contusion, depressed skull fracture, subdural or epidural hematoma, intracerebral hematoma, penetrating head wounds, and seizures within 24 h of injury [77, 78]. Besides acute therapy for first 7 days, there is a relative paucity in evidence to continue pharmacological prophylaxis post-TBI.

Phenytoin (PHT) or valproate (VPA) (loading dose 15–20 mg/kg for either then maintenance dose 2–3 times daily) is the most commonly used drugs to prevent early seizures but not late seizures. Chronic use is associated with numerous side effects [79]. PHT is most widely used and tested and is available in intravenous and oral formulations, serum levels that can be measured. Side effects include hepatotoxicity, rash, fever, and thrombocytopenia. VPA has been studied for early seizures demonstrating a trend toward favorable outcomes with VPA therapy but the study was not adequately powered to detect a significant change [80]. A phase III study sponsored by the USA NINDS evaluating VPA against PHT for seizures post-TBI was recently completed, but the results not yet released. VPA has a similar side effect profile compared to PHT.

Levetiracetam (LEV) is an anticonvulsant which binds synaptic vesicle glycoprotein 2A (SV2A) and likely inhibits presynaptic Ca2+ channels [81, 82]. In basic science work, intraperitoneal LEV given daily to rats which suffered TBI led to improved motor function, reduced hippocampal cell loss, decreased contusion volumes, and reduced IL-1β expression [83]. Clinically, a recent phase II trial among 20 pediatric cases of TBI considered LEV as a feasible option to prevent seizures in high-risk patients because of its safety and lack of adverse events [84]. Additional studies would have to compare LEV to PHT, the current standard prophylaxis. A meta-analysis revealed equal efficacy between PHT and LEV; the authors suggested further high quality RCTs be completed before conclusions are drawn [85]. Trials involving EEG to compare outcome after pharmacologic prophylaxis with PHT or LEV demonstrated that epileptiform activity and discharges were not predictive of outcome in either group after TBI [86]. In a retrospective observational study comparing PHT and LEV in 109 patients (89 receiving PHT and 20 on LEV), only one patient in each group suffered a post-traumatic seizure with a trend favoring LEV for its better side effect profile [87]. Interestingly, anticonvulsant therapy was continued past 7 days in that study, discordant with the present guidelines. IV administration of LEV and PHT in a prospective, randomized trial showed an association of LEV with improved long-term outcomes based on the Disability Rating Score and GOS but without an effect on seizure occurrence compared to PHT [87, 88]. Another prospective multicenter comparison of PHT and LEV for early seizure prophylaxis found no significant improvement in outcomes when LEV was administered [89]. Most studies have examined the effect of LEV vs. PHT in early but not late seizure prophylaxis. The literature is in disagreement concerning the efficacy of LEV as a first-line treatment. Yet, LEV is appealing as a first option because it does not require serum monitoring, which PHT demands owing to its nonlinear metabolism. Moreover, LEV does not affect the enzyme cytochrome P450 leading to numerous drug interactions. However, major side effects of LEV are agitation and psychosis, especially in patients with previous history of psychiatric illness or elderly people. Thus, it is unsuitable to use in patients with agitation, delirium, or alcohol withdrawal.

Other anti-epileptics such as phenobarbital (PHB) and carbamazepine (CBZ) are generally avoided because of adverse effects (sedation for PHB and hyponatremia for CBZ) and of their pharmacodynamic profile (CBZ is administered orally) [90]. Topiramate is currently being studied in the PEPTO trial in comparison with PHT for prevention of epilepsy after TBI.

Hyperventilation

The recommendations from BTF were the following:

Level II – Prophylactic hyperventilation (pCO_2 of 25 mmHg or less) is not recommended [9].

Level III – Hyperventilation is recommended as a temporizing measure for the reduction of elevated intracranial pressure (ICP) [9].

Hyperventilation should be avoided during the first 24 h after injury when cerebral blood flow (CBF) is often critically reduced. If hyperventilation is used, jugular venous oxygen saturation (SjO_2) or brain tissue oxygen tension ($pbtO_2$) measurements are recommended to monitor oxygen delivery [9].

Carbon dioxide dilates the cerebral blood vessels, increasing the volume of blood in the intracranial vault and therefore increasing ICP. Patients should be ventilated to normocapnia ($PaCO_2$ 35–45 mmHg). Transcranial Doppler (TCD) assessment and positron emission tomography (PET) confirmed that hyperventilation induces significant constriction of cerebral vessels along with a reduction of cerebral blood flow below the ischemic threshold. One study has shown an improvement in long-term outcome when hyperventilation is not used routinely [38].

Consequently, hyperventilation should be used only for short periods when immediate control of ICP is necessary. An example is the patient who has an acute neurological deterioration (dilated fixed pupil) prior to CT scanning and surgical intervention [38, 39].

Hyperventilation should not be used in the first 24 h (ischemic phase of TBI) and preferably avoided during active ischemia of the brain tissue [40].

Steroids

The recommendations from BTF were the following:

A. Level I – The use of steroids is not recommended for improving outcome or reducing intracranial pressure (ICP). In patients with moderate or severe traumatic brain injury (TBI), high-dose Methylprednisolone is associated with increased mortality and is contraindicated [9].

In the past there have been multiple trials and papers addressing the use of steroids in TBI. Finally the CRASH (Corticosteroid Randomization After Significant Head Injury) trial collaborators reported the results of 10,008 patients with TBI (GCS < 15) randomized to 2 g IV Methylprednisolone followed by 0.4 mg/h for 48 h or placebo. The study was stopped for the deleterious effect of methylprednisolone: the 2-week mortality in the steroid group was 21 % versus 18 % in controls, with a 1.18 relative risk of death in the steroid group (95 % CI 1.09–1.27, $p=0.0001$) [91].

Other Issues

Tiered Management of ICP

Tier 0

- Head of bed up (30–60°)
- Avoid tight neck collar
- Avoid jugular central lines
- Control fever
- PaCO$_2$ target: 35–40 mmHg
- Control pain and sedate if necessary
- Treat alcohol withdrawal
- Maintain CSF drainage if ventriculostomy is in place

Tier 1

- Short-term hyperventilation (<30 min)
- Mannitol: 1 g/kg body weight should be administered. Repeat dosing of 0.25–1 g every 4–6 h can be done, however, attention must be placed upon maintaining an euvolemic state when osmotic diuresis is instituted with Mannitol. The serum sodium and osmolality must be assessed frequently (every 6 h) and additional doses should be held if the osmolar gap >20 to avoid renal damage. Mannitol should be held if there is evidence of hypovolemia, renal failure or need for vasopressors.
- Hypertonic Saline: boluses of 3 % sodium chloride solution may be used. Hypertonic NaCl infusions can be used to raise serum sodium 8–12 mEq > baseline (Targeting sodium 150–155 mEq/L, serum osmolarity 310–325 mosmol/L). Serum sodium and osmolality must be assessed frequently (every 6 h) and additional doses should be held if the serum sodium exceeds 160 mEq/L or serum osm >330 mosmol/L. If hyperchloremia is present, mixed solutions with sodium bicarbonate or acetate can be used.
- Drain additional amount of CSF from ventriculostomy if present and open if clamped.

Tier 2

- Repeat CT and perform craniotomy for enlarging hematomas
- Propofol drip titrated to take the patient to low levels of sedation scales (5–75 mcg/kg/min)
- CPP optimization

Tier 3

- Decompressive craniectomy
- Paralytics
- Induced hypothermia
- Pentobarbiturate/thiopental coma

Neuroprotective Therapy of TBI

To date, no neuroprotective agents or strategies (including induced hypothermia) have been shown to result in improved outcome [92].

Intravenous Progesterone

Based on two positive phase II studies, *intravenous progesterone* was being tested in two pivotal phase III clinical trials as a neuroprotective agent for severe head injury [93, 94]. The PROTECT trial was a multicenter NIH funded randomized controlled double blinded trial that randomized patients with traumatic brain injury to placebo versus progesterone infusion for 72 h starting within 3 h of injury. The trial had a clinical standardized treatment protocol to address all other physiologic variables controlling outcomes in TBI. The trial was placed on hold and terminated in early 2014 for futility reasons, i.e., there was no difference between the treatment and placebo group on interim analysis. The formal results are not yet published. Early results from SYNAPSE trial which addressed a proprietary pharmaceutical progesterone formulation show similar futile effects.

Other agents being investigated include magnesium [95], hyperbaric oxygen [96], cerebrolysin (The CAPTAIN trial), piracetam, and cyclosporine [97] among others [98]. Citicoline was not found to be effective in improving outcomes in a randomized trial of 1,213 patients with TBI [99].

Erythropoietin

Erythropoietin has been postulated to have neuroprotective effects. In a retrospective case control study of 267 patients with severe TBI, matched for both GCS and severity of systemic injuries, in-hospital mortality was lower among 89 patients treated with erythropoietin compared with 178 control patients (8 versus 24 %) [100]. However, a recent randomized clinical trial showed no difference in neurologic outcomes at 6 months in 200 patients with closed head injury [101].

Hyperbaric Oxygen Therapy (HBOT)

Hyperbaric oxygen therapy (HBOT) is another intervention used in early prophylactic treatment of TBI. HBOT encompasses the inhalation of 100 % oxygen at environmental pressures above one atmosphere. Dysregulation of CBF produces an oxygen deficit causing metabolic modifications and ischemia. By increasing the partial pressure of oxygen in blood, independent of that bound to hemoglobin in erythrocytes, HBOT increases oxygen saturation reaching the brain which may potentially decrease tissue damage secondary to ischemia and hypoxia [102]. Yet, since most oxygen is hemoglobin-bound, HBOT-mediated O_2 saturation increase is limited to up to 10 %; a clinically significant amount in many cases. A small trial showed that treatment with 100 % oxygen for 6 h reduced lactate and increased brain tissue oxygenation [103]. More extensive evidence from an early systematic review deemed HBOT's therapeutic benefit inconclusive [104]. Yet, a recent retrospective study found TBI patients treated with HBOT to have improved outcomes when compared to control counterparts [105]. Additionally, prospective studies administering HBOT after patients' conditions stabilized also demonstrated improved outcomes based on GCS and GOS [106]. One large clinical trial examined the efficacy of HBOT followed by normobaric hyperoxia (NBH) treatment for 3 days and found the treatment group to have reductions in ICP, mortality, and cerebral toxicity with improved favorable GOS outcomes [107].

Dos and Don'ts

Dos

- Transfer to trauma center where imaging and neurosurgical capabilities are available.
- Keep SBP >90 mmHg.
- Keep oxygen saturations >90 %.
- Intubate if GCS <9.
- Keep PaO_2 around 100 mmHg.
- Place ICP monitor (if available) if patient's GCS < 9 with abnormal CT or GCS <9 with normal CT if 2 of following are present: age >40, posturing, hypotension. If ICP monitoring is not available then perform frequent imaging of the head in conjunction with frequent neurological examinations if any change of patient's condition occurs.
- Treat intracranial hypertension aggressively using stepwise overlapping approach to prevent any delay of treatment.
- Apply mechanical DVT prophylaxis as soon as the patient arrives in the ICU and start on pharmacological DVT prophylaxis within 48–72 h given hemorrhage size is stable on CT scan and the patient is stable neurologically.
- Use sedation and analgesia concomitantly to for patient's comfort and minimize intracranial hypertension.
- Correct hyponatremia.
- Maintain normothermia.
- Early nutrition.
- Moderate glycemic control.
- Apply seizure prophylaxis for 7 days post injury.

Don'ts

- Apply tight neck collar
- Put head of bed flat

- Block internal jugular flow by big vascular access catheters that can promote jugular thrombosis
- Allow persistent hypotension
- Allow persistent hypoxemia
- Allow persistent fever
- Allow persistent intracranial hypertension
- Use mannitol if hypotensive or in acute kidney injury or on pressors
- Use steroids
- Use empiric antibiotics without evidence of infection
- Use prolonged or prophylactic hyperventilation
- Use prolonged sedation or paralytics that can eliminate your neurological examination

References

1. Faul MXL, Wald MM, Coronado VG. Traumatic Brain Injury in the United States: Emergency Department Visits, Hospitalizations, and Deaths. Atlanta: Centers for Disease Control and Prevention, National Center for Injury Prevention and Control; 2010.
2. Rutland-Brown W, Langlois JA, Thomas KA, Yongli LX. Incidence of traumatic brain injury in the United States, 2003. J Head Trauma Rehabil. 2006;21:544–8.
3. Lu J, Marmarou A, Choi S, Maas A, Murray G, Steyerberg EW. Mortality from traumatic brain injury. Acta Neurochir Suppl. 2005;95:281–5.
4. Ghajar J, Hariri RJ, Narayan RK, Iacono LA, Firlik K, Patterson RH. Survey of critical care management of comatose, head-injured patients in the United States. Crit Care Med. 1995;23:560–7.
5. Hesdorffer DC, Ghajar J, Iacono L. Predictors of compliance with the evidence-based guidelines for traumatic brain injury care: a survey of United States trauma centers. J Trauma. 2002;52:1202–9.
6. Zaloshnja E, Miller T, Langlois JA, Selassie AW. Prevalence of long-term disability from traumatic brain injury in the civilian population of the United States, 2005. J Head Trauma Rehabil. 2008;23:394–400.
7. Finkelstein E, Corso P, Miller T. The incidence and economic burden of injuries in the United States. J Epidemiol Community Health. 2007;61(10):926.
8. Haas B, Jurkovich GJ, Wang J, Rivara FP, Mackenzie EJ, Nathens AB. Survival advantage in trauma centers: expeditious intervention or experience? J Am Coll Surg. 2009;208:28–36.
9. Brain Trauma Foundation; American Association of Neurological Surgeons; Congress of Neurological Surgeons. Guidelines for the management of severe traumatic brain injury. J Neurotrauma. 2007;24 Suppl 1:S1–95.
10. Chesnut RM, Marshall LF, Klauber MR, et al. The role of secondary brain injury in determining outcome from severe head injury. J Trauma. 1993;34:216–22.
11. Fearnside MR, Cook RJ, McDougall P, et al. The Westmead Head Injury Project outcome in severe head injury: a comparative analysis of pre-hospital, clinical and CT variables. Br J Neurosurg. 1993;7:267–79.
12. Johnston J, Steiner L, Chatfield D, et al. Effect of cerebral perfusion pressure augmentation with dopamine and norepinephrine on global and focal brain oxygenation after traumatic brain injury. Intensive Care Med. 2004;30:791–7.
13. Eskandari R, Filtz MR, Davis GE, Hoesch RE. Effective treatment of refractory intracranial hypertension after traumatic brain injury with repeated boluses of 14.6% hypertonic saline. J Neurosurg. 2013;119:338–46.

14. Oddo M, Levine JM, Frangos S, Carrera E, Maloney-Wilensky E, Pascual JL, Kofke WA, Mayer SA, LeRoux PD. Effect of mannitol and hypertonic saline on cerebral oxygenation in patients with severe traumatic brain injury and refractory intracranial hypertension. J Neurol Neurosurg Psychiatry. 2009;80:916–20.
15. Scalfani MT, Dhar R, Zazulia AR, Videen TO, Diringer MN. Effect of osmotic agent on regional cerebral blood flow in traumatic brain injury. J Crit Care. 2012;526:e7–12.
16. Cottenceau V, Masson F, Mahamid E, Petit L, Shik V, Sztark F, Zaaroor M, Soustiel JF. Comparison of effects of equiosmolar doses of mannitol and hypertonic saline on cerebral blood flow and metabolism in traumatic brain injury. J Neurotrauma. 2011;28:2003–12.
17. Soukup J, Zauner A, Doppenberg EM, Menzel M, Gilman C, Bullock R, Young HF. Relationship between brain temperature, brain chemistry and oxygen delivery after severe human head injury: the effect of mild hypothermia. Neurol Res. 2002;24:161–8.
18. Bukur M, Kurtovic S, Berry C, Tanios M, Ley EJ, Salim A. Pre-hospital hypothermia is not associated with increased survival after traumatic brain injury. J Surg Res. 2012;175:24–9.
19. Rubiano AM, Sanchez AI, Estebanez G, Peitzman A, Sperry J, Puyana JC. The effect of admission spontaneous hypothermia on patients with severe traumatic brain injury. Injury. 2013;44:1219–25.
20. Childs C, Lunn KW. Clinical review: brain-body temperature differences in adults with severe traumatic brain injury. Crit Care. 2013;17:222.
21. Clifton GL, Valadka A, Zygun D, Coffey CS, Drever P, Fourwinds S, Janis LS, Wilde E, Taylor P, Harshman K, et al. Very early hypothermia induction in patients with severe brain injury (the National Acute Brain Injury Study: Hypothermia II): a randomised trial. Lancet Neurol. 2011;10:131–9.
22. Suehiro EMDPD, Koizumi H, Kunitsugu I, Fujisawa H, Suzuki M. Survey of brain temperature management in patients with traumatic brain injury in the Japan Neurotrauma Data Bank. J Neurotrauma. 2013. doi:10.1089/neu.2013.3057.
23. Zhao QJ, Zhang XG, Wang LX. Mild hypothermia therapy reduces blood glucose and lactate and improves neurologic outcomes in patients with severe traumatic brain injury. J Crit Care. 2011;26:311–5.
24. Fox JL, Vu EN, Doyle-Waters M, Brubacher JR, Abu-Laban R, Hu Z. Prophylactic hypothermia for traumatic brain injury: a quantitative systematic review. CJEM. 2010;12:355–64.
25. Brain Trauma Foundation, American Association of Neurological Surgeons, Congress of Neurological Surgeons, et al. Guidelines for the management of severe traumatic brain injury. IV. Infection prophylaxis. J Neurotrauma. 2007;24 Suppl 1:S26–31.
26. Kim J, Gearhart MM, Zurick A, et al. Preliminary report on the safety of heparin for deep venous thrombosis prophylaxis after severe head injury. J Trauma. 2002;53:38–42.
27. Norwood SH, McAuley CE, Berne JD, et al. Prospective evaluation of the safety of enoxaparin prophylaxis for venous thromboembolism in patients with intracranial hemorrhagic injuries. Arch Surg. 2002;137:696–701.
28. Phelan H. Pharmacologic venous thromboembolism prophylaxis after traumatic brain injury: a critical literature review. J Neurotrauma. 2012;29(10):1821–8.
29. Brain Trauma Foundation, American Association of Neurological Surgeons, Joint Section on Neurotrauma and Critical Care. Indications for intracranial pressure monitoring [review]. J Neurotrauma. 2007;24S:S37–44.
30. Narayan RK, Kishore PR, Becker DP, et al. Intracranial pressure: to monitor or not to monitor? A review of our experience with severe head injury. J Neurosurg. 1982;56:650–9.
31. Chesnut R, Videtta W, Vespa P, Le Roux P; The Participants in the International Multidisciplinary Consensus Conference on Multimodality Monitoring. Intracranial Pressure Monitoring: Fundamental Considerations and rationale for monitoring. Neurocrit Care. 2014;21 Suppl 2:64–84.
32. Le Roux P, Menon DK, Citerio G, Vespa P, Bader MK, Brophy GM, Diringer MN, Stocchetti N, Videtta W, Armonda R, Badjatia N, Böesel J, Chesnut R, Chou S, Claassen J, Czosnyka M, De Georgia M, Figaji A, Fugate J, Helbok R, Horowitz D, Hutchinson P, Kumar M, McNett M, Miller C, Naidech A, Oddo M, Olson D, O'Phelan K, Provencio JJ, Puppo C,

Riker R, Robertson C, Schmidt M, Taccone F. Consensus summary statement of the International Multidisciplinary Consensus Conference on Multimodality Monitoring in Neurocritical Care: a statement for healthcare professionals from the Neurocritical Care Society and the European Society of Intensive Care Medicine. Intensive Care Med. 2014;40(9):1189–209.

33. Brain Trauma Foundation, American Association of Neurological Surgeons, Joint Section on Neurotrauma and Critical Care. Recommendations for intracranial pressure monitoring technology [review]. J Neurotrauma. 2007;24S:S45–54.
34. Clark WC, Muhlbauer MS, Lowrey R, et al. Complications of intracranial pressure monitoring in trauma patients. Neurosurgery. 1989;25:20–4.
35. Brain Trauma Foundation, American Association of Neurological Surgeons, Joint Section on Neurotrauma and Critical Care. Intracranial pressure treatment threshold [review]. J Neurotrauma. 2007;24S:S55–8.
36. Kaufman AM, Cardozo E. Aggravation of vasogenic edema by multiple dose mannitol. J Neurosurg. 1992;77:584–9.
37. Brain Trauma Foundation, American Association of Neurological Surgeons, Joint Section on Neurotrauma and Critical Care. Hyperosmolar therapy [review]. J Neurotrauma. 2007;24S:S14–20.
38. Marion DW, Puccio A, Wisniewski SR, et al. Effect of hyperventilation on extracellular concentrations of glutamate, lactate, pyruvate, and local cerebral blood flow in patients with severe traumatic brain injury. Crit Care Med. 2002;30:2619–25.
39. Muizelaar JP, Marmarou A, Ward JD, et al. Adverse effects of prolonged hyperventilation in patients with severe head injury: a randomized clinical trial. J Neurosurg. 1991;75:731–9.
40. Kiening KL, Hartl R, Unterberg AW, et al. Brain tissue pO. Neurol Res. 1997;19:233–40.
41. Roberts I. Barbiturates for acute traumatic brain injury. Cochrane Database Syst Rev. 2000;(2):CD000033.
42. Schreckinger M, Marion DW. Contemporary management of traumatic intracranial hypertension: is there a role for therapeutic hypothermia? Neurocrit Care. 2009;11(3):427–36.
43. Marion D, Bullock RW. Current and future role of therapeutic hypothermia. J Neurotrauma. 2009;26:455–67.
44. Coplin WM, Cullen NK, Policherla PN, et al. Safety and feasibility of craniectomy with duraplasty as the initial surgical intervention for severe traumatic brain injury. J Trauma. 2001;50:1050–9.
45. Guerra WKW, Piek J, Gaab MR. Decompressive craniectomy to treat intracranial hypertension in head injury patients. Intensive Care Med. 1999;25:1327–9.
46. Kunze E, Meixensberger J, Janka M, et al. Decompressive craniectomy in patients with uncontrollable intracranial hypertension. Acta Neurochir Suppl. 1998;71:16–8.
47. Litofsky NS, Chin LS, Tang G, et al. The use of lobectomy in the management of severe closed-head trauma. Neurosurgery. 1994;34:628–32.
48. Munch E, Horn P, Schurer L, et al. Management of severe traumatic brain injury by decompressive craniectomy. Neurosurgery. 2000;47:315–22.
49. Cooper DJ, Rosenfeld JV, Murray L, Arabi YM, Davies AR, D'Urso P, Kossmann T, Ponsford J, Seppelt I, Reilly P, Wolfe R, DECRA Trial Investigators; Australian and New Zealand Intensive Care Society Clinical Trials Group. Decompressive craniectomy in diffuse traumatic brain injury. N Engl J Med. 2011;364(16):1493–502.
50. Rosner MJ, Rosner SD, Johnson AH. Cerebral perfusion pressure: management protocol and clinical results. J Neurosurg. 1995;83:949–62.
51. Feldman Z, Kanter MJ, Robertson CS, Contant CF, Hayes C, Sheinberg MA, Villareal CA, Narayan RK, Grossman RG. Effect of head elevation on intracranial pressure, cerebral perfusion pressure, and cerebral blood flow in head-injured patients. J Neurosurg. 1992;76(2):207–11.
52. Aries MJ, Czosnyka M, Budohoski KP, Steiner LA, Lavinio A, Kolias AG, Hutchinson PJ, Brady KM, Menon DK, Pickard JD, Smielewski P. Continuous determination of optimal cerebral perfusion pressure in traumatic brain injury. Crit Care Med. 2012;40(8):2456–63.

53. Carmona Suazo JA, Maas AI, van den Brink WA, van Santbrink H, Steyerberg EW, Avezaat CJ. CO2 reactivity and brain oxygen pressure monitoring in severe head injury. Crit Care Med. 2000;28:3268–74.
54. Gopinath SP, Valadka AB, Uzura M, Robertson CS. Comparison of jugular venous oxygen saturation and brain tissue PO2 as monitors of cerebral ischemia after head injury. Crit Care Med. 1999;27:2337–45.
55. Meixensberger J, Jaeger M, Väth A, Dings J, Kunze E, Roosen K. Brain tissue oxygen guided treatment supplementing ICP/CPP therapy after traumatic brain injury. J Neurol Neurosurg Psychiatry. 2003;74:760–4.
56. Sarrafzadeh AS, Kiening KL, Callsen TA, Unterberg AW. Metabolic changes during impending and manifest cerebral hypoxia in traumatic brain injury. Br J Neurosurg. 2003;17: 340–6.
57. Soehle M, Jaeger M, Meixensberger J. Online assessment of brain tissue oxygen autoregulation in traumatic brain injury and subarachnoid hemorrhage. Neurol Res. 2003;25:411–7.
58. van Santbrink H, Maas AI, Avezaat CJ. Continuous monitoring of partial pressure of brain tissue oxygen in patients with severe head injury. Neurosurgery. 1996;38:21–31.
59. van Santbrink H, van den Brink WA, Steyerberg EW, Carmona Suazo JA, Avezaat CJ, Maas AI. Brain tissue oxygen response in severe traumatic brain injury. Acta Neurochir (Wien). 2003;145:429–38.
60. Valadka AB, Goodman JC, Gopinath SP, Uzura M, Robertson CS. Comparison of brain tissue oxygen tension to microdialysis based measures of cerebral ischemia in fatally head-injured humans. J Neurotrauma. 1998;15:509–19.
61. van den Brink WA, van Santbrink H, Steyerberg EW, Avezaat CJ, Suazo JA, Hogesteeger C, et al. Brain oxygen tension in severe head injury. Neurosurgery. 2000;46:868–78.
62. Dings J, Meixensberger J, Jager A, Roosen K. Clinical experience with 118 brain tissue oxygen partial pressure catheter probes. Neurosurgery. 1998;43:1082–95.
63. Maas AI, Fleckenstein W, de Jong DA, van Santbrink H. Monitoring cerebral oxygenation: experimental studies and preliminary clinical results of continuous monitoring of cerebrospinal fluid and brain tissue oxygen tension. Acta Neurochir Suppl. 1993;59:50–7.
64. Manley G, Knudson MM, Morabito D, Damron S, Erickson V, Pitts L. Hypotension, hypoxia, and head injury: frequency, duration, and consequences. Arch Surg. 2001;136:1118–23.
65. Menzel M, Doppenberg EMR, Zauner A, Soukup J, Reinert MM, Bullock R. Increased inspired oxygen concentration as a factor in improved brain tissue oxygenation and tissue lactate levels after severe human head injury. J Neurosurg. 1999;91:1–10.
66. Tolias CM, Reinert M, Seiler R, Gilman C, Scharf A, Bullock MR. Normobaric hyperoxia—induced improvement in cerebral metabolism and reduction in intracranial pressure in patients with severe head injury: a prospective historical cohort-matched study. J Neurosurg. 2004;101:435–44.
67. Majdan M, Mauritz W, Wilbacher I, Brazinova A, Rusnak M, Leitgeb J. Barbiturates use and its effects in patients with severe traumatic brain injury in five European countries. J Neurotrauma. 2013;30:23–9.
68. Young B, Ott L, Norton J, et al. Metabolic and nutritional sequelae in the non-steroid treated head injury patient. Neurosurgery. 1985;17:784–91.
69. Brain Trauma Foundation, American Association of Neurological Surgeons, Joint Section on Neurotrauma and Critical Care. Nutrition [review]. J Neurotrauma. 2007;24S:S77–82.
70. Jeremitsky E, Omert L, Dunham C, Wilberger J, Rodriguez A. The impact of hyperglycemia on patients with severe brain injury. J Trauma. 2005;58:47–50.
71. Van Beek J, Mushkudianai N, Steyerberg E, et al. Prognostic value of admission laboratory parameters in traumatic brain injury: results from the IMPACT study. J Neurotrauma. 2007;24:315–28.
72. Vespa P, Boonyaputthikul R, McArthur DL, et al. Intensive insulin therapy reduces microdialysis glucose values without altering glucose utilization or improving the lactate/pyruvate ratio after traumatic brain injury. Crit Care Med. 2006;34:850–6.

73. Costello LA, Lithander FE, Gruen RL, Williams LT. Nutrition therapy in the optimisation of health outcomes in adult patients with moderate to severe traumatic brain injury: findings from a scoping review. Injury. 2014;45(12):1834–41.
74. Glotzner FL, Haubitz I, Miltner F, Kapp G, Pflughaupt KW. Seizure prevention using carbamazepine following severe brain injuries. Neurochirurgia. 1983;26:66–79.
75. Pechadre JC, Lauxerois M, Colnet G, Commun C, Dimicoli C, Bonnard M, Gibert J, Chabannes J. Prevention of late post-traumatic epilepsy by phenytoin in severe brain injuries. 2 years' follow-up. Presse Med. 1991;20:841–5.
76. Temkin NR, Dikmen SS, Winn HR. Management of head injury. Posttraumatic seizures. Neurosurg Clin N Am. 1991;2:425–35.
77. Temkin NR, Dikmen SS, Wilensky AJ, Keihm J, Chabal S, Winn HR. A randomized, double-blind study of phenytoin for the prevention of post-traumatic seizures. N Engl J Med. 1990;323:497–502.
78. Yablon SA. Posttraumatic seizures. Arch Phys Med Rehabil. 1993;74:983–1001.
79. Bratton SL, Chestnut RM, Ghajar J, McConnell Hammond FF, Harris OA, Hartl R, Manley GT, Nemecek A, Newell DW, Rosenthal G, et al. Guidelines for the management of severe traumatic brain injury. XIII. Antiseizure prophylaxis. J Neurotrauma. 2007;24:S83–6.
80. Ma CY, Xue YJ, Li M, Zhang Y, Li GZ. Sodium valproate for prevention of early posttraumatic seizures. Chin J Traumatol. 2010;13:293–6.
81. Lynch BA, Lambeng N, Nocka K, Kensel-Hammes P, Bajjalieh SM, Matagne A, Fuks B. The synaptic vesicle protein SV2A is the binding site for the antiepileptic drug levetiracetam. Proc Natl Acad Sci U S A. 2004;101:9861–6.
82. Vogl C, Mochida S, Wolff C, Whalley BJ, Stephens GJ. The synaptic vesicle glycoprotein 2A ligand levetiracetam inhibits presynaptic Ca2+ channels through an intracellular pathway. Mol Pharmacol. 2012;82:199–208.
83. Zou H, Brayer SW, Hurwitz M, Niyonkuru C, Fowler LE, Wagner AK. Neuroprotective, neuroplastic, and neurobehavioral effects of daily treatment with levetiracetam in experimental traumatic brain injury. Neurorehabil Neural Repair. 2013;27:878–88.
84. Pearl PL, McCarter R, McGavin CL, Yu Y, Sandoval F, Trzcinski S, Atabaki SM, Tsuchida T, van den Anker J, He J, et al. Results of phase II levetiracetam trial following acute head injury in children at risk for posttraumatic epilepsy. Epilepsia. 2013;54:e135–7.
85. Zafar SN, Khan AA, Ghauri AA, Shamim MS. Phenytoin versus Leviteracetam for seizure prophylaxis after brain injury—a meta analysis. BMC Neurol. 2012;12:30.
86. Steinbaugh LA, Lindsell CJ, Shutter LA, Szaflarski JP. Initial EEG predicts outcomes in a trial of levetiracetam vs. fosphenytoin for seizure prevention. Epilepsy Behav. 2012;23: 280–4.
87. Kruer RM, Harris LH, Goodwin H, Kornbluth J, Thomas KP, Slater LA, Haut ER. Changing trends in the use of seizure prophylaxis after traumatic brain injury: a shift from phenytoin to levetiracetam. J Crit Care. 2013;28:e9–13.
88. Szaflarski JP, Sangha KS, Lindsell CJ, Shutter LA. Prospective, randomized, single-blinded comparative trial of intravenous levetiracetam versus phenytoin for seizure prophylaxis. Neurocrit Care. 2010;12:165–72.
89. Inaba K, Menaker J, Branco BC, Gooch J, Okoye OT, Herrold J, Scalea TM, Dubose J, Demetriades D. A prospective multicenter comparison of levetiracetam versus phenytoin for early posttraumatic seizure prophylaxis. J Trauma Acute Care Surg. 2013;74:766–71. discussion 771–3.
90. Torbic H, Forni AA, Anger KE, Degrado JR, Greenwood BC. Use of antiepileptics for seizure prophylaxis after traumatic brain injury. Am J Health Syst Pharm. 2013;70:759–66.
91. Roberts I, Yates D, Sandercock P, Farrell B, Wasserberg J, Lomas G, et al. Effect of intravenous corticosteroids on death within 14 days in 10008 adults with clinically significant head injury (MRC CRASH trial): randomized placebo-controlled trial. Lancet. 2004;364:1321–8.
92. Maas AI, Stocchetti N, Bullock R. Moderate and severe traumatic brain injury in adults. Lancet Neurol. 2008;7:728.

93. Wright DW, Kellermann AL, Hertzberg VS, et al. ProTECT: a randomized clinical trial of progesterone for acute traumatic brain injury. Ann Emerg Med. 2007;49:391.
94. Ma J, Huang S, Qin S, You C. Progesterone for acute traumatic brain injury. Cochrane Database Syst Rev. 2012;(10):CD008409.
95. Arango MF, Bainbridge D. Magnesium for acute traumatic brain injury. Cochrane Database Syst Rev 2008;(4):CD005400.
96. Bennett MH, Trytko B, Jonker B. Hyperbaric oxygen therapy for the adjunctive treatment of traumatic brain injury. Cochrane Database Syst Rev. 2012;(12):CD004609.
97. Mazzeo AT, Brophy GM, Gilman CB, et al. Safety and tolerability of cyclosporin A in severe traumatic brain injury patients: results from a prospective randomized trial. J Neurotrauma. 2009;26:2195.
98. Xiong Y, Mahmood A, Chopp M. Emerging treatments for traumatic brain injury. Expert Opin Emerg Drugs. 2009;14:67.
99. Zafonte RD, Bagiella E, Ansel BM, et al. Effect of citicoline on functional and cognitive status among patients with traumatic brain injury: Citicoline Brain Injury Treatment Trial (COBRIT). JAMA. 2012;308:1993.
100. Talving P, Lustenberger T, Kobayashi L, et al. Erythropoiesis stimulating agent administration improves survival after severe traumatic brain injury: a matched case control study. Ann Surg. 2010;251:1.
101. Robertson CS, Hannay HJ, Yamal J-M, Gopinath S, Goodman JC, Tilley BC; and the Epo Severe TBI Trial Investigators. Effect of erythropoietin and transfusion threshold on neurological recovery after traumatic brain injury: a randomized clinical trial. JAMA. 2014;312(1):36–47.
102. Huang L, Obenaus A. Hyperbaric oxygen therapy for traumatic brain injury. Med Gas Res. 2011;1:21.
103. Menzel M, Doppenberg EM, Zauner A, Soukup J, Reinert MM, Clausen T, Brockenbrough PB, Bullock R. Cerebral oxygenation in patients after severe head injury: monitoring and effects of arterial hyperoxia on cerebral blood flow, metabolism and intracranial pressure. J Neurosurg Anesthesiol. 1999;11:240–51.
104. McDonagh M, Helfand M, Carson S, Russman BS. Hyperbaric oxygen therapy for traumatic brain injury: a systematic review of the evidence. Arch Phys Med Rehabil. 2004;85:1198–204.
105. Sahni T, Jain M, Prasad R, Sogani SK, Singh VP. Use of hyperbaric oxygen in traumatic brain injury: retrospective analysis of data of 20 patients treated at a tertiary care centre. Br J Neurosurg. 2012;26:202–7.
106. Lin JW, Tsai JT, Lee LM, Lin CM, Hung CC, Hung KS, Chen WY, Wei L, Ko CP, Su YK, et al. Effect of hyperbaric oxygen on patients with traumatic brain injury. Acta Neurochir Suppl. 2008;101:145–9.
107. Rockswold SB, Rockswold GL, Zaun DA, Liu J. A prospective, randomized Phase II clinical trial to evaluate the effect of combined hyperbaric and normobaric hyperoxia on cerebral metabolism, intracranial pressure, oxygen toxicity, and clinical outcome in severe traumatic brain injury. J Neurosurg. 2013;118:1317–28.

Chapter 16
Patient Safety in Guillain–Barré Syndrome and Acute Neuromuscular Disorders

Maxwell S. Damian

Introduction

Guillain–Barré syndrome (GBS), or acute inflammatory demyelinating polyradiculoneuropathy (AIDP), typically presents with distal paresthesias, back pain and ascending weakness and loss of deep tendon reflexes. AIDP has an incidence of 10–20 per million populations per year, with around 50 % of cases presenting after a prodromal respiratory or gastrointestinal infection, often due to *Mycoplasma pneumoniae* or *Campylobacter jejuni*. The leading reason for ICU admission is respiratory failure, often compounded by infection due to inadequate airway protection in patients with bulbar weakness. Autonomic dysregulation occurs to some degree in 60 % of patients and includes orthostatic hypotension, diabetes insipidus, ileus, or cardiac arrhythmias; the latter may occasionally necessitate emergency pacing. Dysrhythmia is the second most important life-threatening complication of GBS after respiratory failure. Bedside assessment of postural blood pressures, along with heart rate and rhythm, is therefore essential in all patients. A standard 12-lead electrocardiogram (ECG) is part of the initial neurological assessment. However, the ECG cannot rule out the risk of significant dysrhythmia, as there are no reliable predictors for the individual risk of life-threatening autonomic complications.

Evidence-based specific treatment consists of either IV immunoglobulins (IVIG) 400 mg per kg on 5 consecutive days or 4–6 plasma exchanges (PLEX) of 1.5–2 L each on consecutive or alternate days. Early treatment may be more beneficial. The clinical pattern and effectiveness of IVIG may differ depending on the pattern of antineuronal antibodies (IVIG may be better with GM1-IgG antibodies, GM1b, or GalNac-GD1a), but this is not a practical consideration as results usually become

M.S. Damian, MD, PhD
Department of Neurology, Cambridge University Hospitals, Cambridge, UK
e-mail: msdd2@cam.ac.uk

© Springer International Publishing Switzerland 2015   249
K.E. Wartenberg et al. (eds.), *Neurointensive Care: A Clinical Guide to Patient Safety*, DOI 10.1007/978-3-319-17293-4_16

available after the treatment period. The antibody pattern also influences the clinical subgroup: for instance, patients with anti GD1a/GD1b antibodies tend to have cranial nerve involvement, and the anti-GQ1b antibody is associated with the Miller Fisher syndrome. In daily practice, the choice between IVIG or PLEX depends on local availability and on estimated risk of side effects. For example, IVIG may be more risky in elderly people with vascular and coronary disease, or with heart failure less likely to tolerate the volume infused, but safer than PLEX in septic patients. The dose of IVIG or volume of PLEX is also established by convention rather than based on scientific proof. It is currently unclear whether PLEX in patients who are perceived to fail IVIG treatment actually provides benefit, and there is no rationale to providing early PLEX if IVIG does not show rapid effect. However, in patients in whom immunoglobulin levels fail to increase adequately after a single course of IVIG, a repeat course may improve the result [1].

Most cases reach maximum weakness around day 10 after onset; approximately 30 % of all cases become bedbound, and a third to half of these will become tetraplegic and require intubation and ventilator support. Bedbound patients are most at risk of respiratory failure and cardiac dysrhythmia, and ECG monitoring should be considered in bedbound patients even outside the ICU.

Overall mortality is 5–10 %, mainly due to infection (often through aspiration due to inadequate airway protection) or cardiac arrhythmia. Mortality is much higher in patients requiring ICU treatment, reaching 20 %. A majority of these patients die after discharge from the ICU, which reflects the importance of good step down care unit [2]. Recovery can take up to 2 years, and up to 40 % of patients retain neurological deficits.

Case Scenario

A 53-year-old man presents to the local emergency department having developed tingling in the fingertips followed by weakness in the legs 2 weeks after a gastrointestinal infection. Four days after the onset of weakness, he had lost the ability to walk. He was admitted to a medical ward and within 24 h became unable to sit unaided. The local neurological center was contacted and on the advice of the on-call physician a lumbar puncture was performed, in which the lymphocyte count was slightly elevated at 26 cells/μl and protein mildly elevated at 0.8 g/L. A spinal cord MRI showed a normal lumbar spine (thoracic cord not done as his reflexes were now absent). Nerve conduction studies were requested. As advised, his blood gases were checked regularly; the critical care outreach team assessed him and recommended review if his blood gases deteriorated. IVIG treatment was started after checking IgA levels, and although his condition progressed to include swallowing problems and weak head flexion, 12-h blood gas checks remained stable. The night following day 4 after admission he was found obtunded with severe hypoxic respiratory failure and required emergency transfer to the ICU. During intubation he suffered a brief asystolic cardiac arrest, but awoke rapidly after ventilation was instituted. He was found to have right lower lobe pneumonia. His further course was complicated by episodes of hypotension and bradycardia after he was treated with a beta-blocker for hypertension. He started to improve after four sessions of PLEX in addition to IVIG, as advised by the neurology team in their weekly visit. Nevertheless, he required tracheotomy on day 12 after intubation and the patient spent a total of 5 weeks in the ICU and high dependency unit (HDU). He was discharged to a medical ward after weaning, awaiting rehabilitation. Unfortunately, he suffered a cardiac arrest and died before hospital discharge.

Risk of Patient Safety

1. An elevated cerebrospinal fluid (CSF) cell count should prompt HIV testing, as a GBS-like syndrome with elevated cell count can be a feature of seroconversion.
2. The patient was treated in a general hospital and diagnostic tests were performed according to advice over the phone. This is a recipe for suboptimal investigation, as essential tests such as neurophysiology may be unavailable outside specialist units, or findings may be misinterpreted by the inexperienced physician. For example, in this case a central lesion was not considered because of absent deep tendon reflexes. Such patients should be admitted to a specialist unit with experience in the management of rare neuromuscular diseases.
3. Clinicians unfamiliar with acute neuromuscular disease often rely on blood gas analyses, which tend to become abnormal much later than significant weakness of respiratory muscles can be detected by regular monitoring of vital capacity, inspiratory and expiratory pressures.
4. Critical Care Outreach teams, if used rather than ICU/HDU admission during the progressing phase, must arrange regular visits and provide a detailed and appropriate monitoring protocol to be used by the ward staff between reviews, including plans for escalation.
5. Transfer of patients to the ICU in extremis always signifies inadequate foresight and an inappropriate monitoring regime; near misses need to be reviewed to identify gaps in the patients' supervision as here inadequate respiratory monitoring and probably underrecognition of compromised airway protection.
6. This patient demonstrates numerous signs of autonomic dysfunction and risk of severe dysregulation. Checks of autonomic function need to be part of the daily assessment and risks in routine medical and nursing procedures need to be clear to the treatment team, i.e., hypersensitivity to common drugs; suction and turning; physical exertion or postural change during rehabilitation.
7. The true benefit of adding PLEX to IVIG is not known.
8. More (twice as many) GBS patients die in hospital after discharge from the ICU compared to the acute phase, and the reasons are poorly known. Respiratory infections and cardiac dysrhythmias are suspected; discharge from the ICU to a nonspecialized unit may mean a drop in awareness of risks. Dysautonomia and

cardiovascular instability can continue during rehabilitation, or even reappear as remyelination and axonal function are restored. However, the level of awareness of potential risks is considerably lower on medical wards or nonspecialist rehabilitation units that patients are discharged to after weaning from the ventilator. Treatment on a specialized unit, rather than a general ICU with intermittent specialist review may provide better step down planning.

Safety Barriers

On the ward, patients who are at high risk can be identified by their initial rate of progression and through bedside monitoring protocols. Nursing plans should include a specific plan for the type and frequency of ongoing monitoring required for motor, ventilatory, and cardiac function. Regular neurological assessments need to be documented in a standardized manner that is comparable between different examiners, and use gradings of power such as the Medical Research Council (MRC) score in a way that identifies meaningful changes, whereas statements such as "lower limb power 4/5 MRC" do not. Patients unable to walk 5 m (Hughes scale score ≥3) [3] require intensive monitoring, as they are at risk of respiratory failure, particularly if progression has been rapid, i.e., <1 week from onset. Relatively early admission to ICU is advisable, as cases left until frank respiratory decompensation occurs will be complicated by infection due to inadequate clearing of secretions or failure of airway protection owing to bulbar weakness. Bedbound patients are also most at risk of cardiac dysrhythmia or severe autonomic dysfunction who may need emergency pacing, or demonstrate extreme sensitivity to nursing maneuvers or to commonplace ICU drugs.

Critical care outreach teams need neurological guidance on how to spot patients heading for intubation, even though their respiratory function might still be adequate. Examples are patients who become bedbound within the first week, or patients in whom there is a discrepancy between upright and supine vital capacity indicating early diaphragmatic dysfunction, or patients with significant bulbar symptoms. ICU admission is best planned according to an agreed set of institutional criteria (Fig. 16.1). The rate of progression should allow at-risk patients to be identified.

Monitoring on the ward with hand held devices should include regular surveillance of vital capacity, as well as inspiratory and expiratory mouth pressures. The latter are more specific for respiratory muscle weakness, although more dependent on cooperation. Patients with facial weakness can still provide nasal "sniff" pressures. Nurses monitoring such patients need sufficient training in performing these tests; if not, the values provided may vary widely and are unreliable. Bedside evaluation uses the "20/30/40 rule" [4] where significant ventilatory dysfunction is reflected by the presence of either: forced vital capacity (FVC) <20 mL/kg; peak inspiratory pressure <30 cm H_2O; or peak expiratory pressure <40 cm H_2O. Any of these parameters falling below the 20/30/40 threshold requires critical care review and consideration for ICU admission.

The point of bedside spirometry is to detect significant hypoventilation *prior* to life-threatening hypoxemia. Blood gas analyses are not an adequate form of

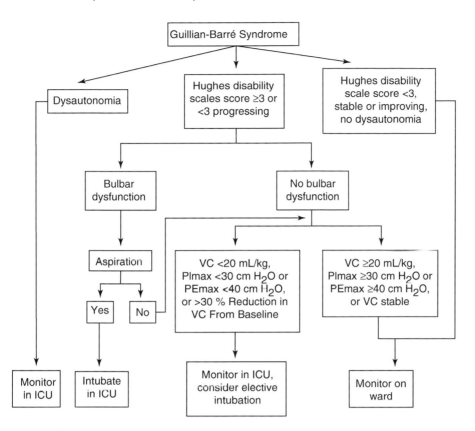

Fig. 16.1 The Mayo Clinic's pathway to ICU admission for GBS (Image courtesy Dr. EFM Wijdicks, with thanks)

monitoring; they are invasive, cannot be performed frequently, and percutaneous oxygen saturations are no substitute. Hypercapnia occurs late and suggests impending respiratory arrest [5]; hypoxemia is even later.

Diaphragmatic failure may be seen in isolation without significant weakness of intercostal and accessory respiratory muscles; patients do not tolerate lying flat and commonly decompensate at night, when reduced central respiratory drive compounds supine mechanical dysfunction. Diaphragmatic paralysis also causes "paradoxical abdominal movement" – indrawing of the abdominal wall on inspiration. In contrast, patients with impaired intercostal muscle function and preserved diaphragmatic function exhibit indrawing of the upper ribcage and intercostal spaces during inspiration due to loss of normal intercostal muscle tone.

Noninvasive bilevel positive airway pressure (BiPAP) ventilation may not be a safe temporizing measure in evolving GBS [6], and early intubation and assist-control (AC) or synchronized intermittent mandatory ventilation (SIMV) with pressure support and positive end-expiratory pressure (PEEP) is advised. Fifty percent of intubated patients require ventilation for over 3 weeks, but there is no clear benefit in early tracheotomy.

Bulbar involvement contributes to respiratory impairment by limiting clearance of secretions, increasing the risk of upper airway obstruction or pulmonary aspiration. Patients with significant impairment of respiratory function due to neuromuscular disease can appear well and only exhibit breathlessness on talking or swallowing. Shallow breathing with increased heart and respiratory rate is not universal, and absence of these features cannot exclude significant ventilatory impairment.

Significant autonomic dysfunction in critical care means orthostatic hypotension and symptomatic dysrhythmia. These patients should have continuous ECG monitoring, and preferably should be monitored in the ICU; emergency external pacing via chest pads must be readily available. Bedside autonomic tests, such as pulse frequency variation, Valsalva, or cold pressor responses, cannot accurately predict which patients are at particular risk; the eyeball pressure test [7] is now considered unsafe. Bradycardia/tachycardia syndrome may predict severe arrhythmia, but its absence does not rule out risk. Apart from dysrhythmia, autonomic dysfunction also causes labile blood pressure, adynamic ileus, or bladder dysfunction. The response to commonly used medications may be excessive in these patients; vasodilators and beta-blockers in particular must be used with caution, likewise neostigmine or metoclopramide in bradycardic patients. The potential for autonomic complications remains even during the rehabilitation phase, as peripheral nerve function is restored patchily to parasympathetic and sympathetic connections. A significant number of the deaths occurring during the recovery phase after discharge from ICU may be due to dysautonomia, but they are inadequately documented.

Younger survivors particularly have a chance of full recovery even after very prolonged ventilation, but 40 % of survivors retain abnormal neurological findings and up to 20 % of all survivors retain a long-term disability. Mortality rates are commonly cited as 5–10 %, but this applies to all cases of GBS. Mortality may reach 20 % in ventilated patients [8]. Mortality varies considerably between units, for reasons which are not yet clear, and bad outcomes may go unrecognised in units with a low volume of cases, which underlines the importance of specialized neuro-ICUs, systematic audits, and national registries. An unselected, nationwide audit surveying the majority of GBS cases admitted to ICU in the UK over a 12-year period found a significantly higher acute hospital mortality than expected, with a majority of deaths occurring after discharge from ICU during the recovery phase [2]. Death is mainly due to infection or cardiac arrhythmia and therefore potentially avoidable.

Dos and Don'ts

Dos

- Patients unable to walk 5 m (Hughes scale score ≥3) require intensive monitoring.
- Establish an institutional monitoring protocol with reproducible criteria for close monitoring, ICU admission, and intubation of patients with neuromuscular disease.

- Patients with autonomic dysregulation should be monitored in the ICU.
- Patients who fail the "20/30/40" rule should be monitored in the ICU and intubated early.
- Further respiratory deterioration, or bulbar dysfunction with risk of aspiration, necessitate intubation, not non-invasive ventilation.

Don'ts

- Don't provide telephone advice without seeing the patient.
- Don't wait for abnormal blood gas analyses to consider ICU admission in neuromuscular disease.
- Don't delay intubation with a trial of NIV in neuromuscular disease.
- Don't rush into early PLEX if IVIG does not show effect early.
- Don't believe there is no risk of cardiac dysrhythmia because "screening tests" are negative of motor signs are improving.

References

1. Kuitwaard K, Gelder J, Tio-Gillen AP, Hop WC, Gelder T, Toorenenbergen AW, et al. Pharmacokinetics of intravenous immunoglobulin and outcome in Guillain–Barré syndrome. Ann Neurol. 2009;66:597–603. doi:10.1002/ana.21737.
2. Damian MS, Ben-Shlomo Y, Howard R, et al. The effect of secular trends and specialist neurocritical care on mortality for patients with intracerebral haemorrhage, myasthenia gravis and Guillain-Barré Syndrome admitted to critical care. Int Care Med. 2013;39:1405–12.
3. Plasma Exchange/Sandoglobulin Guillain-Barré Syndrome Trial Group. Randomised trial of plasma exchange, intravenous immunoglobulin, and combined treatments in Guillain-Barré syndrome. Lancet. 1997;349:225–300.
4. Rabinstein AA, Wijdicks EF. Warnng signs of imminent respiratory failure in neurologic patients. Semin Neurol. 2003;23(1):97–104.
5. Hughes RA, Bihari D. Acute muscular respiratory paralysis. J Neurol Neurosurg Psychiatry. 1993;56(4):334–43.
6. Wijdicks EF, Roy TK. BiPAP in early Guillain-Barré syndrome may fail. Can J Neurol Sci. 2006;33(1):105–6.
7. Flachenecker P, Toyka KV, Reiners K. Cardiac arrhythmias in Guillain-Barre syndrome. An overview of the diagnosis of a rare but potentially life-threatening complication. Nervenarzt. 2001;72(8):610–7.
8. Fletcher DD, Lawn ND, Wolter TD, Wijdicks EF. Long-term outcome in patients with Guillain-Barré syndrome requiring mechanical ventilation. Neurology. 2000;54(12):2311–5.

Chapter 17
Acute Spinal Disorders

Regunath Kandasamy, Wan Mohd Nazaruddin Wan Hassan, Zamzuri Idris,
and Jafri Malin Abdullah

Introduction

Spinal cord injury may result from a number of different etiological factors.
Trauma is the most common source; other causes include degenerative diseases,
inflammatory conditions, impaired vascular supply as well as compression by rapidly enlarging neoplastic, hemorrhagic, or pyogenic mass lesions. A significant
proportion of patients will need to be managed in a critical care setting as they
often have permanent neurological deficits and disability. It is well established that
management strategies strongly influence the outcome of patients [1]. However,
the complex nature of injuries to the spinal cord and vertebral column requires
more than one single absolute management strategy applicable to all patients.
Often the management is based on a heterogeneous combination of patient, physician, and institutional factors. Patient's age and comorbidities, concurrent injuries
as well as physician's experience and available resources all have an impact on
treatment.

The course of a patient's treatment and recovery especially in the acute stage
can be variable and requires constant vigilance with evolving strategies to address
issues that may surface at each juncture. In an Intensive care unit (ICU) setting,
the care of patients is shouldered together by both physician and nursing staff.
Staff with variable levels of training and experience may have different roles in
caring for the patient. Risks to the safety of patients are omnipresent and significant

R. Kandasamy, MBBS, MRCS, MS Neurosurgery • Z. Idris, MBBch, MS Neurosurgery
J.M. Abdullah, FASC, MD, PhD, DSCN, FRCS (✉)
Center for Neuroscience Services and Research, Universiti Sains Malaysia,
Kota Bharu, Kelantan, Malaysia
e-mail: brainsciences@gmail.com

Wan Mohd Nazaruddin Wan Hassan, MD, Master in Medicine
Departments of Anaesthesiology and Intensive Care, Hospital Universiti Sains Malaysia,
Kota Bharu, Kelantan, Malaysia

© Springer International Publishing Switzerland 2015
K.E. Wartenberg et al. (eds.), *Neurointensive Care: A Clinical Guide
to Patient Safety*, DOI 10.1007/978-3-319-17293-4_17

barriers need to be overcome to avoid disastrous results from errors in decision making or judgement, especially by junior or inexperienced staff. Attention to certain core principles of safety, while taking into consideration the varying requirements of each individual patient, forms the basis of this chapter. We acknowledge that acute spinal cord injury may occur in numerous settings; however, for ease of description and to aid understanding, this chapter focuses mainly on patients with traumatic spinal cord injury (SCI) managed in the neurointensive care setting.

Case Scenario

A 43-year-old male patient was involved in an alleged road transport accident. He was thrown off a motorcycle that had skidded while travelling at high speed. The patient was admitted to a district medical center where his post resuscitation Glasgow Coma Scale (GCS) score was noted to be 4/15 (E1, V2, M1). The patient was subsequently intubated and sedated before being transferred to our center for further management. Initial investigations done at the district hospital included radiographs of the chest, pelvis, and cervical spine. The radiographs were reviewed by a medical officer in the district hospital prior to transfer and were reported to be normal.

On arrival at our center, the patient was noted to be ventilated and sedated with midazolam and morphine infusions. His vital signs were stable and GCS remained E1, V1, M1 = 3/15. Both pupils were 3 mm in diameter and reacted briskly to external light. Examination of his chest, abdomen, and extremities revealed no significant abnormality. A per-rectal examination was not performed. A computed tomographic scan showed no intracranial hemorrhage, fracture, or brain swelling.

The patient was subsequently weaned off sedation and extubated. He appeared to be obeying commands and was moving all limbs at that time. Two hours later, the patient suddenly arrested requiring emergency intubation and resuscitation. Upon revision of spontaneous rhythm and stabilization, priapism was noted. Examination revealed generalized hypotonia with loss of the anal and bulbocavernous reflexes. After hemodynamic stabilization CT scan of his brain and spine was performed (Fig. 17.1a). Magnetic resonance imaging (MRI) of his cervical spine was also performed (Fig. 17.1b). The patient underwent a detailed examination and he was labeled as having a Grade A spinal cord injury according to the American Spinal Injury Association (ASIA) scale. He was managed in the Intensive Care Unit and subsequently underwent spine surgery in the form of a C6 corpectomy and fusion. Post operatively the patient's hospital course was complicated with recurrent episodes of pneumonia and he required prolonged ventilator support necessitating a tracheostomy to be performed.

- What were the shortfalls in this patient's management?
- Can you think of any safety barriers that might have helped improve patient safety in this scenario?

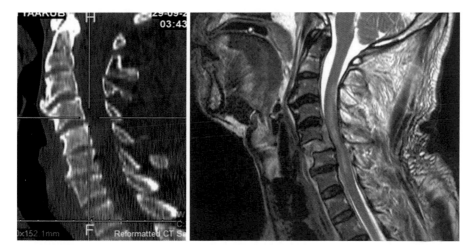

Fig. 17.1 (**a**) A sagittal CT scan of the patient's cervical spine. (**b**) T 2 -weighted sagittal MRI of the same patient

Risks to Patient Safety

Spinal cord injury typically involves a primary mechanical impact followed by a cascade of secondary changes that occur hours to days after the insult. This cascade results in spinal cord edema from vascular compromise, inflammation and impairment in cellular metabolism and ionic hemostasis. Secondary changes are highly sensitive to and influenced by changes in systemic variables such as hypotension, hypoxemia, hyperthermia, hypercoagulability, and catecholamine release [2, 3]. Early detection, treatment and prevention of these conditions form the cardinal principles of neurointensive care management for SCI.

From the time an injury takes place, the patient is immediately at risk of subtle events that may exacerbate and worsen secondary injury. A clear understanding of what the potential risks might be is vital for any preventive or remedial steps to be taken. There are three different phases of care of spinal cord injury. The initial phase includes the pre-hospital and emergency room care, second is the actual care in the intensive care setting and third is the rehabilitative phase. Although this chapter focuses on intensive care, we like to highlight the fact that effective management of a spinal cord injury patient begins from the very first phase where errors can significantly influence the outcome as a whole. The risks to safety in each stage are discussed below.

Pre-hospital and Emergency Room Care

After an episode of trauma, patients are evaluated by first responders who are usually paramedics. First responders need to be well trained to identify patients at risk of spinal cord injury and those who require spinal immobilization. The presence of multisystem injuries predestines for missing of an injury. Synchronous traumatic brain injury (TBI) seen in up to 60 % of patients with SCI has been identified as one co-existing injury which may complicate assessment of patients [4]. The alteration in consciousness of a patient and the requirement of early sedation may result in a patient's neurological deficit being attributed to TBI or to effects of a sedative.

Initial management should always be in accordance with the Advanced Trauma & Life Support (ATLS) guidelines. Airway management in any spinal cord injury can be challenging. When proceeding with the ABCs of resuscitation, manipulation of the neck puts the patient at risk for aggravation of a pre-existing cervical spine injury. Even a short period of neck manipulation or laryngeal compression can lead to disastrous effects such as worsening of the spinal cord injury or even cardiorespiratory collapse. In a conscious patient with an intact airway close monitoring is needed to detect impending respiratory compromise, especially in the setting of a high cervical injury. Failure in anticipation of airway collapse or respiratory failure may result in acute deterioration of the patient necessitating emergency measures. In an emergency situation, the potential for mistakes especially when airway manipulation is performed is also significantly higher.

Early resuscitative care must focus on prevention of hypotension and hypoxemia. Hypotension in the setting of a SCI maybe of hypovolemic or neurogenic etiology. The high incidence of associated injuries in patients with SCI warrants a detailed search for occult sources of hemorrhage before designating that the source is neurogenic in etiology. Possible sources of occult hemorrhage include the abdomen, chest, retroperitoneum, and long bone or pelvic fractures. Once the cause has been established, adequate volume resuscitation is vital prior to the use of vasopressors. Care should be taken to avoid administering an excess of 2,000 mL of crystalloid solutions as this may result in pulmonary edema from associated acute respiratory distress syndrome (ARDS). Hypotension should be avoided (middle artery pressure (MAP) <85 mmHg) due to the possible risk of worsening secondary cord injury.

If spinal cord injury is suspected, examination of patients needs to be conducted in a systematic fashion ensuring an assessment as complete as possible. In patients transferred from one institution to another facility, care must be taken as often significant injuries can be missed and may only be detected at a latter point of time. The documentation of any neurological deficit should be based on a standard system of evaluation to facilitate a clear definition of the extent of injury, the level of injury as well as to monitor for further deterioration. Signs of associated traumatic brain injury should also not be missed as it may co-exist with SCI in about 25 % of patients.

Diagnostic evaluation of the spine usually involves acquisition of an anterior-posterior (AP) and lateral radiographs of the affected region of the spine. In common practice, radiographs are routinely done for evaluation of the cervical spine in patients with altered consciousness or when deemed necessary by the NEXUS (National Emergency X – Radiography Utilization Study) criteria or the Canadian C-Spine rule which have been validated in large clinical trials [5–7]. Radiographs of other spine segments are only performed in the presence of suggestive localizing symptoms.

When interpreting radiographs of a patient with spinal cord injury, one should ensure the technical adequacy of the film and adequate training and experience of the reader. Incomplete radiographs or failure to detect subtle findings are a common cause for missed injury which may pose serious consequences for the patients. When in doubt, a senior staff physician should be consulted.

In centers with CT scanners, it is strongly recommended to proceed with this modality which has been found to be more sensitive and cost effective compared to radiographs for detecting fractures [8, 9]. MRI, however, is more sensitive for detection of ligamentous or other soft tissue injuries as well as lesions such as hematomas, disc rupture, or cord contusion. In patients without fractures on CT, an MRI may be the only modality that demonstrates the extent of injury adequately to facilitate timely treatment. It is also the modality of choice when neurological deterioration occurs due to secondary injury. If clinical suspicion is high in a symptomatic patient, a complete series of imaging including an MRI should be done.

In the presence of any spinal fracture, imaging of the entire spinal axis should be obtained to avoid missing a non-contiguous injury that is known to be present in as many as 28 % of SCI patients.

Other important safety concerns include the risk of pressure ulcers, ileus and urinary retention. Prolonged placement on a spinal board or an unpadded surface can predispose to a pressure ulcer within 2 h. If a patient remains in the emergency department for a prolonged period, the spinal board should be removed as soon as possible and the patient rested on well-padded surfaces. Patient's garments with possible contents especially in the back pockets may also cause undue pressure and should be changed to hospital gowns. Ileus as well as urinary retention is also common and thus nasogastric and bladder drainage tubes need to be inserted to reduce the risk of aspiration and to prevent urinary retention.

Neurointensive Care Phase

The second phase of care in SCI usually takes place in an intensive care unit. There are numerous potential safety risks for the patient, beginning the moment of transfer out of the emergency room. Patients requiring intubation as a part of their airway management are particularly at risk of events such as tube dislodgement or even the depletion of oxygen stores in transport cylinders which can lead to hypoxemia. Attention to proper anchoring of endotracheal tubes as well as all invasive devices is vital before any attempt to move a patient. The provision of analgesics as well as sedative medication can also reduce the potential for dislodgement of devices while ensuring that the patient's spine remains immobilized and comfortable during movement. Overzealous or infrequent ambu-bag ventilation by an inexperienced staff member can also result in impairment in ventilation and unnecessarily increased airway pressure leading to hypocarbia or hypercarbia and barotrauma. The use of a portable ventilator for transport would provide more stable conditions with more regulated ventilation. However, it may not always be available and requires properly trained staff to operate.

During the initial definitive management of the SCI, common areas of risk to patient's safety include the application of traction and immobilization of the spine. The indication for traction must be clearly defined. Application of traction is best done with close monitoring of the patient for acute worsening. Weight should also be increased progressively and any new symptoms of acute worsening should be sought for. Once weight has been applied, an x-ray should be performed and screws need to be tightened on a daily basis. Adequate sedation and analgesia should also be ensured during the procedure. It is important to remember that traction and immobilization are not benign procedures and up to 70 % of patients will experience additional pain, decubitus ulcers impaired chest wall mobility, airway compromise, and raised intracranial pressure [10].

The decision on timing of surgical intervention is dictated by the nature of injury. At present emergency decompression is advocated in selected scenarios such as progressive neurological deterioration, facet dislocation, or bilateral locked facets, or in the presence of epidural hematomas, abscesses, or nerve root impingement with radiculopathy. It is important to be aware of a clear indication for urgent surgery as some studies have shown that early treatment may have a beneficial effect on neurological recovery in patients [11]. Definitive guidelines however are still pending at present. A patient admitted to the ICU for SCI should also be reassessed regularly as there is a potential for secondary neurological deterioration which usually is attributed to cord edema. This condition can benefit from surgical decompression granted that it is detected early. Thus it is always important to regularly reassess a patient with SCI. This is particularly relevant in patients who are sedated and intubated, in whom only subtle signs of deterioration may be seen.

Abnormalities in respiratory function as well as pulmonary complications are also a prominent issue in SCI management. Besides being identified as the leading cause of death and morbidity in patients with SCI, the respiratory failure has been identified as an independent predictor of 3-month mortality [1, 12–14].

The extent of respiratory dysfunction correlates with the level of the injury. A complete injury above the level of C3 usually results in severe apnea with respiratory arrest requiring immediate ventilator support. Injuries between C3-5 have variable degrees of respiratory complications due to a combination of muscle weakness, paradoxical chest movement as well as impaired ability to clear respiratory secretions. Acutely, these patients suffer from markedly reduced lung volumes requiring ventilation, but a significant number can be weaned weeks to months after the injury [15]. The typical time course in these patients begins with an acute phase of worsening over the first 48 h till about the fifth day followed by slow improvement in function. Lesions below C5 rarely lead to respiratory failure in the absence of pulmonary infections. The key concern in this patient population is a lack of effective clearance of respiratory secretions leading to atelectasis and pneumonia. The patients need to be monitored and managed with ventilator strategies avoiding new complications. For example, usage of high PEEP or airway pressure settings causes ventilator-induced lung injury if used injudiciously for prolonged periods. Fluid management should also be titrated to avoid volume overload leading to pulmonary edema.

Patients with SCI usually require prolonged ventilator support. This creates a few potential risks such as reintubation after accidental dislodgement of endotracheal tube (ETT). Once again, difficult intubation must be anticipated and neck immobilization maintained. In the ICU setting when pre-planning is possible the use of video laryngoscopy or fiberoptic intubation may be advisable. Alternatively, an ETT exchanger device or gum elastic Bougie adjunct is beneficial to aid the use of direct laryngoscopy and to minimize neck mobilization. Prolonged ventilator requirements should prompt insertion of a tracheostomy early to facilitate ventilator weaning and trachea-bronchial toilet, either open surgery or percutaneous. Open tracheostomy has the advantage of less blunt force needed during open insertion of the tube. The higher force used during cannulation of a percutaneous tracheostomy may lead to unnecessary spine movements which may aggravate SCI. Open surgery, however, is sometimes performed in an operation theater requiring transport of the patient which may not always be feasible. Both procedures, however, have been found to be safe in SCI patients [16].

Cardiovascular problems related to SCI are most importantly hypotension due to neurogenic or spinal shock. The patients need to be maintained with adequate intravenous fluids and inotropic support to ensure blood pressure (BP) is maintained at a threshold which may not worsen secondary injury. When performing fluid resuscitation, it is important to restrict the high volume as this may result in pulmonary edema and worsen ventilator function. Dehydration on the other hand, while worsening hypotension, can affect renal function leading to acute kidney injury (AKI). Inotropic agents need to be used with caution in this setting as some agents may result in reduction of renal perfusion thus potentiating the AKI. Ideally, invasive monitoring should be utilized to guide fluid management.

Gastrointestinal complications such as aspiration and stress ulcers are common after SCI. Early enteral feeding, if necessary through nasogastric tubes, is important to prevent this complication. For periods of prolonged fasting for surgical procedures, fluids and gastric prophylaxis be ordered accordingly. Acute SCI also carries the risk of gastric distension and ileus, which may lead to aspiration. Placement of orogastric or nasogastric tubes with administration of prokinetic agents may be required in patients.

Bladder drainage is advocated in all SCI patients due to a high likelihood of urinary retention. Furthermore, placement of a Foley catheter also supports the need for close monitoring of fluid status in management of SCI. If a urinary catheter is kept in place for a prolonged period, it is important to always screen for urinary infection in SCI. The urinary tract can sometimes be the source of an occult infection which only becomes obvious when it is disseminated. Patients who are sedated or who have impaired sensation might not be able to complain of symptoms referable to the bladder, thus requiring a high index of suspicion by the treating team.

Metabolic and electrolyte imbalances are common during any acute injury including SCI. Poor glycemic control has been found to predict poor outcome in various forms of trauma. Hyperglycemia may be present in patients who are not known to be previously diabetic. High glucose levels also predispose to infective complications and poor wound healing and thus need to be controlled to acceptable levels. Conversely one should also be vigilant for hypoglycemia which may occur during prolonged fasting. Hypoglycemia also has a potential to worsen any neurological injury and should be addressed quickly. During acute phase of injury, imbalances in sodium, potassium, calcium, and magnesium may all occur and should be tackled appropriately.

Multiple drug requirements in SCI also create issues regarding drug interactions as well as appropriateness of a particular drug type in a particular phase of the injury. For example, when deciding on a sedative agent, the choice will depend on the phase of mechanical ventilation and patient's condition at the time. During the early phase of full mechanical ventilation and neurogenic shock, the choice of midazolam infusion and an opioid are ideal. In the latter phase of weaning these agents may not be appropriate despite their cardiac stability as they cause respiratory depression counteracting the patient's spontaneous breathing effort. Alternatively, propofol infusion may also be used during the acute stage of management. This agent has a faster recovery profile, neuroprotective effects, but it suppresses the cardiovascular system more than other agents. The optimization of inotropic support may overcome this problem. Dexmedetomidine is a central alpha agonist, which does not affect respiration. In acute neurogenic shock state, it can worsen hypotension and bradycardia. Other pharmacological agents utilized in SCI are the high-dose corticosteroids. Corticosteroids became standard practice following the National Acute Spinal Injury Studies (NASCIS) [17]. Recent evidence however suggests that corticosteroids may worsen the outcome after SCI due to increased incidence of complications. It is no longer a standard practice in many neurological centers and recent guidelines have all discouraged their use in SCI [18].

Medical complications after SCI include deep vein thrombosis (DVT) from immobilization as well as pressure sores from a combination of immobility, impaired perfusion, and loss of pain sensation. Both conditions should be screened for and treatment initiated promptly. Early transfer of a patient off a spinal board and care for skin should start right in the emergency department to prevent ulcer formation. A combination of medical anticoagulants as well as mechanical means should be applied as early as possible to reduce the risk of DVT. However in the ICU, patients are best maintained in a rotating spinal bead which eases the administration of nursing care and physiotherapy and allows for any intervention such as traction to be performed with ease. Improper beds without ripple mattresses interfere with nursing care and may also predispose to ulcer formation.

The psychological wellbeing of patients with SCI should not be forgotten. Many patients develop depression (30–40 %), anxiety (20–25 %), or substance related problems (40–50 %) [19, 20]. Every effort should be made to comfort and motivate a patient and to decrease his anxiety. Pharmacological agents should be utilized when necessary and effective communication with the patient and his family is also vital.

Reduction of Safety Barriers

Table 17.1 lists some common measures to reduce safety barriers that may be implemented by any institution involved in the care of patients with SCI. They encompass all staff working with patients and will help promote a safer environment for

Table 17.1 Safety measures

Method	Advantage
Written guidelines	Presence of a well-developed evidence based local guidelines for managing SCI is a vital step for good patient care. Guidelines should include treatment objectives, assessment details as well as decision-making flow charts based on latest available evidence. All staff should be familiarized with the system and adhere to them at all times
Effective teamwork and communication	Good communication from one caregiver to another is important safety measure. Furthermore it helps ensure the continuity of care for a patient. Error reporting is also a part of good communication in order to rectify any problem early without emphasis on placing blame
Skill training	Training of staff in basic skills for managing patients with SCI. Those with prior training should receive refresher sessions at regular intervals to maintain basis as well as updated knowledge
Checklists	Checklist of Items that should be reviewed and adhered to by physicians and nurses at all times
Governance	Audit of complicated cases to ensure improvement of pre-existing treatment policies

patients. The listed methods below when used in unison may have a significant effect in reducing management errors.

Solutions to Potential Risks

In order to reduce potential risks to patients, the described safety measure should be utilized:

Written Guidelines

The following guidelines are aimed at ensuring that patients with SCI are managed by staff of varying knowledge and experience in a manner in which safety is maintained at all times.

Pre-hospital and Emergency Room Care

(a) Spinal cord injury should be suspected in all of the following circumstances:

- Patient with altered consciousness;
- Patients suspected to be under the influence of drugs/alcohol;
- Presence of neck or back pain and tenderness or focal neurological deficits;
- Presence of long bone fractures or distracting injuries.

(b) In potential cases, a rigid collar with a spinal board should be utilized for immobilization and transfer of patient until definitive investigations can be performed. Patients should be rapidly transferred off the spinal board in the Emergency Department onto a firm surface while maintaining alignment of the spine. Care is advised in elderly patients with pre-existent spinal stiffness and rigidity due to degenerative conditions.

(c) Initial evaluation of patients should always be according to the ATLS guidelines – Airway, Breathing, Circulation, etc.

(d) If the patient requires intubation (Table 17.2), it should be performed via rapid sequence intubation only by trained personnel while constantly maintaining inline immobilization of the neck.

(e) Aim to avoid hypotension (middle artery pressure (MAP) >85 mmHg). Other injuries should always be excluded first prior to assigning the cause of hypotension to neurogenic shock.

(f) Management of hypotension related to SCI should involve fluid challenges (up to 2,000 mL) and norepinephrine at 0.05 mcg/kg/min and titrated to maintain MAP >85 mmHg up to 7 days post injury [21].

(g) During secondary survey, a log roll should always be performed by a minimum of five people to ensure that spinal alignment is maintained. Assess for spinal tenderness, step deformities, bruising, as well as loss of rectal tone and reflexes.

(h) Attempts should be made to always reexamine patients brought into a tertiary hospital center in order to detect injuries that might have been overlooked earlier.

(i) Assessment of patients should include motor and sensory function as well as deep tendon reflexes. The level of the injury should be defined as the most caudal segment of spinal cord with normal bilateral motor function (MRC grade >3/5) and sensory function (light touch and pinprick).

(j) Patients should be further classified according to the American Spinal Injury Association (ASIA) classification and the injury defined based on the ASIA Impairment scale [22].

(k) Clearance of the cervical spine is an important management goal and should be done rapidly. Those patients with risk factors for SCI should undergo radiographic investigations.

Table 17.2 Indications for endotracheal intubation in spinal injury

Impaired airway
Altered consciousness (GCS < 8/15), severe maxillofacial injuries, retropharyngeal swelling or hematoma, intoxication with risk of aspiration
Respiratory failure
$PaO_2 < 60$ mmHg
$PaCO_2 > 60$ mmHg
Increased breathing effort with evidence of impending exhaustion
Associated injuries
Traumatic brain injury with raised intracranial pressure or impending herniation,
Multisystem injury with severe hemodynamic instability
Severe burns with possible inhalational injury

(l) Standard cervical spine radiographs (AP, lateral, and open mouth views) should be performed in all patients with suspected trauma.
(m) The radiographs should visualize from the level of C1 to T1.
(n) CT scanning should be performed if the spine is inadequately visualized or when the radiographs are found to be abnormal. In patients with clinical features highly suggestive of injury, a CT of the spine should also be performed. Alternatively dynamic flexion/extension view radiography may be performed in cooperative patients or with experienced senior staff.
(o) Magnetic resonance imaging is indicated in the presence of neurological findings suggestive of cord injury.
(p) All radiological investigations should ideally be reported by a radiologist or medical officer with at least 3 years of experience.
(q) Injury can be ruled out clinically in the absence of neck pain or tenderness, altered consciousness or intoxication, neurological deficit and painful distracting injuries. Normal CT and radiographs in conjunction with negative MRI or dynamic radiographs within 48 h of a SCI can be used to rule out a cervical spine injury.
(r) Clearance of the cervical spine does not indicate absence of injury in other segments of the spinal cord and these should be investigated according to the symptoms of the patient and suspected level of injury.
(s) Always screen for spinal cord injury in patients who suffer from electrocution by high voltage currents as well after diving accidents.
(t) Patients with suspected SCI should receive adequate analgesia and sedation with intravenous opioids and sedatives as indicated.
(u) An indwelling catheter for urinary drainage should be inserted when any form of SCI is suspected.
(v) All members of the managing team should be aware of the diagnosis and this should be communicated effectively to the patient's next of kin.
(w) If available, patients with SCI should be transferred early to specialized SCI centers for further management as it is associated with better outcome [23].

Neurointensive Care Management

To prevent secondary injury and maximize recovery, patients with SCI should ideally be managed in an ICU setting.

(a) Patients should be nursed in a spinal rotator bed.
(b) Immobilization is continued when patients are found undergoing SCI pending definitive treatment.
(c) When traction is indicated it should be performed using a Gardner Wells Tongs device progressively increasing incremental weights in accordance to the level of injury.

   Radiographic and clinical vigilance at frequent time intervals is necessary to prevent worsening of pre-existing injuries. Traction should be reduced or discontinued in the presence of increasing pain or neurological deficits. Traction for prolonged periods is not advised due to the high incidence of complications from prolonged bed rest.

(d) Surgical intervention for SCI is aimed at decompressing neural structures and maintaining mechanical stability. This may be done either using external immobilization device or via open reduction and internal fixation. Patients with incomplete injury or with bilateral cervical facet dislocation are the ideal candidates for reduction. Reduction in a complete SCI may be considered to assist in the nursing and rehabilitative care of the patient.

(e) Airway management: Emergency intubation must be performed via rapid sequence induction with stabilization and alignment of the spine as mentioned before. Cricoid pressure when used should be performed via a double-handed technique to reduce cervical spine movement. This technique utilizes the right hand to apply pressure backwards, upwards, and to the right (BURP), while the left hand supports the back of the neck. Intubation adjunct devices such as the "gum elastic Bougie" are useful in assisting intubation. Video laryngoscopy with a levering laryngoscope or awake fiberoptic intubation is a useful alternative to regular laryngoscopy in order to facilitate visualization of the vocal cord with minimal movement of the neck in elective or semi-urgent circumstances.

(f) Up to 20 % of SCI patients will require a tracheostomy as part of their ICU management. Those patients with pre-existing medical conditions, pre-morbid lung disease, high ASIA levels, and with evidence of pneumonia are particularly suitable for early tracheostomy. Performing this procedure is noted to shorten the ICU stay and improve functional outcome in patients [24] Both open as well as percutaneous tracheostomy have been found to be safe in SCI patients [16].

(g) Ventilator management: SCI patients initially require high ventilator setting with application of adequate pressure support and PEEP. Aim to keep $PaO2 > 60$ mmHg and $PaCO2$ between 35 and 45 mmHg. Weaning is dependent on the response of the patient.

(h) When managing the cardiovascular system, aim to maintain $MAP > 85$ mmHg as well as euvolemia [21]. Adequate fluid resuscitation should be initiated followed by inotropic support during neurogenic shock to prevent secondary injury. Aside from fluid resuscitation, inotropes would often be needed to maintain target BP. The choice of inotropic agents includes either dopamine, phenylephrine, or norepinephrine. However, no clear evidence favoring any agent is available at present. Vigilant monitoring is required. Symptomatic bradycardia should also be treated with vasopressors with combined alpha and beta adrenergic actions unless contraindicated [25].

(i) Gastrointestinal: Enteral feeding should be started as soon as possible and ideally within 12 h of admission. Gastric ulcer prophylaxis must be given if patients need to be fasting for a prolonged period of time. In the presence of high aspirate output from feeding tubes, electrolyte levels should be checked and if normal, prokinetic drugs such as metoclopramide or erythromycin may be utilized. Patients with SCI are often constipated and may require the use of laxatives or enemas to aid bowel clearance. Daily monitoring of frequency of bowel opening together with abdominal distension should be done. Conversely, diarrhea may also occur and in such a case, the electrolytes, feeding regime as well as other medications should be reviewed.

(j) Urine output should ideally be in the range of 0.5–1.0 mL/kg/h. Daily balance charts are mandatory to monitor fluid states. Continuous bladder drainage is usually performed in the acute phase in all suspected SCI. The catheter should be regularly reviewed to rule out kinks or blockage of the tube. Once the patient's hemodynamic status improves and they are no longer on intravenous fluids, the bladder catheter may be weaned off. In patients with a neurogenic bladder, it is necessary to evaluate the volume of residual urine in the bladder if catheter is removed, as either continuous or intermittent drainage may be required. Signs of infection should also always be screened for. The urinary drainage catheter should be replaced at regular intervals and signs of calculi or fistula formation should be looked for.

(k) Thromboembolism prophylaxis- All patients with SCI should have graduated compression stockings applied. In the ICU, pneumatic compression devices are preferred. Thrombosis prophylaxis should be started as soon as possible (within 72 h) if there are no contraindications, such as planned surgery or coagulopathy. Prophylaxis can be started between 48 and 72 h post operatively. Low-molecular-weight heparin (LMWH) is the current agent of choice [25].

(l) Glycemic Control. All patients admitted to the ICU after SCI should receive glucose monitoring. Maintain blood glucose levels <10 mmol/L. In the acute phase, insulin drips can be started to achieve the target range.

(m) Once a patient has been admitted with SCI, early involvement of a physiotherapist and occupational therapist is advised. Patient should be nursed in a rotator bed and turned at regular intervals. Patients with evidence of neuropathic pain or spasticity are treated with agents such as gabapentin, pregabalin, and baclofen to relieve symptoms.

(n) To reduce patient stress and anxiety, early education of the patient and family knowledge is needed. Patients should be referred to a neuropsychologist early for motivation and for help in planning goals and targets. Patient problems and concerns should be heard and addressed as best as possible. Mood stabilizers may sometimes be needed.

Effective Teamwork and Communication

All members of the health care team need to be informed of any major issues in the management of patients. In order to promote such circumstances, a sign-out meeting or combined rounds are ideally held every morning for all residents and consultants to discuss and be updated of the progress of a patient. Nursing staff should also perform sign-out rounds during the beginning of each shift.

Interdisciplinary rounds, involving physicians as well as nursing and rehabilitation teams, case management and social workers, should be done at least once a week to ensure all aspects of management are reviewed, planned, and discussed.

Skill Training

Regular courses training staff in basic skills pertaining to SCI Care should be conducted. Accreditation should be given to staff once they acquired such skills and only then they would be suited to manage patients with SCI.

Checklists

Checklists will ensure no step in treatment is overlooked or missed. Each center should have its own series of checklists for SCI patients admitted to the ICU.

Governance

Audits should be conducted monthly to review morbidity and mortality related to SCI.

Discussion of Risk/Benefit Ratios in the Management of SCI

The risk/benefit ratio of vital aspects of SCI management will be discussed in Table 17.3.

Summary

Risks to patients with SCI are omnipresent in the pre-hospital as well as intensive care phase of treatment. The first step in managing these risks is the awareness of their exact etiology, nature as well as their causative factors. Subsequently, by adhering to safety barriers and evidence-based guidelines, these risk factors may be minimized and complications reduced. A team-based approach by all members of the health care team together with effective communication holds the key to safe and optimal patient management in SCI.

Dos and Don'ts

Pre-hospital and Emergency Care Phase

Dos

- Always systematically evaluate patients to avoid missing injuries
- Immobilize patients early when spine injury is suspected
- Exercise caution during neck manipulation for airway management
- Provide fluid and inotropic resuscitation to prevent hypotension
- Ensure technical adequacy of all radiological investigations before making any conclusions based on them
- Insert bladder drainage and gastric tubes early in patients requiring them

Don'ts

- Do not rush to transfer a patient without adequate pre-hospital resuscitation
- Do not keep patient immobilized for prolonged periods especially on rigid spinal boards
- Do not intubate without inline immobilization
- Do not assume that hypotension is due to SCI without ruling out other causes first
- Do not hesitate to consult a senior colleague is unsure about findings on radiological investigations

Neurocritical Care Phase

Dos

- Manage SCI patients in designated ICU setting
- Adequately secure the ET tubes or other adjunctive airway devices to prevent dislodgement and hypoxemia
- Provide adequate sedation/analgesia as indicated
- Perform traction under close monitoring and always perform a check x-ray after the procedure
- Be aware of indications for emergent surgical management of SCI
- Regularly reassess a patient's neurological status
- Start early enteral feeding
- Administer thromboembolism prophylaxis
- Perform early tracheostomy when indicated
- Address psychological issues pertaining to the patient
- Communicate effectively

Table 17.3 Discussion of the risk/benefit ratio in the management of SCI

Risk stratification	Identification of patients at risk of SCI is vital due to the significant morbidity and mortality related to this condition. Early studies have estimated that between 2 and 5 % of patients sustaining blunt trauma have associated injuries to the cervical spine [26]. In conscious patients, neck tenderness, focal neurological deficits, and distracting injuries have been validated as a highly sensitive method of detecting SCI particularly of the cervical spine [6]. In unconscious patients, such as those with suspected head injury, often a higher index of suspicion needs to be exercised. The presence of severe head injury was noted to be significantly associated with cervical SCI (odds ratio 8.5) by *Hackl et al.* In persistently unconscious patients and those with focal neurological deficits the Odds Ratios to have an associated SCI were 14 and 58 respectively [27]. The need for stratifying patients with potential SCI identification is related to the need for immobilization as well as early transfer to a specialized center for SCI management. A systematic review of literature by *Parent et al.* has revealed a significant reduction in the length of stay and decreased overall mortality following early transfer to specialized centers caring for SCI patients [23]
Immobilization	When SCI is suspected, the generally accepted standard of care is that the neck should be immobilized using a rigid collar and hard spinal board [28]. A Cochrane review by *Kwan et al.* did not find any conclusive evidence of improved outcome with immobilization [10]. Immobilization has been found to limit spine movement to only 5 % of normal range with the hope of reducing any further worsening of an unstable SCI. Immobilization is, however, associated with complications such as pressure sore formation as well as difficulty in mouth opening and airway management. *Goutcher et al.* noted that an excess of 20 % of patients had a mouth opening of less than or equal to 20 mm when wearing a rigid collar. Airways were also noted to become grade III or IV on laryngoscopy evaluation in patients who are immobilized with a collar [29]. Despite these findings, collars are still widely used possibly due to a lack of other convenient and suitable options [30]

Table 17.3 (continued)

Airway management	Practice patterns of airway management have evolved with the advent of advanced intubation adjunctive devices. Currently awake fiberoptic intubation and video laryngoscopy are the most preferred options to use when intubating an SCI patient. The choice of which one to utilize would depend on a physician's familiarity with the risk and benefit analysis of each method. Fiberoptic intubation is useful in conscious cooperative patients in an elective or semi-urgent situation. It however can become challenging if patients are anxious and uncooperative or if there are blood and other secretions in the airway [30]. Video laryngoscopy is advantageous due to its indirect nature and angulation that results in less force used during laryngeal viewing and tube insertion. The degree of mouth opening required is also less using this modality and this is particularly advantageous in patients with rigid collar mobilization. This modality though not requiring patient cooperation, still can be challenging in an emergency situation or if the airway is blocked with secretions. The alternative in emergency situations would be to use direct laryngoscopy. This method has been found to be safe and effective if done by experienced persons [31]. *Ong et al.* have noted in a prospective study that direct laryngoscopy was faster in normal airways and at least equivalent to fiberoptic and video laryngoscopy in difficult airways [32]. Further studies reviewing differences in operator experience as well using actual patients are still required to make this comparison more valid
	Tracheostomy is often necessary when patients require prolonged ventilation in the ICU. *Branco et al.* have noted that one-fifth of patients with SCI will require tracheostomy. Independent risk factors predicting the need for tracheostomy include patients requiring intubation at the scene or in the emergency department, complete cervical SCI at C1-C4 or C5-C7 levels, Injury severity score $\geq$16, facial fracture, and thoracic trauma [33]. Tracheostomy when performed early (<7 days) has been found to be associated with favorable effects in patients with traumatic SCI [16]

(continued)

Table 17.3 (continued)

Blood pressure targets	Evidence from multiple historical cohorts have noted that maintaining MAP > 85 mm for 7 days maybe associated with better functional outcome [21]. However, there is concern regarding complications that may arise such as worsening of ischemic heart disease, hypertension, renal insufficiency, and pulmonary edema. Thus management should be guided by invasive devices to avoid overzealous BP management. Additionally, it has been noted by *Kong et al.* that despite the application of strict targets for MAP, patients with cervical SCI and thoracic SCI were found to have 18.4 % and 35.9 % of their BP readings respectively below 80 mmHg despite being managed in specialized ICU settings. This highlights the point that constant vigilance is as important as target setting in effective hemodynamic management of patients with SCI [34]
Steroids in SCI	High-dose methylprednisolone was found to result in significantly improved motor function and sensation in patients with complete and incomplete SCI by the National Acute Spinal Cord Injury (NASCIS) II and III [35–37] Following these studies, steroid therapy became widely used in acute SCI. In recent times however, the findings of these studies have received criticism due to flaws in randomization, statistical analysis, and clinical end points used [38]. Steroid therapy was found to be associated with an increased risk of infection and avascular necrosis. Thus at present the use of steroids are no longer recommended in SCI due to lack of medical evidence in support and their association with complications
Timing for surgery	At present, no defined standard exists regarding the timing of decompression and stabilization in SCI. Emergency decompression of the spinal cord has been suggested in the setting of progressive neurologic deterioration, facet dislocation, or bilateral locked facets. Surgery can also be done for spinal nerve impingement with progressive radiculopathy and in patients with extradural lesions such as epidural hematomas and for cauda equina syndrome
	Studies from the 1960s and 1970s showed no improvement with emergent surgical decompression. In the late 1990s, two authors reported improved neurologic outcomes with early stabilization. *Gaebler et al.* reported that early decompression and stabilization procedures within 8 h of injury allowed for a higher rate of neurologic recovery [39]. *Mirza et al.* also reported that stabilization within 72 h of injury in cervical spinal cord injury improved neurologic outcomes [40]. *Vaccaro et al.,* however, noted in their prospective randomized controlled trial that no significant difference was seen between patients who underwent early or late surgery [41]
	Preliminary data from the Surgical Treatment for Acute Spinal Cord Injury Study (STASCIS) has found that early surgery may be associated with better outcome. It was noted that 24 % of patients who underwent decompressive surgery within 24 h experience a 2-grade or better improvement on the ASIA scale, compared with only 4 % of those in the delayed-treatment group. Furthermore, the study found that cardiopulmonary and urinary tract complications were higher in the delayed group compared to 48.6 % [11]. The final results of this study will hopefully help guide decisions for timing of surgery in future

Table 17.3 (continued)

Gastrointestinal management	It is accepted practice that early (within 72 h) enteral feeding improves outcome in critically ill patients. However, therapeutic interventions or patient condition may often not allow the early initiation of feeding. *Rowan et al.* have noted that enteral feeding can be safely initiated in patients in the acute phase SCI without significant complications [42]. Despite the general acceptance of the importance of early feeding, one randomized study has noted no significant difference in infection rates, nutritional status, feeding complications, and length of hospital stay between SCI patients receiving early and late feeding. The possible explanation for this finding maybe related to the fact that patients in this study also received high-dose steroid therapy which may negate any positive infection reduction effects mediated by early feeding
Bladder drainage	Drainage of the urinary bladder is generally indicated in patients with SCI particularly after trauma. Options for drainage include an indwelling Foley catheter, suprapubic cystostomy, intermittent catheterization, or combined consecutive methods. Intermittent catheterization has been found to be associated with the shortest time from injury to established micturition. Incidence of complications was also higher when indwelling Foley catheters were used compared to other methods of drainage [43]. Despite this finding, Foley catheters are still widely used due to the ease of insertion, especially in an acute setting. Increasing popularity of intermittent catheterization has been noted, but it has still not superseded the use of indwelling catheters as yet. Some authors now advocate the consecutive use of an indwelling catheter in the acute setting with conversion to intermittent catheterization as soon as possible
Thromboembolism prophylaxis	Thromboembolism prophylaxis is accepted as the standard of care for patients in the acute stage after SCI. Level I evidence exist that support the usage of mechanical prophylaxis such as a compression stockings or pneumatic devices in both legs of all patients for at least the first 2 weeks after acute SCI. In addition to mechanical methods, administration of an adjuvant thromboprophylactic drug such as low-molecular-weight heparin within the first 72 h is recommended if there are no contraindications such as active bleeding or coagulopathy. When a thromboembolism is diagnosed, patients will definitely require therapeutic anticoagulant therapy. In view of the risk of bleeding associated with this therapy, there is a need to weigh the potential benefits and risks for each patient in the process of decision making [25]

Don'ts

- Do not manage SCI patients in general wards
- Do not allow ETT dislodgement or occlusion to occur especially during patient transfer
- Do not wait for the patient to complain of pain before administering analgesia
- Do not perform traction without adequate monitoring

- Do not delay surgery in SCI cases if emergent intervention is indicated
- Do not assume that neurological deficits remain static after the injury
- Do not withhold feeding unnecessarily
- Do not miss electrolyte and glycemic abnormalities
- Do not delay thromboembolism prophylaxis including anticoagulant medications
- Do not delay physiotherapy

References

1. Stevens RD, Bhardwaj A, Kirsch JR, Mirski MA. Critical care and perioperative management in traumatic spinal cord injury. J Neurosurg Anesthesiol. 2003;15:215–29.
2. Oyinbo CA. Secondary injury mechanisms in traumatic spinal cord injury: a nugget of this multiply cascade. Acta Neurobiol Exp (Wars). 2011;71:281–99.
3. Rossignol S, Schwab M, Schwartz M, Fehlings MG. Spinal cord injury: time to move? J Neurosci. 2007;27:11782–92.
4. Macciocchi S, Seel RT, Thompson N, Byams R, Bowman B. Spinal cord injury and co-occurring traumatic brain injury: assessment and incidence. Arch Phys Med Rehabil. 2008;89:1350–7.
5. Hoffman JR, Wolfson AB, Todd K, Mower WR. Selective cervical spine radiography in blunt trauma: methodology of the National Emergency X-Radiography Utilization Study (NEXUS). Ann Emerg Med. 1998;32:461–9.
6. Hoffman JR, Mower WR, Wolfson AB, Todd KH, Zucker MI. Validity of a set of clinical criteria to rule out injury to the cervical spine in patients with blunt trauma. N Engl J Med. 2000;343:94–9.
7. Stiell IG, et al. The Canadian C-spine rule for radiography in alert and stable trauma patients. JAMA J Am Med Assoc. 2001;286:1841–8.
8. Holmes JF, Akkinepalli R. Computed tomography versus plain radiography to screen for cervical spine injury: a meta-analysis. J Trauma Injury Infect Crit Care. 2005;58:902–5.
9. Blackmore CC, Ramsey SD, Mann FA, Deyo RA. Cervical spine screening with CT in trauma patients: a cost-effectiveness analysis 1. Radiology. 1999;212:117–25.
10. Kwan I, Bunn F, Roberts I. Spinal immobilisation for trauma patients. Cochrane Database Syst Rev. 2001;(2):CD002803.
11. Fehlings MG, et al. Early versus delayed decompression for traumatic cervical spinal cord injury: results of the Surgical Timing in Acute Spinal Cord Injury Study (STASCIS). PLoS One. 2012;7:e32037.
12. De Vivo MJ, Stuart Krause J, Lammertse DP. Recent trends in mortality and causes of death among persons with spinal cord injury. Arch Phys Med Rehabil. 1999;80:1411–9.
13. Frankel H, et al. Long-term survival in spinal cord injury: a fifty year investigation. Spinal Cord. 1998;36:266–74.
14. Claxton AR, Wong DT, Chung F, Fehlings MG. Predictors of hospital mortality and mechanical ventilation in patients with cervical spinal cord injury. Can J Anaesth. 1998;45:144–9.
15. Wicks A, Menter R. Long-term outlook in quadriplegic patients with initial ventilator dependency. Chest J. 1986;90:406–10.
16. Ganuza JR, et al. Effect of technique and timing of tracheostomy in patients with acute traumatic spinal cord injury undergoing mechanical ventilation. J Spinal Cord Med. 2011;34:76–84.
17. Bracken MB. Steroids for acute spinal cord injury. Cochrane Database Syst Rev. 2012;1, CD001046.
18. Walters BC, et al. Guidelines for the management of acute cervical spine and spinal cord injuries: 2013 update. Clin Neurosurg. 2013;60:82–91.
19. Kennedy P, Rogers BA. Anxiety and depression after spinal cord injury: a longitudinal analysis. Arch Phys Med Rehabil. 2000;81:932–7.

20. Kolakowsky-Hayner SA, et al. Post-injury substance abuse among persons with brain injury and persons with spinal cord injury. Brain Inj. 2002;16:583–92.
21. Casha S, Christie S. A systematic review of intensive cardiopulmonary management after spinal cord injury. J Neurotrauma. 2011;28:1479–95.
22. American Spinal Injury Association, American Paralysis Association. International standards for neurological and functional classification of spinal cord injury. Chicago: American Spinal Injury Association; 1996.
23. Parent S, Barchi S, LeBreton M, Casha S, Fehlings MG. The impact of specialized centers of care for spinal cord injury on length of stay, complications, and mortality: a systematic review of the literature. J Neurotrauma. 2011;28:1363–70.
24. Harrop JS, Sharan AD, Scheid Jr EH, Vaccaro AR, Przybylski GJ. Tracheostomy placement in patients with complete cervical spinal cord injuries: American Spinal Injury Association Grade A. J Neurosurg Spine. 2004;100:20–3.
25. Furlan JC, Fehlings MG. Cardiovascular complications after acute spinal cord injury: pathophysiology, diagnosis, and management. Neurosurg Focus. 2008;25:E13.
26. Crosby ET, Lui A. The adult cervical spine: implications for airway management. Can J Anaesth. 1990;37:77–93.
27. Hackl W, Hausberger K, Sailer R, Ulmer H, Gassner R. Prevalence of cervical spine injuries in patients with facial trauma. Oral Surg Oral Med Oral Pathol Oral Radiol Endod. 2001;92:370–6.
28. Ahn H, et al. Pre-hospital care management of a potential spinal cord injured patient: a systematic review of the literature and evidence-based guidelines. J Neurotrauma. 2011;28:1341–61.
29. Goutcher C, Lochhead V. Reduction in mouth opening with semi-rigid cervical collars. Br J Anaesth. 2005;95:344–8.
30. Austin N, Krishnamoorthy V, Dagal A. Airway management in cervical spine injury. Int J Crit Illn Inj Sci. 2014;4:50.
31. Stephens CT, Kahntroff S, Dutton RP. The success of emergency endotracheal intubation in trauma patients: a 10-year experience at a major adult trauma referral center. Anesth Analg. 2009;109:866–72.
32. Ong JR, et al. Comparing the performance of traditional direct laryngoscope with three indirect laryngoscopes: a prospective manikin study in normal and difficult airway scenarios. Emerg Med Australas. 2011;23:606–14.
33. Branco BC, et al. Incidence and clinical predictors for tracheostomy after cervical spinal cord injury: a National Trauma Databank review. J Trauma Acute Care Surg. 2011;70:111–5.
34. Kong C, et al. A prospective evaluation of hemodynamic management in acute spinal cord injury patients. Spinal Cord. 2013;51:466–71.
35. Bracken MB, et al. Methylprednisolone and neurological function 1 year after spinal cord injury: results of the National Acute Spinal Cord Injury Study. J Neurosurg. 1985;63:704–13.
36. Bracken MB, et al. Administration of methylprednisolone for 24 or 48 hours or tirilazad mesylate for 48 hours in the treatment of acute spinal cord injury: results of the Third National Acute Spinal Cord Injury Randomized Controlled Trial. JAMA. 1997;277:1597–604.
37. Bracken MB. Steroids for acute spinal cord injury. Cochrane Database Syst Rev. 2002;3, CD001046.
38. Sayer FT, Kronvall E, Nilsson OG. Methylprednisolone treatment in acute spinal cord injury: the myth challenged through a structured analysis of published literature. Spine J. 2006;6:335–43.
39. Gaebler C, Maier R, Kutscha-Lissberg F, Mrkonjic L, Vecsei V. Results of spinal cord decompression and thoracolumbar pedicle stabilisation in relation to the time of operation. Spinal Cord. 1999;37:33–9.
40. Mirza SK, et al. Early versus delayed surgery for acute cervical spinal cord injury. Clin Orthop Relat Res. 1999;359:104–14.
41. Vaccaro AR, et al. Neurologic outcome of early versus late surgery for cervical spinal cord injury. Spine. 1997;22:2609–13.
42. Rowan C, Gillanders L, Paice R, Judson J. Is early enteral feeding safe in patients who have suffered spinal cord injury? Injury. 2004;35:238–42.
43. Wyndaele J, De Sy W, Claessens H. Evaluation of different methods of bladder drainage used in the early care of spinal cord injury patients. Spinal Cord. 1985;23:18–26.

Chapter 18
Care for Complications After Catastrophic Brain Injury

Vera Spatenkova and Nehad Nabeel Mohamed AL-Shirawi

Introduction

The target of neurocritical care is maintenance of intracranial and systemic (extracranial) homeostasis including prevention, timely detection, and treatment of all systemic complications (Table 18.1). These systemic complications could potentially cause secondary brain damage, thereby influencing the mortality and outcome of neurocritically ill patients.

Due to the variety of cases admitted to the neurointensive care unit (NICU), nontraumatic subarachnoid hemorrhage will be taken as an example to describe the complications associated with catastrophic brain injury.

Case Scenario

A 34-year-old woman weighing 74 kg with a subarachnoid hemorrhage (SAH) of Hunt and Hess grade I, modified Fisher grade 2, from a gigantic aneurysm of the left internal carotid artery underwent coiling. Three days after SAH, she had polyuria 4.5 L/day, serum sodium (SNa^+) was 130 mmol/L, measured serum osmolality (SOsm) amounted to 265 mmol/kg (hypoosmolar hyponatremia), serum urea was 2.4 mmol/L, serum creatinine 58 umol/L, specific urine weight was low with 1,005 kg/m^3, and electrolyte-free water clearance (EWC) was 0.016 mL/s (not an abnormal

V. Spatenkova, MD, PhD (✉)
Neurointensive Care Unit, Neurocenter, Liberec, Czech Republic
e-mail: vera.spatenkova@nemlib.cz

N.N.M. AL-Shirawi, MRCP
King Abdulla Medical City, Makka, Kingdom of Saudi Arabia

© Springer International Publishing Switzerland 2015
K.E. Wartenberg et al. (eds.), *Neurointensive Care: A Clinical Guide to Patient Safety*, DOI 10.1007/978-3-319-17293-4_18

Table 18.1 Systemic	Systemic complications
complications in neurocritical care	Hyp-/hyperoxia
	Hypo-/hypercapnia
	Hyperthermia
	Hypo-/hypertension
	Anemia
	Coagulopathy
	Hypo-/hyperglycemia
	Hypo-/hypernatremia
	Hypomagnesemia
	Hypophosphatemia
	Hypothyreosis
	Hypocortisolism
	Panhypopituitarism
	Uremia
	Hepatic encephalopathy
	Sepsis

response to the antidiuretic hormone (ADH), ADH-renal axis). She received desmopressin acetate (DDAVP) 10 ug/day. The next day, her SNa$^+$ was 128 mmol/L, SOsm amounted to 263 mmol/kg. (Free water polyuria without an abnormal response to the ADH-renal axis in hypoosmolar hyponatremia was not an indication for desmopressin administration, because it decreases SNa$^+$). Therapy with fludrocortisone was administered over the next few days and the patient's fluid balance and serum sodium returned to normal values.

Metabolic Complications

Acid-Base Disorders

Acidosis, Acidemia – Arterial pH <7.35

Respiratory acidosis with an increase in carbon dioxide (*hypercapnia* defined as partial pressure of arterial carbon dioxide (PaCO$_2$) >45 mmHg/6 kPa) due to hypoventilation in relation to an increase in CO$_2$ production by shivering, and fever poses a risk for cerebral vasodilation, increasing cerebral blood volume (vascular compartment), and intracranial hypertension. Respiratory acidosis can represent a primary or secondary compensation of metabolic alkalosis.

Metabolic acidosis is defined by a decrease in bicarbonate (HCO$_3^-$<22 mmol/L) and base excess (BE<−3 mmol/L). Risk factors for metabolic acidosis include (1) a decrease of the strong ion difference (SID) from increasing chloride (hyperchloridemia – infusion of unbuffered hypertonic sodium chloride), an increase in strong anions (ketoacidosis in diabetes mellitus, starvation and alcoholism, lactic acidosis, intoxication), dilution by water (hyponatremia); (2) an increase in nonvolatile weak acids (hyperphosphatemia).

Alkalosis, Alkalemia – Arterial pH >7.45

Respiratory alkalosis is caused by a decrease in $PaCO_2$ (hypocapnia defined as $PaCO_2 < 35$ mmHg, 4.6 kPa) due to hyperventilation in relation to CO_2 production (decreased in hypothermia), which puts the patient at risk for cerebral vasoconstriction and hypoxemia. Respiratory alkalosis can represent a primary or secondary compensation of metabolic acidosis. *Metabolic alkalosis* is a consequence of an increase of HCO_3^- (>26 mmol/L) and BE (>3 mmol/L). Risk factors encompass (1) an increase in SID with chloride depletion (hypochloridemia) or water deficit (concentrated alkalosis, hypernatremia), and (2) a decrease in nonvolatile weak acid (hypoalbuminemia, hypophosphatemia).

Discussion of Risks for Patient's Safety

Acid-base disorders pose a higher risk for patient's safety if they occur acutely and consist of combination of both acidosis and alkalosis along with a massive electrolyte disorder. In a combined acidosis–alkalosis disorder, the blood pH does not necessarily change. Before starting treatment it is important to determine the cause of the disturbance. Respiratory disorders are caused by a disturbance of CO_2 elimination. Metabolic disorders are a result of a change to the amount of acidifying and alkalizing substances. Safe management of metabolic disorders requires calculation of parameters such as SID, anion gap, corrected chloride, unmeasured anions, and measurement of lactate. Early recognition of these disorders necessitates regular checks of the acid-base-status, evaluation, and early treatment initiation once a trend toward a disorder becomes obvious.

Protocol to Overcome Barriers to Patient's Safety

- Obtain arterial blood gas measurement, capnometry (end tidal CO_2), in all mechanically ventilated patients.
- Target value of pH 7.35–7.45.
- Adjust mechanical ventilation to target value of pCO_2 (35–45 mmHg, 4.6–6 kPa).
- Hyperventilation causing hypocapnia ($pCO_2 < 35$ mmHg, 4.6 kPa) is only permitted for <30 min in patients with intractable intracranial hypertension as a bridge to more definite relief of increased intracranial pressure.
- Elimination of medications for suppression of respiratory drive in awake patients.
- Prevention/treatment of metabolic acid-base disorders: ketoacidosis in diabetes mellitus with fluid replacement and insulin, lactic acidosis – goal-directed therapy of the sepsis, consideration for renal replacement therapy [1].

Hypo- and Hypernatremia

Sodium is the main extracellular cation maintaining the effective osmolality of extracellular fluid (ECF). Sodium changes in the ECF are balanced by a shift of water between ECF and intracellular fluid (ICF) spaces. Hyponatremia leads to intracellular edema, and hypernatremia results in dehydration of the cells. Dysnatremias are common and serious complications in neurocritical care. Hyponatremia occurs more frequently, but hypernatremia is prognostically more serious. Serum sodium (SNa^+) >160 mmol/L is an independent risk factor for higher mortality (2,3). Risk factors for dysnatremias include (1) brain injury, (2) administration of medications during neurocritical care, (3) iatrogenic conditions.

Hyponatremia

Hyponatremia is defined as *SNa+ <135 mmol/L* (mild 134–130, moderate 129–125, severe 125 mmol/L). Hypoosmolar hyponatremia leads to brain swelling. Clinical signs of hyponatremia comprise seizures (convulsive or nonconvulsive), alterations of consciousness such as delirium, somnolence to coma.

The first step in the management of hyponatremia is measurement of serum osmolarity (SOsm) utilizing an osmometer. The calculated osmolality is not accurate, especially in the presence of an unmeasured osmotic substance such as mannitol and alcohol. Hyponatremia is not always associated with hypoosmolality (hypotonicity); it can be normoosmolar or hyperosmolar (hypertonicity). Hyperglycemia (an increase of glucose >5.5 mmol/L (100 mg/dL) lowers serum sodium by 1.6 mmol/L) (1) Hyperglycemia, (2) Increased urea concentration, (3) Mannitol, (4) Alcohol cause hyperosmolar hyponatremia, so does increased urea concentration, mannitol, alcohol).

Hyponatremia is caused by

1. Sodium loss – renal: hypoaldosteronism, cerebral salt wasting (CSW), or extra-renal: gastrointestinal tract (vomiting, diarrhea);
2. Free water retention – renal: syndrome of inappropriate secretion of ADH (SIADH, iatrogenic drug-associated SIADH – desmopressin acetate administration in normal response of the ADH-renal axis), hypocortisolism (corticosteroids in brain tumor), or extrarenal: polydypsia, infusion of hypotonic saline. CSW and SIADH are the most common causes for hyponatremia in neurocritical care, especially in the patient with subarachnoid hemorrhage.

Safe management requires measured and calculated renal function parameters from a 24-h urine collection to diagnose extrarenal losses of sodium (urine Na 10 mmol/L), natriuresis in CSW and ADH-renal axis response, the organism's compensatory response to hypotonicity (EWC 0.116 mL/s) in polydypsia, hypotonic saline or abnormal response in SIADH (EWC 0.006 mL/s). The appropriate therapy is geared toward the cause: fluid replacement with isotonic saline in cerebral salt wasting syndrome and fluid intake restriction in SIADH always ensuring euvolemia. SNa$^+$ needs to be checked at close intervals during sodium correction to avoid rapid alterations posing the patient at risk for pontine or extrapontine osmotic demyelination syndrome, the maximal change recommended is 6–8 mmol/L SNa$^+$ per day.

Hypernatremia

Hypernatremia is defined as *SNa+ >150 mmol/L* (mild 151–155, moderate 156–160, severe 160 mmol/L). Clinical signs result from brain dehydration and include confusion, seizures, and coma. Hypernatremia arises during an increase in the concentration of sodium in ECF in relation to water. Risk factors encompass the following:

(1) Sodium retention – extrarenal: use of salt, infusion of hypertonic saline.
(2) Free water loss – renal: free water diuresis in central or nephrogenic diabetes insipidus (DI), osmotic diuresis in glycosuria, urea, mannitol, furosemide (more water than sodium is lost from lower reabsorbtion of ions in the ascending loop of Henle and distal tubule), renal failure, or extrarenal: loss of water from the gastrointestinal tract in diarrhea, from the skin in sweating, fever, burns. Hypernatremia is always hyperosmolar (hypertonicity). Central DI (CDI) is rare in neurocritical care. Most hypernatremias have multifactorial causes: osmotherapy, forced diuresis, renal failure. The treatment is according to the mechanism, in CDI intravenous desmopressin should be given according to the specific gravity of urine <1.005. The safety threshold of SNa$^+$ correction to avoid osmotic demyelination syndrome (ODS) is 6–8 mmol/L/day.

Discussion of Risks for Patient's Safety

Dysnatremias are some of the most frequent and serious complications in neurocritical care. Daily monitoring of serum sodium should be part of the daily care of every patient with acute brain disease. Standardized sodium management in neurocritical care includes target values of SNa$^+$ to define therapy, such as SNa$^+$ <135 mmol and 155–160 mmol/L.

This protocol can reduce the iatrogenic causes of dysnatremias, ensure maintenance of fluid balance without use of hypotonic saline, and prevent administration of desmopressin in normonatremia and polyuria with low specific urine weight (normal response the ADH-renal axis). Diagnostic management of hyponatremia is more difficult in clinical practice than of hypernatremia. The first step is measurement of SOsm, followed by assessment of the ADH-renal axis and volume status.

Protocol to Overcome Barriers to Patient's Safety

- Daily assessment of SNa^+ in neurocritical care patients.
- Definition of hyponatremia as SNa^+ <135 mmol/L; hypernatremia SNa^+ >150 mmol/L.
- Maintain fluid balance: fluid intake of 40 mL/kg weight/day in BMI <25; in BMI >25, use adjusted body weight, calculate output from diuresis, drainage, water loss caused by fever (200 mL per 1 °C above 37 °C) or sweating.
- Thiazide should not be used in hypo/normonatremia; it can be used in hypernatremia (non-CDI).
- Desmopressin is the causal therapy of CDI and should not be used in polyuria from a normal of ADH-renal axis response, that is, in hypo/normonatremia.
- Therapy according to set target levels of SNa^+. Check SNa^+ 4–6 h, maximum increase in sodium is 6–8 mmol/L/day [2, 3].

Dos and Don'ts in Metabolic Disorders

Dos

- Keep the target value of pH 7.35–7.45
- Regularly measure serum lactate
- Avoid hypophosphatemia
- Avoid hypomagnesemia
- Actively search for hypo-/hypernatremia
- Measure serum osmolality by osmometer in hyponatremia
- Maintain fluid balance with the aim of keeping euvolemia by SVV or PPV
- Prevent ODS by not exceeding the planned target levels of SNa^+ and checking SNa^+ at frequent intervals

Don'ts

- Give hypotonic saline in normo-/hyponatremia
- Administer desmopressin in normonatremia
- Use thiazide in normonatremia in patients at risk for hyponatremia

Renal Complications

Acute kidney injury (AKI) is associated with increased morbidity and mortality. Poor renal function is an independent risk factor for mortality. AKI is classified according to the RIFLE criteria (*R*isk – *I*njury – *F*ailure – *L*oss – *E*nd stage kidney disease, ESKD) from increased serum creatinine level (R 1.5×, I 2×, F 3×) or decreased glomerular filtration rate (GFR, creatinine clearance from urine, R >25 %, I >50 %, F >75 %) and urine output (R <0.5 mL/kg/h×6 h, I <0.5 mL/kg/h×12 h, F <0.3 mL/kg/h×24 h or anuria×12 h).

Risk factors for AKI include (1) prerenal: hypovolemia, hypotension; (2) renal: acute tubular necrosis (ATN) from sepsis, ischemia, antibiotics (aminoglycosides, amphotericin), contrast agents, myoglobin, nonsteroidal anti-inflammatory drug (NSAID); (3) postrenal: obstruction.

Risk of renal failure: uremic encephalopathy, hyperkalemia, hyperphosphatemia, metabolic acidosis.

Polyuria defined as diuresis >3,500–4,000 mL/day is common in neurocritical care and carries the risk of water and sodium imbalance. It can be caused by osmotic (mannitol, glycosuria, urea) or water diuresis (DI). There are three mechanisms of kidney injury: prerenal, renal, and postrenal.

Discussion of Risks for Patient's Safety

In neurocritical care, there are several potential risk factors for renal failure. Their accumulation must be avoided, especially contrast-induced nephropathy by repeated administration of contrast agents in management of acute brain disease; hypovolemia and hypotension; or nephrotoxic antibiotics. Safe management is geared at maintenance of fluid balance – the measurement of all parts of fluid intake and output including insensible losses from fever, sweating, vomiting, drainage. The volume status can be assessed by stroke volume variation (SVV) or pulse pressure variation (PPV). Oliguria and azotemia are reversible, but need active and rapid management.

Protocol to Overcome Barriers to Patient's Safety

- Maintenance of fluid balance by measurement of intake and output (diuresis, drainage, vomiting, gastric tube, water loss caused by sweating or fever-200 mL per 1 °C above 37 °C), and replacement or induction of diuresis. Urine output should be assessed hourly in oliguria.
- Daily measurement of blood and urine biochemical parameters. Creatinine clearance should be measured from a 24 h urine collection in AKI.
- Avoidance of oliguria: check the urinary catheter's position, palpate bladder or sonography of bladder and ureters to assess for mechanical obstruction as a cause.
- Avoid polyuria: diagnostic management of water or osmotic diuresis.
- Safe fluid replacement in oliguria: start early, avoid hypotonic saline, set the rate according to SVV or PPV recorded by arterial catheter to eliminate fluid overload.

Dos and Don'ts in Renal Disorders

Dos

- Avoid hypovolemia by following SVV or PPV
- Avoid hypotension
- Determine the cause of polyuria if it is a compensatory response to higher fluid or osmotic intake or an abnormal response to brain damage – the ADH-renal axis according EWC

Don'ts

- Use nephrotoxic medications: thiazides → hyponatremia, furosemide → hypernatremia
- Allow accumulation of risk factors for renal failure
- Use NSAIDs in a risk patient of AKI

Gastroenterological Complications

Catastrophic brain injury carries a risk of gastrointestinal bleeding from peptic stress ulcers or erosions, vomiting, and diarrhea from multifactorial causes. Risk factors for *peptic stress ulcers* are traumatic brain injury, mechanical ventilation, polytrauma, shock, administration of corticosteroids (brain tumor), nonsteroidal anti-inflammatory drugs (NSAIDs), previous peptic ulcer disease. These risks can be minimized by early enteral nutrition and prophylaxis with H2 antagonists or proton pump inhibitors. *Vomiting* is a sign of intracranial hypertension and has a potential risk of water and sodium imbalances. *Diarrhea* may be a result of antibiotic therapy (*Clostridium difficile*) or tube feeding.

Discussion of Risks for Patient's Safety

Incidence of stress ulcers in neurocritical care has been reduced by effective gastric prophylaxis (H2 antagonists and proton pump inhibitors) and early enteral feeding. The protective agents, however, increase the incidence of pneumonia. The greatest risk of potential bleeding stems from unknown gastric or duodenal ulcers, for example, in chronic alcohol abuse.

Vomiting and diarrhea may affect the maintenance of sodium and water homeostasis and should be treated quickly. Diarrhea from *Clostridium difficile* colitis can be diagnosed quickly by the detection of the toxin.

Protocol to Overcome Barriers to Patient's Safety

- Initiation of early enteral nutrition as most effective prophylaxis of stress ulcers.
- Additional administration of H2 antagonists and proton pump inhibitors.
- Acute management of vomiting and diarrhea is essential to reduce sodium and water imbalances [4].

Dos and Don'ts in Gastroenterological Complications

Dos

- Avoid hypovolemia in vomiting, diarrhea, gastrointestinal bleeding
- Use peptic stress ulcer prophylaxis during administration of corticosteroids, chronic alcoholism
- Order diagnostic test to detection of toxin *Clostridium difficile* in diarrhea

Don'ts

- Apply extended drugs peptic stress ulcer prophylaxis
- Allow accumulation of risk factors for stress ulcer: NSAIDs with antiplatelet agents

Hematological Complications

Anemia

Anemia reduces cerebral oxygen delivery. Risks for the development of anemia include neurosurgical procedures, traumatic injuries, blood sampling without returning blood to the system, sepsis, malnutrition. The optimal hemoglobin level is not defined. Blood transfusions carry a risk of immunosuppression resulting in infections, of pulmonary edema, and of transfusion-related acute lung injury (TRALI).

Coagulopathy

Coagulopathy may increase (1) intracranial hematomas in thrombocytopenia or drug-related coagulopathy – antiplatelet agents, warfarin, heparin (heparin-induced thrombocytopenia, HIT), thrombolytic agents, liver failure, NSAIDs, or lead to (2) thrombotic complications (deep venous thrombosis, pulmonary embolism).

Discussion of Risks for Patient's Safety

The target level of hemoglobin (Hb) concentration is not well established, the restrictive strategy (Hb <7 g/dL) used in critically ill patients is not recommended for neurocritically ill patients. Blood transfusion for maintaining optimal tissue oxygenation carries the risk of infections and pulmonary complications. The management of coagulopathy needs to be balanced between the risk of intracranial hemorrhage and effective protection against pulmonary embolism.

Protocol to Overcome Barriers to Patient's Safety

- Maintenance of Hb level 8–9 g/dL, hematocrit >30%, thrombocytes >75–100×10^9/L.
- Safe blood management: returning blood to the system after blood sampling, nutrition, infection control.
- Correction of drug-related coagulopathy to the target level of laboratory results: international normalized ratio (INR) 1.4 factor, repeated testing according to the half-life of drugs.
- In management of thrombocytopenia, exclude HIT with an immunoassay test [5].

Dos and Don'ts in Hematological Complications

Dos

- Use returning blood systems for blood sampling
- Repeat coagulation tests in drug-related coagulopathy according to half-life of drugs
- Exclude HIT in thrombocytopenia during heparin therapy
- Use prophylaxis of venous thromboembolic disease

Don'ts

- Apply restrictive transfusion strategy of hemoglobin target <7 g/dL
- Allow accumulation of risk factors for bleeding: NSAIDs with anticoagulant therapy

Cardiac Complications

Case History

A 60-year-old previously healthy female presented to the emergency department with sudden onset of severe headache associated with neck pain. Neurologic examination was completely normal. Computed scan of the head revealed subarachnoid hemorrhage and cerebral angiography disclosed a right middle cerebral artery aneurysm. Electrocardiography (ECG) showed sinus rhythm with a heart rate of 70/min, with ST segment elevation in leads V1–V4 with T-wave inversion in the same leads. Chest radiography did not show any evidence of pulmonary edema. Troponin I level was 2.6 mcg/L. The patient underwent surgical clipping on the second day. The operation was uneventful. Postoperative ECG showed significant T-wave inversion in V1–V6. The patient developed severe shortness of breath and the chest radiograph revealed pulmonary edema. She was intubated and kept on positive pressure ventilation. After intubation, her blood pressure dropped and she was started on dopamine and norepinephrine to maintain her blood pressure. Once the blood pressure was stabilized, furosemide infusion was started with subsequent improvement of the pulmonary edema on the chest x-ray. Echocardiography showed severe hypokinesia in the anterior and apical regions with an ejection fraction of 40%. The diagnosis of acute congestive heart failure due to Tako-Tsubo cardiomyopathy was made. Patient was extubated on the seventh postoperative day. Follow-up echocardiography confirmed the return of left ventricular function to normal.

Discussion

Subarachnoid hemorrhage (SAH) is well known to be associated with cardiac complications. These changes are due to increased central sympathetic output that results in stunning of the myocardium. Table 18.2 lists the cardiac complications associated with SAH [6–9].

In patients with subarachnoid hemorrhage, cardiac complications are thought to be more common in elderly patients (above 50 years), female gender (up to 90%), patients with previous history of hypertension or coronary artery disease, smokers, and patients with poor Hess and Hunt (HH) classifications.

Studies have shown that patients with SAH with these cardiac manifestations typically have normal coronary arteries on cardiac catheterization. These changes are thought to be due to catecholamine-mediated cardiac stunning.

The development of cardiac complications significantly affected the prognosis after SAH even when correcting for HH grade. Patients with SAH who develop significant cardiac complications are at increased risk of delayed cerebral ischemia,

Table 18.2 Cardiac complications associated with SAH

Complication	Frequency
ECG changes	Common (50–100 %)
T-wave inversions Peaked P waves ST segment elevations/depression QT prolongation Q waves	
Echocardiographic changes	Common (50 %)
Regional wall motion abnormalities Global left ventricular impairment	
Elevated troponin level	Common (50 %)
Arrhythmias	Uncommon (5 %)
Atrial flutter/atrial fibrillation (76%) Ventricular arrhythmias (16%) Junctional rhythm (16%) Supraventricular tachycardia (12%)	
Left ventricular dysfunction (Tako-Tsubo cardiomyopathy)	Uncommon (1–2 %)
Myocardial infarction	Uncommon (1%)

which is probably related to the decreased cardiac output. In addition, patients with SAH who develop cardiomyopathy were found to have increased length of ICU stay and mortality [8, 10].

Neurogenic stunned myocardium associated with SAH (Tako-Tsubo cardiomyopathy) is characterized by the following features:

1. Transient nature (left ventricular dysfunction is fully reversible)
2. Not caused by a primary defect in myocardial perfusion (normal coronary arteries)
3. Echocardiographic evidence of regional wall motion abnormalities or global hypokinesia
4. Elevated cardiac enzymes level (creatine kinase(CK)-MB, troponin I or T)

It is very important to differentiate between neurogenic stunned myocardium (NSM) and true myocardial infarction (MI). Sometimes, coronary angiography is required to differentiate between the entities. Table 18.3 lists suggested criteria for NSM and MI [8, 10]. Management of cases of stunned cardiomyopathy is summarized in Table 18.4.

Early surgical clipping is considered to be the mainstay of treatment of aneurysmal subarachnoid hemorrhage. However, this intervention may be delayed in patients with severe cardiac dysfunction. Less invasive procedures such as endovascular coiling might be more appropriate in such patients.

Patients Safety Protocol

1. All patients who present to the NICU should have ECG and chest radiography done at baseline.
2. Continuous ECG, heart rate, blood pressure and pulse oximetry monitoring should be available to all patients in the NICU.

Table 18.3 Criteria for differentiation between NSM and MI

1. No previous history of cardiac problems
2. New-onset left ventricular dysfunction (ejection fraction less than 40%)
3. Cardiac wall motion abnormalities on echocardiogram that do not correlate with the coronary vascular distribution performance on ECG
4. Cardiac troponin levels less than 2.8 ng/mL

Table 18.4 Management of Tako-Tsubo cardiomyopathy

1. Admission to neurointensive care unit
2. Neurologic and cardiac monitoring
3. Positive inotropic agents such as dobutamine or milrinone
4. Vasopressors to maintain mean arterial blood pressure
5. Intra-aortic balloon pump counterpulsation (in some cases)

3. QT interval should be measured in all patients at risk as prolonged QT interval is associated with serious ventricular arrhythmias.
4. Patients who develop cardiopulmonary symptoms or ECG findings suggestive of heart failure or ischemia should have echocardiography and cardiac enzymes done to diagnose neurogenic stunned cardiomyopathy.
5. Efforts should be made to differentiate between neurogenic stunned cardiomyopathy and actual myocardial infarction because of the difference in prognosis and management.

Dos and Don'ts for Cardiac Complications

Dos

- Twelve-leads ECG for all patients admitted to the NICU
- Delay surgical clipping of the ruptured aneurysm for patients with severe cardiac manifestations
- Troponin level for all patients with ECG changes
- Consider less invasive procedures such as endovascular coiling in patients with significant cardiac complications
- Consider intraaortic balloon pump conterpulsation in cases with severe myocardial stunting

Don'ts

- Postpone surgical clipping in patients with minimal ECG changes

Pulmonary Complications

Case History

A 25-year-old male was brought to the emergency department (ED) by ambulance after having been found comatose at home. Upon arrival, his vital signs were: heart rate = 110/min, BP = 170/95 mmHg, and SpO_2 = 87% on room air. His Glasgow coma scale was 5 and pupils were 3 mm with sluggish reaction to light. The patient was immediately intubated and kept on mechanical ventilation with the following settings: tidal volume (VT) of 450 mL, respiratory rate (RR) of 14 (breaths/min), inspired oxygen concentration (FIO_2) of 100%, and positive end expiratory pressure (PEEP) of 5 cm H_2O. The postintubation chest x-ray showed diffuse bilateral alveolar infiltrates suggestive of pulmonary edema. CT scan of the brain revealed massive subarachnoid hemorrhage with brain edema. The diagnosis of severe subarachnoid hemorrhage (HH of 5) with neurogenic pulmonary edema was made. The patient underwent external ventricular drain (EVD) insertion for the purpose of intracranial pressure monitoring.

The patient was admitted to neurointensive care unit, where he received pharmacologic therapy aiming at reduction of ICP. Despite all measures, the patient's ICP remained high and his condition continued to deteriorate. Brain death was diagnosed 48 h after hospital admission.

Discussion

Pulmonary complications in patients with subarachnoid hemorrhage include pulmonary edema and pneumonia. There are three causes of pulmonary edema in those patients. The majority of cases are due to volume overload associated with triple H therapy or secondary to cardiomyopathy. However, neurogenic pulmonary edema (NPE) resulting from acute brain insult may occur but remains underdiagnosed. In one study, pulmonary edema occurs in 23% of patients with SAH with mortality rates between 7 and 10% [10].

NPE is diagnosed as bilateral pulmonary edema following acute brain insult without associated heart failure, significant volume overload, or other obvious cause of hypoxemia. The onset of NPE is usually acute (within hours) but in some patients it may develop over several days. With correct management it is usually reversible within 24 h.

The underlying pathophysiology of NPE is thought to be increased sympathetic outflow associated with acute brain insult. This leads to severe systemic vasoconstriction and hypertension, forcing intravascular fluid into the pulmonary bed. Some more recent studies have shown that the pulmonary edema fluid is rich in protein, which is suggestive of pulmonary capillary leakage as a result of the sympathetic surge.

Table 18.5 Management of pulmonary edema

1. Rapid treatment of underlying central nervous system insult including rapid control of intracranial pressure
2. Mechanical ventilation (invasive/noninvasive)
3. Hemodynamic support and monitoring
4. Use of diuretics with caution

Neurogenic pulmonary edema should be treated symptomatically. The management is similar to the therapy of cardiogenic pulmonary edema. Early intubation is recommended. The use of diuretics in patients with SAH should be exercised with extreme caution as these patients need to be euvolemic to decrease the risk of delayed cerebral ischemia [11]. Table 18.5 summarizes the management of pulmonary edema in patients with SAH [10].

Patients Safety Protocol

1. Every effort should be made to differentiate between different causes of new pulmonary infiltrates/effusions as the treatment plan is completely different.
2. Patients in the NICU are at high risk for nosocomial pneumonia including aspiration pneumonia. Early diagnosis and appropriate management are key points in improving patient's outcome.
3. Early intubation and mechanical ventilation should be considered in patients with severe respiratory compromise.

Dos and Don'ts for Pulmonary Complications

Dos

- Baseline chest x-ray for all patients admitted to NICU
- Apply ventilator-associated pneumonia (VAP) bundle to all patients who are mechanically ventilated
- Use diuretics with caution in patients with neurogenic pulmonary edema (NPE) to avoid systemic hypotension that results in cerebral hypoperfusion
- Patients at risk of fluid overload (such as elderly, patients with underlying cardiac or renal dysfunction) should be monitored closely when applying triple H therapy to minimize the risks of pulmonary edema

Don'ts

- Avoid use of PEEP more than 15 cm H_2O
- Avoid use of permissive hypercapnia or prone positioning especially without concurrent ICP monitoring

Infectious Complications

Case History

A 28-year-old male patient was admitted to our hospital following a motor vehicular accident. His Glasgow Coma Scale on arrival was 8/15 on admission. A computerized tomography scan (CT) of the brain showed multiple skull fractures, bilateral temporal lobe contusions, subarachnoid hemorrhage and severe brain edema. The CT scan of his cervical spine showed fractures of the fourth and fifth cervical spine vertebras with mild displacement. He underwent craniotomy on the day of admission for elevation of depressed skull fracture. Eighteen days later, the patient had a halo vest applied followed by surgical tracheostomy on the next day. The patient was weaned off mechanical ventilation successfully and was transferred to the neurosurgical ward 7 days later. Three days later, he was found with a decrease of his level of consciousness and the emergence of fever, a new CT scan of the brain was performed. Hydrocephalus was diagnosed. An external ventricular drainage of the cerebrospinal fluid (CSF) was inserted. The CSF sample showed an increased cell count with decreased glucose and elevated protein. CSF specimen was cultured on MacConkey agar and *Acinetobacter baumannii* was identified using API system 20NE strip. The patient was started on meropenem 1 g q 8 h, ciprofloxacin 400 mg q 12 h, and vancomycin 1 g q 12 h intravenously. Two days later, the CSF culture showed heavy growth of acinetobacter species, which was sensitive only to colistin. Intravenous colistin (2.5 million units q 12 h) was started. After 5 days of intravenous colistin, the CSF culture continued to be positive for acinetobacter. The antimicrobial regimen was changed to intrathecal colistin (3.2 mg via EVD daily). Three days later, the CSF culture was negative.

Discussion

Patients admitted to the neurointensive care unit commonly encounter nosocomial infections, most of these are nosocomial pneumonias. Risk factors for developing infections in the NICU include the following:

1. Presence of catheters and drains
2. Defect in cellular immunity in some patients admitted to the NICU such as patients with head injury
3. Use of steroids

Nosocomial infections that affect patients admitted to the neurointensive care unit include pneumonia including ventilator-associated pneumonia (VAP), catheter-related bloodstream infections, urinary tract infections, pseudomembranous colitis secondary to *Clostridium difficile* and external ventricular drain related meningitis. Table 18.6 shows the different types of nosocomial infections in the neurointensive care unit.

One of the most common procedures in the neuro-intensive care unit is external ventricular drain insertion. EVD-related meningitis is a major complication.

Table 18.6 Nosocomial infections in the neurointensive care unit

Type	Pathogens	Diagnosis	Treatment
Respiratory Early (<3 days)	S. aureus Haemophilus influenzae Streptococcus pneumoniae Gram-negative rods	Chest x-ray ABG Blood cultures Sampling of lower respiratory tract secretions	IV beta-lactam + IV macrolide or IV fluoroquinolone
Late	Pseudomonas Acinetobacter MRSA		IV antipseudomonal beta-lactam + IV antipseudomonal quinolone + IV vancomycin
Bloodstream infection	S. epidermidis S. aureus Enterococcus Klebsiella Enterobacter Candida	2 sets of blood cultures (from catheter and distant site)	IV vancomycin (consider IV beta-lactam or third-generation cephalosporins if you suspect gram-negative rods)
Urinary tract infection	E. coli Pseudomonas Enterococcus Acinetobacter Klebsiella Proteus	Urine culture	Third-generation cephalosporin
	C. albicans		Fluconazole
	C. glabrata		Voriconazole
Gastrointestinal infection	Clostridium difficile	Clostridium difficile toxin in stool Colonoscopy	Oral or IV metronidazole Oral vancomycin
Ventricular-drain-related infections	S. epidermidis S. acnes S. aureus Pseudomonas Acinetobacter		Vancomycin + IV antipseudomonal beta-lactam or third-generation cephalosporin Consider IV colistin is multidrug-resistant agents are suspected

Abbreviations: *Chest x-ray* chest radiograph, *ABG* arterial blood gas, *IV* intravenous, *S. Staphylococcus*, *E. Escherichia*, *C. Candida*, *MRSA* methicillin-resistant *Staphylococcus aureus*

The incidence ranges between 2 and 27%. The other possible infectious complications of EVD insertion include skin and soft tissue infections, cerebritis, brain abscess, subdural empyema, osteomyelitis, endocarditis, intraabdominal abscess formation, and sepsis. Risk factors for EVD-related meningitis are as follows:

1. Duration of EVD presence more than 11 days
2. High frequency of EVD manipulation such as sampling and irrigation
3. Intraventricular hemorrhage
4. Nonadherence to strict surgical technique used for insertion of EVD [12]

The most common etiological agents identified in EVD-related meningitis are *Staphylococcus epidermidis*, *Staphylococcus aureus*, gram-negative bacteria, and rarely anaerobes and *Candida* species. Every effort should be made to differentiate between catheter contamination, colonization, and true meningitis. Contamination is defined as isolated CSF culture in the absence of abnormal findings on CSF chemistry and cell count. EVD catheter colonization is defined as multiple positive CSF cultures with abnormal CSF profile but no clinical signs of infection such as fever. EVD-related meningitis includes positive CSF culture, abnormal CSF results, and clinical signs such as fever and reduced level of consciousness [12].

Early appropriate antibiotic treatment of EVD-related meningitis is associated with reduced morbidity and mortality. Initial antibiotic therapy depends on many factors including prevalence of methicillin-resistant stains of staphylococcus, comorbid diseases such as renal impairment, and immune status of the patient. The majority of EVD-related infections caused by coagulase-negative staphylococcus can be treated with antibiotics without removal of the catheter. If the catheter is not removed, longer duration of therapy (10–14 days) rather than 7 days should be considered. It is recommended to remove the EVD in case of infection caused by other organisms, especially gram-negative rods and fungi [12].

Patients Safety Protocol

- Avoid prophylactic EVD exchange as it is not proven to decrease the risk of EVD-related meningitis.
- Avoid the use of prophylactic antibiotics as it might increase the risk of infection with multiresistant organisms.
- If available, use antimicrobial-impregnated EVD or silver-coated catheters as they have been shown to reduce the risk of catheter-related meningitis.
- Avoid repeated unnecessary manipulation.
- Remove the EVD catheter as soon as possible as the risk of meningitis increases with prolonged duration of insertion.
- As soon as EVD-related meningitis is diagnosed, the appropriate antibiotic regimen should be started taking into consideration all modifying factors.
- EVD can be retained with prolonged antibiotic therapy (10–14 days) only in case of infection with coagulase-negative staphylococcus.
- EVD should be removed or exchanged in case of infection with all other organisms.

Dos and Don'ts for Infectious Complications

Dos

- Observe CSF characteristics on routine basis
- Send CSF sample for gram stain and culture when infection is suspected

- Use antibiotic-impregnated or silver-coated catheter
- In case of suspected or proven EVD-related meningitis, start early appropriate antibiotics
- Use longer duration of antibiotic therapy in CNS infection if the EVD catheter is retained
- Remove the EVD catheter in all other EVD-related meningitis

Don'ts

- Avoid prophylactic catheter exchange
- Avoid prophylactic antibiotics
- Avoid unnecessary manipulation

References

1. Seder DB, Riker RR, Jagoda A, Smith WS, et al. Emergency neurological life support: airway, ventilation, and sedation. Neurocrit Care. 2012;17:S4–20.
2. Aiyagari V, Deibert E, Diringer M. Hypernatremia in the neurologic intensive care unit: how high is too high? J Crit Care. 2006;21:163–72.
3. Qureshi AI, Suri MF, Sung GY, et al. Prognostic significance of hypernatremia and hyponatremia among patients with aneurysmal subarachnoid hemorrhage. Neurosurgery. 2002;50: 749–55.
4. Kellum JA, Bellomo R, Ronco C. The concept of acute kidney injury and the RIFLE criteria. Contrib Nephrol. 2007;156:10–6.
5. Kramer AH, Zygun DA. Anemia and red blood cell transfusion in neurocritical care. Crit Care. 2009;13(3):R89.
6. Frontera JA, Parra A, Shimbo D, Fernandez A, Schmidt JM, Peter P, et al. Cardiac arrhythmias after subarachnoid hemorrhage: risk factors and impact on outcome. Cerebrovasc Dis. 2008;26:71–8.
7. Mayer SA, Fink ME, Homma S, Sherman D, LiMandri G, Lennihan L, et al. Cardiac injury associated with neurogenic pulmonary edema following subarachnoid hemorrhage. Neurology. 1994;44:815–20.
8. Lee VH, Oh JK, Mulvagh SL, Wijdicks EF. Mechanisms in neurogenic stress cardiomyopathy after aneurysmal subarachnoid hemorrhage. Neurocrit Care. 2006;5:243–9.
9. Muroi C, Keller M, Pangalu A, Fortunati M, Yonekawa Y, Keller E. Neurogenic pulmonary edema in patients with subarachnoid hemorrhage. J Neurosurg Anesthesiol. 2008;20:188–92.
10. Wartenberg KE, Mayer SA. Medical complications after subarachnoid hemorrhage: new strategies for prevention and management. Curr Opin Crit Care. 2006;12:78–84.
11. Diringer MN, Bleck TP, Claude Hemphill 3rd J, Menon D, Shutter L, Vespa P, et al. Critical care management of patients following aneurysmal subarachnoid hemorrhage: recommendations from the neurocritical care society's multidisciplinary consensus conference. Neurocrit Care. 2011;15:211–40.
12. Beer R, Lackner P, Pfausler B, Schmutzhard E. Nosocomial ventriculitis and meningitis in neurocritical care patients. J Neurol. 2008;255:1617–24.

Chapter 19
Neuroimaging in the Neuro-ICU

Sharon Casilda Theophilus, Regunath Kandasamy, Khatijah Abu Bakar,
and Jafri Malin Abdullah

Introduction

A number of imaging modalities can be performed for patients in a neurointensive
care setting. These range from simple radiographs to magnetic resonance images
(MRIs) capable of detailed information on soft tissue structures with great accuracy.
The indications and uses of each of these are discussed below.

Radiographs

X-rays are used as a preliminary investigation for some CNS-related conditions.
The commonest example would be patients who have sustained some form of traumatic brain or spine injury with suspected fractures or dislocation. Radiographs
serve as a screening tool and can sometimes dictate the need for further imaging in
patients presenting after an injury. The CT scan, however, has superseded the radiographs when it is available. The simple radiograph, nevertheless, remains a valuable
utility in the ICU, for example, in search for a foreign body or to assess the course
of a ventriculoperitoneal shunt. When produced through an image intensifier, x-ray
images may be useful following traction and attempted reduction of cervical spine

S.C. Theophilus, MD (USU), MS Neurosurgery (USM)
Department of Neurosurgery, Sultanah Aminah Johor Bahru, Johor Bahru, Johor, Malaysia

R. Kandasamy, MBBS, MRCS, MS Neurosurgery
J.M. Abdullah, FASC, MD, PhD, DSCN, FRCS (✉)
Center for Neuroscience Services and Research, Universiti Sains Malaysia,
Kota Bharu, Kelantan, Malaysia
e-mail: brainsciences@gmail.com

K.A. Bakar, MD (UKM), MMed Radiology (UM)
Department of Radiology, Sultanah Aminah Johor Bahru, Johor Bahru, Johor, Malaysia

© Springer International Publishing Switzerland 2015   299
K.E. Wartenberg et al. (eds.), *Neurointensive Care: A Clinical Guide
to Patient Safety*, DOI 10.1007/978-3-319-17293-4_19

fractures pending definitive therapy. X-rays can be performed quickly and simply with minimal risk of radiation exposure to patients and staff. However, the lack of detailed structural imaging and the availability of superior alternative modalities have made this modality become less utilized than it was before [1].

Computed Tomography

Since its introduction in the 1970s, this imaging modality has grown in terms of the clarity of images produced as well as the extent of its usage. The majority of hospitals around the world are equipped with a CT scan machine to facilitate rapid investigation of patients. CT is the gold standard of evaluation for patients who have sustained traumatic brain injury (TBI) and its use has revolutionized treatment. CT scans of the brain or spine can be performed rapidly with or without contrast. It allows immediate detection of conditions such as intracranial bleeding, fractures, cerebral edema, and pneumocephalus. It also has great value in patients presenting with altered sensorium who might be suspected to have a cerebrovascular accident, which maybe either hemorrhagic or ischemic. The addition of angiography also allows quick visualization of arteries located mainly in the vicinity of the circle of Willis, to detection of aneurysmal dilatations or arteriovenous malformations as well as sinus thrombosis. Reconstructed views are also helpful to visualize craniofacial bony abnormalities [1].

Doppler Sonography/Ultrasound

Doppler sonography is a useful tool to assess both intracranial as well as extracranial large vessels. Conditions such as carotid stenosis as well intracranial proximal vasospasm can be detected easily at the bedside using this modality. The Doppler sonographic examinations, however, are subject to interobserver variations and thus need to be done by an experienced person and repeated regularly to obtain accurate results. Transcranial ultrasonography (TCD) is particularly useful in neonates with patent fontanelles where the ventricular anatomy as well as any obvious space occupying lesions can be delineated. In adults with sufficient bone windows, midline shift can also be followed sonographically in space-occupying lesions. Once again, both investigations require a fair level of experience and skills to interpret with accuracy [1].

Magnetic Resonance Imaging (MRI)

This modality is particularly useful to visualize the detailed soft tissue structures in the brain as well as spinal cord. In neurocritical care, it is often not performed due to the patient being required to be transported to the MRI suite, as well as due to

MRI-incompatible metallic devices attached to the patient. Furthermore, the pro-longed duration of this investigation degrades MRI down from first line for patients in a neurocritical care setting [1].

Case Scenario

A 20-year-old male patient was involved in an alleged road traffic accident. He was riding a motorcycle that collided with a car. On admission his Glasgow Coma Scale Score was E4, V4, M6 = 14/15 with pupils that were bilaterally 3 mm in diameter and reactive to light. Both primary and secondary surveys were reported to be nor-mal except for a fracture of his right femur. He was observed in the Emergency Dept. and subsequently admitted in the Orthopedics Unit for further treatment of his fracture after basic chest, pelvic, and cervical radiographs were found to be unre-markable. No CT of the brain was done prior to admission. After a duration of 6 h, he was noted to have a deterioration in consciousness and his GCS score was docu-mented as E2, V2, M5 = 9/15. His pupils remained 3 mm and reactive to light. An urgent CT of the brain revealed a left frontotemporoparietal convexity acute subdu-ral hemorrhage resulting in midline shift. He was immediately referred to the neu-rosurgery team. The patient subsequently underwent a decompressive craniectomy, clot evacuation, and placement of an ICP monitor. Postoperatively patient was man-aged in the ICU with cerebral resuscitation with intracranial pressure (ICP) moni-toring. Around 6 h after surgery, his ICP levels increased to 35 mmHg in spite of adequate sedation. A portable CT scan was done and it showed minimal residual subdural blood measuring 3 mm in thickness, and mass effect with midline shift had corrected. It was noted that the patient's pCO2 was 50 mmHg, after adjustment of ventilation, ICP was below 20 mmHg and subsequently maintained for 24 h and cerebral protection was then weaned off.

It was noted that definite fixation of the fractured femur was not done yet after the craniotomy and the patient was again reviewed by the orthopedic team and planned for surgery. Patient went in for an interlocking nail insertion for his right femur on posttrauma day 3. He was weaned off sedation thereafter, and his GCS at the time was noted to be E2, V3, M6 = 11/15. A repeat CT of the brain was done and it showed no changes from the previous CT scan done postcraniotomy.

On posttrauma day 4, the patient suddenly developed an episode of focal seizures with secondary generalization. Postictally, his GCS was E2, V1, M6 = 9/15 and a CT scan was repeated once again. The findings were similar to those seen in both previous postoperative scans. He was managed further by optimization of his antiepileptic medication and the seizures did not recur. Patient seemed to have a good postoperative recovery until the postoperative day 8 when he was noted to have serious discharge from the craniotomy wound. An urgent contrasted CT scan of the brain was obtained. The contrasted scan showed no signs of intracranial infection. Daily dressing was done for the wound and the patient was discharged well on postcraniotomy day 10.

- What were the shortfalls in this patient's management?
- Were all his imaging studies indicated and what were the associated risks?
- What safety barrier could be put in place to reduce risks to patients?

Risks to Patient's Safety

Delay in Performing CT Scan

Patient was initially admitted with a GCS score of 14; however, no head CT was done. Thus, the diagnosis of traumatic brain injury was missed initially and only detected upon deterioration of consciousness. In the case of this patient, a CT scan should have ideally been performed on admission. Below is the recommendations by the "Mild TBI Clinical Policy Adult guidelines 2008 in regard to indications for a CT scan" [2].

"*Level A recommendations*: A non-contrast head CT is indicated in head trauma patients with loss of consciousness or posttraumatic amnesia only if one or more of the following is present: headache, vomiting, age >60 years, drug or alcohol intoxication, deficits in short-term memory, physical evidence of trauma above the clavicle, post-traumatic seizure, GCS score <15, focal neurologic deficit, or coagulopathy" [2, 3].

"*Level B recommendations*: A non-contrast head CT should be considered in head trauma patients with no loss of consciousness or posttraumatic amnesia if there is a focal neurologic deficit, vomiting, severe headache, ≥65 years old, physical signs of a basilar skull fracture, GCS score <15, coagulopathy, or a dangerous mechanism of injury" [2, 3].

Forgoing CT scanning at the time of admission even though his GCS was 14 put him at risk. Delayed surgery in this patient could have worsened his long-term functional and cognitive outcome or potentially resulted in death if there had been an extreme delay. The duration of hospital stay as well as the cost of treatment for this patient also has increased due to the fact that early treatment could have potentially reduced the need for prolonged intensive care management.

Multiple Repeated Head CTs and Risk of Radiation Exposure to Patient

This patient had a total of 5 CT brain and the question is whether repeated CT was really necessary. This patient was exposed to multiple episodes of radiation. In this case, fluctuating neurological symptoms was the reason for repeat scans. Rise in ICP is also another justified cause for repeat CT. Seizures and an infected wound is also a clear indication for a repeat scan.

We do have to consider that the initial repeat CT postcraniotomy showed good evacuation of the clot, hence the argument whether a repeated scan was needed after orthopedic surgery and after the patient had a seizure. However, fluctuating neurological symptoms warrant a repeat scan unless there is a clear explanation.

Patient was not started on prophylactic antiepileptic drugs (AED), which is a level II recommendation for early posttraumatic seizure prophylaxis. An AED could have potentially prevented the seizure and hence the repeat CT scan.

As the above measures were not identified and managed appropriately, the patient did have to undergo multiple exposures to radiation. The risk of radiation exposure is outweighed by the risk of increased ICP, seizures, or an infected wound that could lead to meningitis, which are all immediately life-threatening [4].

Intrahospital Transfer for CT Versus Portable CT

This patient was cared for in the neurointensive care unit. He underwent ICP monitoring for his brain injury. His lower limbs were placed on skin traction while awaiting definitive orthopedic surgery. Multiple transports of this patient for CT scans are associated with many risks. He had to be connected to a portable ventilator and also needed multiple drug infusion pumps to be carried along. The presence of skin traction aggravated the transport. The patient was unstable and often needed inotropic support. The staff transferring him needs to be highly trained and a physician's presence is required. The portable head CT scanner reduces all the above-described risks tremendously making it safe for a critically ill patient to undergo immediate imaging [4, 5].

Time needed for transportation of patients to and from the radiology department was approximately 85 min in comparison with 15 min with a portable CT for this patient. Time for CT scanning was the same: 2 min.

Safety Barriers

Despite the potential benefits of using a portable head CT scanner (Fig. 19.1), concerns about its safety are bound to occur. We reviewed the safety of our portable head CT scanner (CereTom, NeuroLogica Corporation, Danvers, MA, USA) with regard to its radiation safety, need for shielding as wall scatter of radiation.

Radiation Exposure and Shielding

An operator at a distance of 2 m from the CereTom's isocenter could perform over 26 scans per day, for 250 days per year without any additional lead protection based on the ALARA (As Low As Reasonably Achievable) standard (500 mRem/ year per operator) with a typical brain scan protocol (15 Rotations $\times$ 2 s per rotation $\times$ 7 mA = 210 mAs). The CereTom covers are coated with 0.5-mm laminated lead providing maximum scatter reduction. There are an additional three externally mounted 0.5-mm lead curtains (two in front, one at the back) provided, adding shielding to the gantry. Thus, no additional lead shielding is required [6, 7].

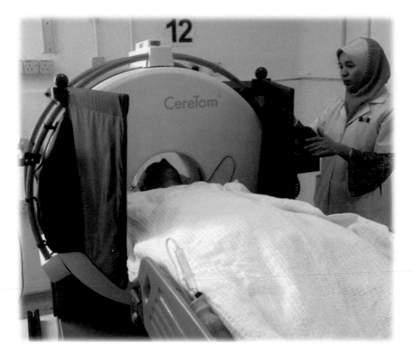

Fig. 19.1 A simulated patient undergoing a CT scan of his brain in the mobile CT scan unit

Scatter Radiation Plot

The scatter map was measured using a 15.9 cm diameter×14 cm length CTDI (Computed Tomography dose index) cylindrical phantom (Fig. 19.2). A scan board and Stryker patient table were used. A typical ACR (American College of Radiology) standard brain protocol was applied. Scatter dose varies between scanners up to 10%. Dose numbers represented are air doses and not organ doses, which is similar to the skin dose. The scatter dose is dependant on the object being scanned and the peak kilovoltage (kVp) setting. Scatter dose scales match linearly with the milliampere second (mAs) technique. Absorption of scatter by the patient will reduce external scatter rates [6, 8]. Figure 19.2 is a scatter plot of a routine CT Brain.

Discussion of Risk/Benefit Ratios

Appropriate Use of Imaging

Presently ongoing debates on the misuse of CT facilities in spite of multiple, validated, evidence-based guidelines advising the appropriate use of computed tomography (CT) to differentiate mild traumatic brain injury (MTBI) from clinically important brain

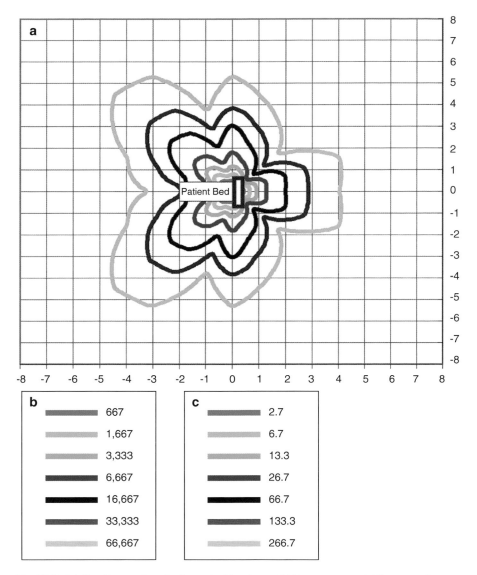

Fig. 19.2 (**a**) CereTom scatter plot for typical head scan (**b**) Scans per year (**c**) Scans per day

injury and to prevent overuse are controversial. Misuse of CT scanning potentially exposes patients to unnecessary ionizing radiation, risks, and costs. A study by Melnick ER et al. showed that 10–35% of CTs obtained in the emergency department (ED) for MTBI did not adhere to guideline recommendations. This study also showed that successful implementation of existing guidelines could decrease CT use in MTBI by up to 35%, leading to a significant reduction in radiation-induced cancer and health care costs [9, 10].

Repeated CT Scanning

A prospective study by Connon et al. concluded that no patient from their study with a "routine" repeat CT required a change in management. Considering the costs and potential risks of routine repeat CT, and lack of demonstrable benefit, the need for routine CT should take into account the costs and potential risks of routine repeat CT with lack of demonstrable benefits. On the other hand, in patients with deteriorating neurological status, especially in younger and more severely head-injured patients, repeat CTB is clearly indicated [4]. A similar prospective study conducted by Brown et al. noted that serial head CT is routinely performed after TBI without neurologic change and there is no alteration to their management after repeat head CT, unless these patients have neurologic deterioration before the repeat head CT [5]. Another study was conducted by Bee TK et al. in an attempt to better allocate scarce resources. They concluded that there is a benefit in routine follow-up CT scans for MTBI (minimal traumatic brain injury), as it led to higher levels of medical management or neurosurgical intervention in patients with worsening CT findings. These patients are best kept in an ICU setting until head CT demonstrates stable conditions [11].

Exposure to Radiation

Radiation dose (in gray or mGy) is proportional to the amount of energy that an irradiated body part is expected to absorb. The Sievert (Sv) unit is the effective dose that can induce cancer. Dose radiation estimated from a CT of the brain is 1–2 m Sv (effective dose) and 56 mGy (absorbed dose). Integral dose is directly proportional to the number of sections in an examination.

In portable CT scanners, examination factors are changed to reduce the dose as the scanning is done within a small radius. Hence, it explains the increase in image noise and the decrease in quality with portable CT scanners. In this patient, the total dose radiation is estimated around 4–8 mSv and 160–240 mGy, which remains in a safe range.

Role of Portable CT

It is a great challenge to transport critically ill patients from the intensive care unit (ICU). Generally, when transporting patients from ICUs for any mode of imaging, the inherent risks of intrahospital transport are well known. In the decision to obtain a CT in a critically ill patient, the benefit should outweigh these risks. Therefore, the request for a CT in an ICU patient with minimal or no neurological deterioration or in a patient who is doing well clinically after surgery is debatable. These risks and consequences are addressed with the availability of a portable CT scanner. Pearce K et al. studied the use of a portable head CT scanner (CereTom) in the ICU to assess its feasibility, safety, and radiological quality. This study concluded that the vast majority of portable CT scans were performed after an intracranial procedure (24%), when there was neurological deterioration (16%), or in routine follow-up (16%). The portable CT scanner proved to have adequate diagnostic quality. Common complications arising from intrahospital transportation such as accidental disconnection of an intravenous line, interruptions in mechanical ventilation and inadvertent extubations were not encountered in portable CT scanning [12]. Pearce K et al. also noted the average total time to perform a portable head CT scan was 19.5 ± 3.5 min. The actual scan time was 2.5 ± 0.7 min [12]. In conclusion, the portable CT scanner (CereTom) is safe, easy to use, and provides adequate radiological quality for diagnostic decisions [12].

From our experience, the apparent benefits from the use of portable CT include the following:

1. A CT can be safely done without an interruption of monitoring and drug infusions during transfer and without manipulation of ventilator settings. During the transport complications due to endotracheal tube dislodgement, empty oxygen tanks or ventilator failure can cause secondary cerebral insults. Patients being transported also need continuous monitoring, and it is always a risk during use of technical equipment [12].
2. A CT can be ordered immediately and reviewed at the time of scanning or shortly thereafter, assisting in prompt diagnosis and early treatment [12]. In neurocritical care, this capability can make a difference in minimizing insults to the brain, as time is a factor in prognostication.
3. There is definitely greater satisfaction among the ICU nurses as they remain in a familiar environment and monitoring of patients is not compromised. An intrahospital transfer requires at least two staff members including a physician. For portable CT, there is only one staff nurse involved. Reducing the number of staff members and risks that can be encountered during transport both to patient and staff makes portable CT a welcome addition to the neurocritical care unit. All of these have potential economic benefits beyond that of improved patient outcome. Ultimately, time, energy, and costs are saved. All that is required is good communication and teamwork between the radiology staff, technicians, ICU nurses, and the treating physicians. Preparing a good flowchart as a standard protocol in the neurocritical ICU helps to facilitate the process [12].
4. Patients in the neurocritical ICU, frequently need CTs of the head and usually on a short notice. A portable CT in this instance has proven to be invaluable. Carrlson et al. reviewed their initial experience with a portable CT at a tertiary trauma center; they noted that the average time to perform a CT scan (from time of request to transmission into image archiving and communication system) was 12.6 min (range 7.8–47 min). Image quality was judged to be excellent by the entire neurosurgical faculty in the intensive care unit. Their experience suggests that mobile CT is extremely useful in care of patients with severe traumatic brain injury and is useful for any high-volume neurosurgery department in the country [13].

5. The use of portable CT technology in obtaining diagnostic imaging in the neuro-critical care unit reduces both costs and risk associated with transport. It is economical in providing patient care [2, 12–14]. The portable CT is only limited by its dedication to head scans, for other CT scans such as chest and abdomen patients still have to be transported. However, the use of the portable CT in the neurocritical care unit is justifiable as imaging of the head is the most commonly ordered examination. On the other hand, the use of a dedicated brain scanner in the ICU reduces congestion in the CT suite as most head CTs are urgent [13, 14]. It improves the work environment of both the radiologists and radiographers and improves the relationship between the physicians managing the patient in the neurocritical care unit.

6. Portable computed tomography scanners have a scan plane selected by means of gantry translation rather than by translation of the patient table [13]. This allows a patient who is positioned on a radiolucent surface to fit within the inner diameter of the portable CT gantry. Other features of the portable CT include being equipped with wheels, fitting into standard-sized elevators, drawing power from common electrical wall outlets and a translating gallery [6, 7, 13, 15].

7. Finally, we take into account the radiation exposure for a portable CT scanner. The radiation exposure from a head CT using the portable CT scanner as we have mentioned earlier is 1–2 msV. The worldwide average dose annually from our environment to humans is about 2.4 msV. The lowest annual dose at which any increase in cancer is clearly evident is more than 100 msV. The recommended limit for radiation workers every 5 years is 100 msV [16].

Therefore, there is minimal risk of radiation exposure to the patient and staff and it remains within the recommended limit.

The portable CT scanner used in the neurocritical care unit is the CereTom (Neurologica: Danvers, MA), a second-generation portable CT scanner. The CereTom is lighter in weight and can be easily moved by a single operator. It runs on batteries and is charged from a standard three-prong outlet. The following parameters are used for CT scanning of patients: electrical capacity of 120 kV, 7 mA with standard sharpness, and standard resolution (4-s scan) (CT Dose Index) CTDIw = 80 mGy. The portable CT scanner can sustain its battery power up to five patients. More patients can be scanned in a given period if the device is plugged into a standard electrical outlet between scans [6].

The portable scan produces three 5-mm axial sections per 2-s scan to a maximum of 46 images in total, and an additional reconstruction for 2.5-mm intervals data acquisition. Although this increases image noise, it is still a highly reliable scanner able to produce good quality images for diagnosis and management plan. The advantage of the CereTom is its capability to image smaller fields in order to generate higher quality images. The disadvantage is its limitation to the region of the head excluding the neck [6, 7, 13, 15]. The CereTom has various imaging capabilities such as CT with contrast, CT angiography, and CT perfusion, which provides clinicians the ability to address nearly every neurological or neurovascular question in the setting of a neurocritical care unit. The CereTom is rapidly becoming an absolute requirement for any modern neurological medical center [2, 6, 12, 13, 15].

Contrasted CT in an Intensive Care Unit

The patient discussed was subjected to a portable CT contrasted scan 2 weeks post-craniotomy when he presented with wound discharge to rule out intracranial infection. We should be aware of risks that can arise from administrating contrast agents.

Side effects of intravenous contrast include nausea and vomiting. Rapid infusion of contrast causes a warm feeling in the arm and sometimes severe pain. Extravasated contrast can cause serious skin injury to require skin grafting. Katayama H et al. concluded the risk of developing anaphylactic shock in iodinated contrast is 0.2% and in noniodinated contrast is 0.04%. Anaphylactic symptoms include urticaria, bronchospasm, laryngeal edema, and hypotension [16]. Clearance of contrast is renal. Patients with preexisting renal impairment have an increased risk of worsening renal function and may even require hemodialysis. When diagnosing a contrast-induced nephropathy, the increase in serum creatine has to be more than 25% or an absolute increase of 0.5 mg/dL [16].

Risk factors for developing anaphylactic shock include asthma, history of previous allergy to contrast, history of any kind of allergy or skin reaction to food, drugs, or environment, very young or elderly patients. These are given steroids prior to their scan with contrast although there is no clear benefit of this policy. Interestingly, a recent survey revealed that, although the use of nonionic contrast media has increased, the use of premedication with steroids is being increasingly used. This is unnecessary, as the risk of allergic reactions is low with nonionic contrast media and application of steroids places the patient at an additional risk of side effects.

Solutions to Potential Risks

Transportation

Portable CT scanning prevents interruption of continuous intracranial and systemic monitoring, accidental disconnection of an intravenous line, or from mechanical ventilation [6, 7, 12, 13, 15].

Radiation

Radiation emitted from the portable scanner was shown to be at an angle of 45° and to spread outward 10 ft. During a routine scan, the radiation dose to the patient's head was expected to range between 1 and 2 mSv. Measurements taken at 6 and 10 ft away in front of the scanner demonstrated radiation exposure free in air of 50 and 139 2R, respectively (129 kVp at 7 mA for 3 min). Radiation badges were not worn by the staff as studies concluded that staff members were not exposed to radiation [7, 8, 13, 15].

The average patient effective dose for a routine head CT examination on the CereTom is thus ~1.7 mSv. This radiation exposure is typical for CT performed on any CT scanner [7, 13, 15].

Radiation Safety Precautions

(a) Because the scanner is internally shielded with lead in the covers, approximately 2 m away from the scanner is a safe distance for staff. Because the scanner and workstation communicate wirelessly, the radiological staff often operates the scanner from outside the patient's room, which is definitely a safe distance. There are also lead curtains that hang off the system to cut down scatter off the patient [6, 7].
(b) The dose to the patient is comparable to that of a CT in a fixed scanner. There are noise reduction algorithms that can be implemented to further reduce the dose and/or protocol based on the patient's condition [6, 7].

Safe Contrast Usage

If contrast is to be used during a scan, the following precautions and guidelines should be adhered to:

(a) Before any contrasted scan, the patient's kidney function should be checked to ensure the iodine can be processed correctly.
(b) The most common contrast agent used is iodine based such as Iohexol (Omnipaque). It is offered in 300 mg/mL, 320 mg/mL, or 350 mg/mL concentrations. The higher the concentration the more dense the liquid and the better vascular image can be obtained by CT angiogram.
(c) In a CT angiography study, it is most common to use 80–100 mL of contrast at a rate of 5 mL/s. The amount of contrast can vary from adult to pediatric patients.
(d) For a CT perfusion study (brain), it is most common to use 40–50 mL of contrast at a rate of 5 mL/s. The scan takes typically 30–40 s to complete [13, 14].
(e) To minimize the risk for contrast-induced renal injury, the patient should receive adequate hydration prior to and after application of contrast media. Selected patients may benefit from a sodium bicarbonate infusion.

Additional Issues with Portable CT

Artifacts and Related Factors

(a) Movement artifacts: Movement can contribute to significant artifacts during scanning. In noncooperative confused patients, this may pose a challenge. Thus, adequate sedation and restrains should be used to minimize the artifacts during image acquisition. Well-written guidelines regarding sedative dosing is a must to ensure no unnecessary complications arise from the use of sedatives during scanning [6, 7].

(b) Metal artifacts: Metal artifacts may occur from internal and external sources such as bolts, plating, clips, lines, monitors, or electroencephalography arrays on the patient's head. It is best to minimize the amount of metal in the scan plane as much as possible prior to the scan to reduce this source of artifacts [7].

Safety and Security of CT Image Data

(a) The scanner workstation receives all images from the gantry and stores them until they are deleted by the end user. Most often these images are sent to the Picture Archival and Communication System (PACS) network in the hospital where they are permanently stored and archived. It is also possible to print to film or archive to external media [6].

(b) The images on the workstation are encrypted on the hard drive itself and can only be accessed through the application [6].

(c) The workstation is password protected to prevent any unauthorized access to the system, protecting patient data [6].

Summary

Any imaging study requiring transportation of the patient from the ICU should be carefully checked for its indication. The portable CT scanner in the setting of the neurocritical care unit saves cost, reduces the risks of transporting patients, and keeps the intensive care staff safe and happy. Physicians are able to acquire immediate images and treat patient promptly. The portable CT scanner is a light, easily maneuvered machine with minimal risks of radiation exposure, making it the best choice for management of patients with intracranial pathology in the neurocritical care unit enabling improved patient safety and outcome.

Dos and Don'ts

Dos

- Repeat CT of the brain only if there is a deterioration in neurological status or Glasgow Coma Scale
- Carefully evaluate the indication for each imaging study requiring transportation of the patient
- Perform all repeat CT in the neurointensive care using a portable CT
- Ensure the portable CT lead curtains are in place during scanning

Don'ts

- Don't stand within 2 m (6 ft) from patient during scanning with a portable CT
- Don't use the portable CT if imaging of any other organ is also required (Portable CT only capable to scan till C3)
- Don't remove the portable CTs lead curtains from machine
- Don't repeat CT routinely unless indicated

References

1. Making the best use of clinical radiology services: referral guidelines. 6th ed. Royal College of Radiologists (Great Britain) Amy Davis, 20 Oct 2007.
2. Neuroimaging and decision making in Adult Mild Traumatic Brain Injury in Acute Setting, American college of emergency surgeons (ACEP) CDC Panel. Ann Emerg Med 2008; 52:714–48.
3. Haydel MJ, Preston CA, Mills TJ, et al. Indications for computed tomography in patients with minor head injury. N Engl J Med. 2000;343(2):100–5.
4. Connon FF, Namdarian B, Ee JL, Drummond KJ, Miller JA. Do routinely repeated computed tomography scans in traumatic brain injury influence management? A prospective observational study in a level 1 trauma center. Ann Surg. 2011;254(6):1028–31.
5. Brown CV, Weng J, Oh D, Salim A, Kasotakis G, Demetriades D, Velmahos GC, Rhee P. Does routine serial computed tomography of the head influence management of traumatic brain injury? A prospective evaluation. J Trauma. 2004;57(6):1340.
6. CereTom Brochure pdf-2013 Neurologica corp., a subsidiary of Samsung electronic company ltd.
7. Rumboldta Z, Hudaa W, Allb JW. Review of portable CT with assessment of a dedicated head CT scanner. Am J Neuoradiol. 2009;30:1630–6.
8. McCormick M. Radiation exposure: a quick guide to what each level means. Guardian Datablog 15 March 2011.
9. Hammell CL, Henning JD. Prehospital management of severe traumatic brain injury. BMJ. 2009;338:b1683.
10. Melnick ER, Szlezak CM, Bentley SK, Dziura JD, Kotlyar S, Post LA. CT overuse for mild traumatic brain injury. Jt Comm J Qual Patient Saf. 2012;38(11):483–9 (ISSN: 1553–7250).
11. Bee TK, Magnotti LJ, Croce MA, Maish GO, Minard G, Schroeppel TJ, Zarzaur BL, Fabian TC. Necessity of repeat head CT and ICU monitoring in patients with minimal brain injury. J Trauma. 2009;66(4):1015–8.
12. Peace K, Wilensky EM, Frangos S, MacMurtrie E, Shields E, Hujcs M, Levine J, Kofke A, Yang W, Le Roux PD. The use of a portable head CT scanner in the intensive care unit. J Neurosci Nurs. 2010;42(2):109–16.
13. Carlson AP, Yonas H. Portable head computed tomography scanner–technology and applications: experience with 3421 scans. J Neuroimaging. 2012;22(4):408–15.
14. Agrawal D, Sahoo S, Satyarthee GD, Gupta D, Sinha S, Misra MC. Initial experience with mobile computed tomogram in neurosurgery intensive care unit in a level 1 trauma center in India. Neurol India. 2011;59(5):739–42. JPN Apex Trauma Centre, All India Institute of Medical Sciences, New Delhi, India.
15. Stevens GC, Rowles NP, Foy RT, Loader R, Barua N, Williams A, Palmer JD. The use of mobile computed tomography in intensive care: regulatory compliance and radiation protection. J Radiol Prot. 2009;29(4):483–90.
16. Katayama H. Adverse reactions to contrast media. What are the risk factors? Invest Radiol. 1990;25 Suppl 1:S16–7.

Chapter 20
Brain Death

Michael A. Kuiper, Gea Drost, and J. Gert van Dijk

> *The boundaries which divide Life from Death are at best*
> *shadowy and vague. Who shall say where the one ends, and*
> *where the other begins? Edgar Allan Poe, 1844 (in: The*
> *Premature Burial)*

Introduction

It is important to acknowledge that brain death is not just a theoretical construct with the exclusive purpose of accommodating organ donation. Some, however, view the 1968 definition of brain death by the Harvard ad hoc committee as such, and while this paper indeed made organ retrieval possible from patients in irreversible apneic coma, doing so was not the primary goal of the paper [1]. The authors stated: *"Our primary purpose is to define irreversible coma as a new criterion for death. There are two reasons why there is need for a definition: (1) Improvements in resuscitative and supportive measures have led to increased efforts to save those who are desperately injured. Sometimes these efforts have only partial success so that the result is an individual whose heart continues to beat but whose brain is irreversibly damaged. The burden is great on patients who suffer permanent loss of intellect, on their families, on the hospitals, and on those in need of hospital beds already occupied by these comatose patients. (2) Obsolete criteria for the definition of death can lead to controversy in obtaining organs for transplantation."*

The first of these two items clearly aimed to end a continuation of measures that have no value at all for the patient with irreversible brain damage. This cessation of

M.A. Kuiper, MD, PhD (✉)
Intensive Care Department, Medical Center Leeuwarden, Leeuwarden, The Netherlands
e-mail: mi.kuiper@wxs.nl

G. Drost, MD, PhD
Department of Neurology, University Medical Center Groningen,
Groningen, The Netherlands

J.G. van Dijk, MD, PhD
Department of Neurology, Leiden University Medical Center, Leiden, The Netherlands

© Springer International Publishing Switzerland 2015   313
K.E. Wartenberg et al. (eds.), *Neurointensive Care: A Clinical Guide*
to Patient Safety, DOI 10.1007/978-3-319-17293-4_20

purposeless treatment may be seen as the essential consequence of brain death, and making brain death equal to death formed the conditio sine qua non for organ donation and subsequent transplantation.

During history, different criteria to establish death have been used, from putrefaction to death on neurological criteria. After Harvey published his "De Motu Cordis" in 1628, in which he had given the heart the central role in the circulation of the blood, and hence life, a cardiorespiratory standard of establishing death became dominant. From the eighteenth century on through the mid-twentieth century, the following standard of death was used: a person was declared dead when the heart stopped beating and breathing ceased, usually without doctors having any chance to prevent this from happening; the lack of ability to do so also negated any choice in the matter. Since the early 1950s the development of mechanical ventilators made it possible to manipulate death as a direct consequence of organ support in intensive care departments; hence, the question about what defines the end of human life has become more pressing and more intricate. While respiration was supported the circulation could remain intact, while all signs of function of the brain could disappear [2, 3]. During the 1960s, criteria were sought to recognize those who were beyond hope and who could consequently be taken off the ventilator [4]. This eventually led to the Harvard ad hoc committee definition of irreversible coma in 1968 [1]. Although Henry Beecher, president of the ad hoc committee, stated that they could not define death [5], the resulting paper is widely accepted as the one that defined brain death and through that death itself. According to the paper, death should be declared before the respirator was to be turned off, not only to prevent causing death by termination of ventilation, but also to make organ donation possible with an intact circulation [5].

As said, the first reason to define brain death was to identify those patients who had no chance of regaining brain activity and in whom it was therefore justifiable to stop treatment and take them off the ventilator. The ad hoc committee followed this with a connection with organ donation, stating that "*Obsolete criteria for the definition of death can lead to controversy in obtaining organs for transplantation*" [1]. In a letter from the Dean of the Harvard Medical School, Robert Ebert, to the transplant surgeon, Dr Joseph Murray, dated January 4, 1968, he stated that "*Dr. Beecher's presentation (on the ethical problems created by the hopelessly unconscious man) re-emphasized to me the necessity of giving further consideration to the problem of brain death. With its pioneering interest in organ transplantation, I believe the faculty of the Harvard Medical school is better equipped to elucidate this area than any other single group*" [6]. That the need for organs was closely related to the definition of death in 1968 became clear from a draft version dated April 11, 1968: "*The question before this committee cannot be simply to define brain death. This would not advance the cause of organ transplantation since it would not cope with the essential issue of when a surgical team is authorized – legally, morally and medical – in removing a vital organ*" [6].

Presently we have two windows to look at death: a circulatory-respiratory window and a neurological window. Although there are two windows, or "two entrances," there is just one "exit": death. In all cases the brain will ultimately have irreversibly stopped functioning, causing the death of the individual. *"Individuals die, but their cells continue to metabolize"* as Beecher stated [5] *"and who are we to know when the exact moment is that death occurs?"*

In many Western countries, protocols for the determination of brain death (or brain stem death, as in the UK) were developed after the Harvard declaration and have gained rapid and wide acceptance.

Case Scenario

In this case scenario we will pay attention to problems that may present in making the diagnosis of brain death. These problems will be addressed in the later parts of this chapter.

A 35-year-old male endured traumatic brain injury in a traffic accident. He was intubated in the street by the emergency physician and admitted to the emergency room (ER) of a tertiary trauma center in order to be evaluated and treated for his injuries. He was in a deep coma, without opening of the eyes on stimuli, with abnormal flexor posturing of the left arm, and an extensor response of the right arm. A CT scan of the brain showed a very severe traumatic concussion of the brain with intracerebral and subarachnoid hemorrhages. The evaluation of the clinical situation and the CT scan prompted the decision to not perform surgery of the skull and brain, and he was admitted to the ICU where he was ventilated. Soon thereafter he did not respond to any stimulus anymore, and after sedative effects had worn off, neurological examination revealed the absence of brain stem reflexes. The medical team decided there were no options for treatment, so the primary responsible physician, in this case the treating intensivist, organized a meeting with the family of the patient and informed them about the condition and prognosis of the patient. The family had been expecting this outcome, as there had never been any progress during treatment. They were informed that their family member could become an organ donor. The treating physician emphasized the seriousness of the present condition and the bleakness of prognosis, and arranged for another meeting the following day to discuss the possibility of organ donation. The next day the same physician confirmed the diagnosis and prognosis and discussed organ donation. The family declared that in the past the patient had indicated to support organ donation, as did they; if the condition was beyond hope, they would want him to become an organ donor.

The same afternoon, a consultation by a neurologist was requested, and he confirmed the absence of responses to painful stimuli and the absence of brain stem reflexes. During nursing care, movements of the legs had been noted, which was confirmed during neurological examination. The neurologist diagnosed these movements as spinal reflexes and not as meaningful responses. An electroencephalogram (EEG) was performed, which showed no electrical activity ("iso-electric EEG"). An apnea test was performed, which showed no respiratory efforts and the expected increase in partial pressure of carbon dioxide (pCO_2), and consequently the diagnosis of brain death was made and a death certificate was signed.

The local transplant coordinator informed the surgical team about the presence of a potential donor, and preparations were made to remove the transplantable organs. The patient was moved to the operating theater. Meanwhile, however, the leg movements had become so prominent that the transplant surgeon doubted that the patient was in fact brain dead and informed the neurologist of this suspicion. The neurologist reexamined the patient in the operating room and reached the same conclusion as earlier that day: there were no responses to pain, no brain stem reflexes, and the observed leg movements were considered spinal reflexes. Although the neurologist was completely convinced that the diagnosis of brain death was sound, the transplant surgeon did not and refused to perform surgery to remove the transplantable organs. The patient was moved back to the ICU, where a meeting was held with the family to explain the course of events. A decision was agreed upon to convert the heart-beating organ donation procedure into a nonheart beating organ donation ("Donation after Circulatory Death"; DCD). The patient was extubated. He did not make any breathing efforts, and after a few minutes, circulation stopped. After 5 min of circulatory arrest, he was declared dead and taken to the operating room for organ donation.

Patient Safety

Safety in relation to brain death includes two major issues: the first concerns the interests of the future donor, i.e., how certain is the diagnosis of brain death, and the second concerns the interests of the organ recipient. It may be thought that the latter consideration should not affect the diagnosis of brain death at all, and indeed the interest of an organ recipient should never affect the decision-making process in evaluation for brain death. Further reflection reveals that donation does affect brain death, but in another way: in many countries brain death is only formally diagnosed when there is a possibility of organ donation. In patients who are not suitable as organ donors, the process of determination of brain death is hardly ever completely carried out: the presence of catastrophic brain injury, the clinical symptoms thereof, with its subsequent prognosis of poor outcome will suffice to justify limitation or withdrawal of treatment. The additional steps of ancillary testing and an apnea test are then only carried out with an expectation for organ donation.

Diagnosis of Brain Death

Brain death occurs as a result of severe brain injury, most often associated with elevated intracranial pressure. Inadequate perfusion of the brain, resulting from increased intracranial pressure, results in a cycle of cerebral ischemia and edema, further increasing intracranial pressure, or could result from an insufficient systemic circulation as in circulatory arrest. Diagnosing brain death requires the irreversible absence of consciousness and the absence of brain stem reflexes including the absence of spontaneous respiratory efforts. The overall function of the whole brain is assessed. However, no clinical or ancillary test can establish under such circumstances that every brain cell has died, and indeed this is not likely to be the case. There is however no believable documented case of a person who fulfilled the preconditions and criteria for brain death who showed any return of brain function.

Brain death may never be considered proven without evidence of intracranial pathology. There must be evidence of brain pathology (e.g., traumatic brain injury, intracranial hemorrhage, hypoxic encephalopathy) consistent with the irreversible loss of neurological function. There are conditions that can mimic the clinical presentation of brain death but lack the required preconditions for making the diagnosis and therefore lack the required irreversibility; examples are the clinical condition shortly after circulatory arrest and subsequent cardiopulmonary resuscitation, Locked-in syndrome, and acute severe Guillain-Barré syndrome [7].

Other problems can occur, as presented in the case scenario, in establishing the absence of consciousness, absence of brain stem reflexes, and absence of respiration. Absence of consciousness, which in brain death means a deep unresponsive coma with bilateral absence of motor responses, speech, and eye opening, is diagnosed by applying painful stimuli. If there is a response to a painful stimulus, the patient is not brain dead. A diagnostic problem may occur if spinal reflexes are elicited, as presented in the case scenario. Over the years, there have been various reports of spinal reflexes [8–10]. In the case description, representing a combination of several well-documented cases in the Netherlands, these spinal reflexes mimicked normal motor responses to such a degree that even experienced transplant surgeons were not convinced that these movements were spinal reflexes.

Whereas spinal reflexes can cause confusion, they are in fact not very relevant to brain death. Brain stem reflexes are in contrast of utmost importance: they must all be absent to diagnose brain death. A problem can occur if, in a patient in deep apneic coma and without brain stem reflexes, one forgets to check the first step, i.e., to ensure that there is evidence of inconvertible brain damage. For instance, a deep coma without brain stem reflexes and without respiratory efforts may exist in the early stages after circulatory arrest, only to change into a state of responsiveness after hours to days. Another source of confusion is the presence of the ciliospinal reflex. This consists of dilation of the pupil in response to ipsilateral pain applied to the neck, face, and upper trunk. The pathway of this reflex lies beneath the brain stem and is not in conflict with the requirement of absent brain stem function, but when this reflex is not properly appreciated it may lead to confusion in patients fulfilling criteria for brain death [11].

The absence of respiration in ventilated patients can be ascertained by performing an apnea test. In some patients, this may be done by disconnecting the ventilator while applying high flow oxygen into the endotracheal tube and observing for respirations. In other, unstable, patients, disconnection from the ventilator may lead to rapid deoxygenation and, if not acted upon, to bradycardia and cardiac arrest. To prevent this from happening, these patients need to stay on positive pressure ventilation. The positive intrathoracic pressure often prevents deoxygenation, even without breathing efforts. We need to make sure that in the event of an apnea test, auto-triggering of the ventilator circuit does not occur. Flow triggering of the mechanical ventilator may sometimes lead to auto triggering, resulting in mechanical ventilation of the patient, suggesting respiratory efforts even when there are none [12, 13]. Continuous flow or pressure triggering may be preferred in order not to misdiagnose auto-cycling of a mechanical ventilator as respiratory efforts. Modern ventilators have flow triggering as the preferred mode of pressure support (or other modes of spontaneous breathing), so one needs to be careful when performing the apnea test in a patient connected to the ventilator.

So, there are several important issues to take into account in the diagnosis of brain death. In addition to the careful execution of the tests, the sequence of testing is important. We need to adhere to the correct order of tests, primarily to make sure that there is severe brain damage explaining the clinical condition.

There are many differences between countries in mandating additional, ancillary, or conformational tests, e.g., electroencephalogram (EEG), evoked potentials, scintigraphy, blood flow studies, such as conventional CT- or MRI angiography, etc. In some protocols a transcranial Doppler ultrasound is required.

In most protocols, such ancillary tests are followed by the apnea test as the last and final step as a test of one of the most basic functions of the brain stem. Another reason for performing the apnea test last is that it can sometimes lead to clinical instability with hypoxia, bradycardia, hypotension, and cardiac arrest.

There are differences in duration of the required observational period before formal brain death confirmation is allowed. Many protocols require at least several hours, but some do not specify a duration at all. As the return of brain function may be delayed for more than several hours after resuscitation from cardiorespiratory arrest, it is recommended that clinical testing for brain death is delayed for at least 24 h following the return of spontaneous circulation in cases of acute hypoxic-ischemic brain injury. However, in some countries brain death may be determined earlier than that by demonstration of absent cerebral blood flow.

Despite many national protocols being derived from protocols from other countries, there is international variability in adapting brain death guidelines. Algorithms of preclinical testing and preconditions in order to demonstrate irreversibility (e.g., causes of primary or secondary brain injury, absence of sedatives, neuromuscular blocking agents, acid-base or endocrine disturbances, hypothermia, hypotension, and others) differ from country to country. There are also differences in the order of tests concerning the apnea test, specification and certification of the diagnosing physicians in terms of amount of physicians required, specialization, and clinical experience, ancillary tests, observation period, and legal provisions of organ transplantation and brain death. Uniformity is only to be found in the required presence of a clear cause of brain damage and demonstration of absent brain stem function.

Imminent Brain Death

Not all patients with severe acute brain damage fulfill the criteria of brain death. Possible criteria have been proposed to identify a patient with a reasonable probability to become brain dead: imminent brain death. A patient who fulfills the criteria of imminent brain death is a mechanically ventilated, deeply comatose patient, with irreversible catastrophic brain damage of known origin. This state has to be considered in relation to criteria to determine irreversibility and futility in acute neurological conditions. A condition of imminent brain death requires either a Glasgow Coma Score of 3 and the progressive absence of at least three out of six brain stem reflexes. Imminent brain death can be used as a point of departure for potential heart-beating organ donor recognition in the intensive care unit [14].

Definition of Death

Shemie et al. published a report on international guideline development for the determination of death, resulting from an international invitational forum, supported by the WHO [15], and including an operational definition of human death which is "the permanent loss of capacity for consciousness and loss of all brainstem functions, as a consequence of permanent cessation of circulation or catastrophic brain injury." As said, Henry K. Beecher, anesthesiologist and president of the Harvard ad hoc committee stated that only a very bold man would attempt to define death; the present definition will surely cause criticism, but regardless of that a great merit of the definition proposed by Shemie et al. is that it aims to steer away from terms that suggest the death of only one organ, such as brain death or cardiac death. While medical philosophers and bioethicists will surely scrutinize the proposed definition of death, the authors should be applauded for their effort to compose a definition that aims at reuniting the "two deaths" and return to "one death." Another advantage of the paper is the emphasis that is placed on the clinical evaluation in confirming death.

There are, however, also some problems with the definition. In the context of death determination, "permanent" refers to loss of function that cannot resume spontaneously and will not be restored through "intervention" [16, 17]. The word "permanent" is used instead of "irreversible," permanent referring to a condition that regardless of its duration could in theory be reversed. The term "irreversible" determines that function cannot be restored no matter what. This is an important notion: with our current technology, many organs can be replaced or their function supported, but not all: the brain cannot be replaced. It may therefore be concluded that the word "permanent" refers not directly to the brain but merely to the circulation. The circulation can in many circumstances be restarted or supported by means of cardiopulmonary resuscitation (CPR) or extracorporeal life support (ECLS), when this is required. However, there are circumstances where maintaining the circulation is technically possible but not be desirable, such as in catastrophic brain injury with a poor prognosis. The word "permanent" brings about the possibility of choice. We could also say that the word "irreversible" refers to a condition or diagnosis and the word "permanent" refers to prognosis.

Regardless of whether the concept of brain death was originally intended to delineate when it was warranted to stop or limit therapy in patients on mechanical ventilation, now the proposed definition and operational criteria of brain death are intricately related to establishing death in relation to organ donation. Two problems need to be addressed: the acceptance of brain death as death of the individual and the limited time available to declare death after cessation of circulation and respiration.

The first is the acceptance of brain death as death. The case of Jahi McMath may help to illustrate the problems: the case concerns a 13-year-old girl who was declared brain dead. This happened after massive blood loss and consequent cardiac arrest, the result of surgery at UCSF Benioff Children's Hospital Oakland, USA, on December 9, 2013, aimed at relieving sleep apnea. Her family rejected brain death as equal to death of the individual and made efforts to maintain her (or her remains, depending on the point of view) on life support and to have her transferred to another facility to continue medical support. Alameda County Superior Court Judge Evelio Grillo ruled that the child must be kept on a ventilator until a court-approved doctor could assess whether there was any chance of recovery. Despite the confirmation of brain death by an independent child neurologist, the Judge ruled that Jahi could be transferred to an undisclosed facility, which happened on January 5, 2014, and where she remains to the time of writing (November 2014). The Alameda County Coroner issued but has not publicly released a death certificate, marking December 12, 2013, as the date of her death but not listing a cause of death, pending an autopsy. Her family has issued optimistic reports on her condition, claiming she is sleeping. She has even received, in absence, a graduation diploma from her school.

The story of Jahi McMath teaches us that even in countries with clear laws defining brain death, as the USA, there is opposition against the concept of brain death, which is not always accepted as death of the individual [16, 17]. Shemie et al. stated in his WHO forum paper on the definition of death that "For the purposes of this forum, death was fundamentally considered a biological event" and that "… legal, ethical, cultural and religious perspectives on death were not included." Still, the problem remains that cerebral function is only one "biological event," but there are other biological functions: circulation remains present while ventilation continues in brain death, as do hormonal and other processes. Cultural and religious aspects are not to be ignored either: there are countries in which brain death is not accepted as death and in countries where brain death is legally accepted, it might not be universally accepted in the general population. The opposition against brain death as death of the individual does not exist in the case of death on circulatory-respiratory grounds; someone who would not accept circulatory death as death of the individual would not be taken seriously, and a family insisting to take such a patient from hospital with the claim of continuing care at home would not be considered to be of sound mind. However, in the case of the brain dead Jahi McMath, her relatives were allowed to take her from the hospital and to transport her elsewhere to continue ventilation and restart enteral feeding [16]. This sad story reverts the situation to where it started in the late 1950s: brain death is of use as a criterion to stop treatment in someone who is beyond hope and also in fact beyond harm.

This societal opposition could also form an argument against abandoning the dead-donor rule (DDR), which states that the donor needs to be dead before organ donation can occur, and removing of vital organs may not cause death. Truog and Miller and others have proposed to abolish the dead-donor rule and to accept alternative reasoning based on the principles of autonomy and nonmaleficence. The result would be that those who are dying, but not yet dead could become organ donors [17]. There is at least one major problem with this approach. While establishing death, whether on neurological or circulatory criteria in potential organ donors is difficult enough, abandoning the DDR requires a certain prognostication of impending death. While we may have philosophical and semantic problems in this regard, prognosticating outcome in those with severe brain injury is prone to error [18]. Even if we would doubt the concept of brain death, we need to admit that there is no documented case of a person who regained brain function (or "survived") after a technically correct diagnosis of brain death, fulfilling preconditions and criteria thereof. This makes brain death at least the best predictor of death of the individual.

Marlise Muñoz was a 33-year-old American woman who probably suffered a pulmonary embolism and subsequent circulatory arrest. On November 28, 2013, she was declared brain dead. Because she was 14 weeks pregnant, doctors at a Texas hospital kept her body on a respirator in the intensive care unit despite brain death and in conflict with the wishes of her husband. The decision of the physicians to do so was based on the legal notion that Texas law restricts the application of advance directives in pregnant patients. Muñoz's husband, who, just like his wife, was a paramedic, argued that the law was not applicable because his wife was legally dead, so there was no decision to make that would require advance directives. The judge agreed that the law did not apply to people who are dead. Following this judgment the hospital was ordered to remove mechanical ventilation, and her circulation stopped on January 26, 2014.

This case illustrates that a legal diagnosis of brain death is necessary to prevent harm, perhaps not so much for the brain dead patient, who is not beyond hope and harm, but for the family and relatives of the deceased person.

As already stated, criteria used to establish (brain) death differ across the globe. In many countries, laws on determination of death leave the determination to the physician. Legally a person is dead when a doctor declares that person to be dead. The law usually does not provide specific criteria for the determination of death, which may be wise, as otherwise laws might have to be updated frequently.

The debate should not center on the probably unsolvable riddles of whether we can define "life" and "death"; it should be centered on the question whether current practices of establishing death and organ donation are sound, ethically justifiable and acceptable. If one would argue that consciousness is needed to be alive, one could also argue that a lack of consciousness and a subsequent lack of possible harm would justify certain medical decisions.

Therefore, we probably need to retain the DDR, even if there is no definition of death that is philosophically sound, as we will be even less certain than we have to rely on the prognosis of impending death.

The changing practice of organ donation and transplantation does not in any way reduce our responsibility to perform organ donation with the utmost care and respect for the organ donor. Quite the contrary: all changes in donation guidelines need to be weighed anew against ethical and moral considerations. This respect is expressed in the diagnosis of death. If there is doubt about what death is, the burden is on the medical community to examine all doubts and facts, and to seek consensus and agreement on diagnosing death. While this is a daunting task, it is not one we should refrain from performing. We as a society are obliged to carefully balance the interests of both organ donors and organ recipients [19]. In this process we need to take into account the possibility of legislative amendments in order to legitimize changes in organ donation practices that we as a society see as justifiable [20]. In some countries, like the USA, the UK, Belgium, and the Netherlands, the possibility of DCD was introduced based on these notions. The case scenario reflects this possibility. Such considerations also affect the time that physicians breach the subject of organ donation to the relatives, which will typically have to be done before the patient has been declared dead. While DCD increases the potential number of organ donors, it has also introduced new practical, judicial, and ethical problems [20].

While the philosophical debate on the definitions of life and death is extremely interesting and needed, we need to be aware of the practical problems intensive care physicians and neurologists are confronted with. We need operational criteria to guide us in our daily practice, and while the debate on life and death continues, we make decisions based on the best available guidelines [21].

Summary

Brain death is a concept of death based on neurological criteria. In the late 1950s, brain death has been introduced to identify patients on the mechanical ventilator with intact circulation but without any signs of central nervous function and without spontaneous respiration. In these patients, treatment could be limited or withdrawn, as it was recognized that they could not improve. In 1968 irreversible apneic coma was defined as death, and this made organ donation in heart beating, brain dead patients possible. This definition has gained wide, albeit not complete, acceptance. Various problems in making the diagnosis of brain death clinically and in the use of ancillary tests have been documented. Ethical and judicial problems have been identified and need constant attention; in order to maintain a careful balance between the respects, we owe the patient who becomes brain dead and the great need for organs to help patients who need them.

Protocol

Brain death is determined by:

- Fulfilling preconditions
- Clinical testing if preconditions are met

- Absence of electrical activity of the brain by EEG
- Apnea test
- Imaging (4 vessel digital subtraction angiography, computed tomography angiography, magnetic resonance angiography, single photon emission computer tomography (SPECT), or transcranial Doppler ultrasound that demonstrates the absence of intracranial blood flow

Preconditions

- Normothermia (temperature >35 °C).
- Normotension (as a guide, systolic blood pressure >90 mmHg, mean arterial pressure (MAP) >60 mmHg in an adult).
- Exclusion of effects of sedative drugs.
- Absence of severe electrolyte, metabolic, or endocrine disturbances.
- Intact neuromuscular function.
- Ability to adequately examine the brain stem reflexes.
- Ability to perform apnea testing; this may be prevented by severe hypoxic respiratory failure or a high cervical spinal cord injury.

Clinical Neurological Investigation

If fulfillment of preconditions has been established, we need to perform a clinical investigation, showing no signs of activity of the brain or brain stem: no motor response to stimuli, no brain stem reflexes, and no respiratory efforts.

The clinical criteria are as follows:

- Irreversible absence of consciousness (coma)
- Absence of reactions to pain stimuli
- Absence of pupillary reactions
- Absence of corneal reflexes
- Absence of oculocephalic reflexes
- Absence of oculovestibular reflexes
- Absence of reaction from trachea and pharynx (cough reflex)
- Absence of spontaneous breathing

EEG

- Absence of electrical activity of the brain

Apnea Test

- Formalized testing of absence of breathing/respiratory efforts with disconnection of the patient from mechanical ventilation and demonstration of an increase in partial pressure of carbon dioxide by 20 mmHg

Cerebral Blood Flow

In several countries brain death can be determined if the preconditions cannot be met by demonstrating the absence of intracranial blood flow. There is a great variety in the type of test advocated for this purpose, and no specific recommendation can be given in this chapter. A general recommendation is to use the best test available that local specialists have experience with.

The following do not preclude determination of brain death:

- Spinal reflexes – these can be either spontaneous or elicited by stimulation, including a painful stimulus applied to limbs or sternum, tactile stimulation applied to palmar or plantar areas, neck flexion, limb elevation or hypoxia (such as during ventilation disconnection). Spinal reflexes are not to be confused with a pathological flexion or extension responses. For a complete list of spinal reflexes, see Jain and De Georgia [9].
- Absence of diabetes insipidus.

The following are incompatible with the presence of brain death:

- Decerebrate or decorticate posturing
- True extensor or flexor motor responses to painful stimuli
- Epileptic seizures

(Protocol based on the ANZICS statement of death and organ donation, 2013) [22]

COI Statement The authors state that there is no conflict of interest in regard to this chapter.

References

1. Beecher HK, Ad Hoc Committee of the Harvard Medical School to Examine the Definition of Brain Death. A definition of irreversible coma. Special communication: report of the Ad Hoc Committee of the Harvard Medical School to Examine the Definition of Brain Death. JAMA. 1968;205:337–40.
2. Wertheimer P, Jouvet M, Descotes J. À propos du diagnostic de la mort de système nerveux. Dans les comas avec arrêt respiratoire traités par respiration artificielle. Presse Med. 1959;67:87–8.
3. Mollaret P, Goulon M. Le coma dépassé (mémoire préliminaire). Rev Neurol (Paris). 1959;101:3–15.

4. Rosoff SD, Schwab RS. The EEG in establishing brain death. A 10-year report with criteria and legal safeguards in the 50 states. Electroencephalogr Clin Neurophysiol. 1968;24:283–4.
5. Beecher HK. Definitions of "life" and "death" for medical science and practice. Ann N Y Acad Sci. 1970;169:471–4.
6. Giacomini M. A change of heart and a change of mind? Technology and the redefinition of death in 1968. Soc Sci Med. 1997;44:1465–82.
7. Vargas F, Hilbert G, Gruson D, et al. Fulminant Guillain-Barré syndrome mimicking cerebral death: case report and literature review. Intensive Care Med. 2000;26(5):623–7.
8. Bueri JA, Saposnik G, Mauriño J, et al. Lazarus' sign in brain death. Mov Disord. 2000;15:583–6.
9. Jain S, De Georgia M. Brain death-associated reflexes and automatisms. Neurocrit Care. 2005;3:22–6.
10. Saposnik G, Maurino J, Saizar R, et al. Spontaneous and reflex movements in 107 patients with brain death. Am J Med. 2005;118:311–4.
11. Ikeda H, Aruga T, Hayashi M, Miyake Y, Sugimoto K, Mastumoto K. Two cases in which the presence of ciliospinal response led to indecisiveness in the evaluation of brain death. No To Shinkei. 1999;51:161–6.
12. Speelberg B, van Wezel HB. Continuous pressure is preferred to flow triggering of respiration in the apnea test following the protocol for brain death determination. Ned Tijdschr Geneeskd. 1998;142:1392–3.
13. McGee WT, Mailloux P. Ventilator autocycling and delayed recognition of brain death. Neurocrit Care. 2011;14:267–71.
14. de Groot YJ, Jansen NE, Bakker J, Kuiper MA, et al. Imminent brain death: point of departure for potential heart-beating organ donor recognition. Intensive Care Med. 2010;36:1488–94.
15. Shemie SD, Hornby L, Baker A, Teitelbaum J, Torrance S, Young K, Capron AM, Bernat JL, Noel L, The International Guidelines for Determination of Death Phase 1 Participants, in Collaboration with the World Health Organization. International guideline development for the determination of death. Intensive Care Med. 2014;40:788–97.
16. Magnus DC, Wilfond BS, Caplan AL. Accepting brain death. N Engl J Med. 2014. doi:10.1056/NEJMp1400930
17. Truog RD, Miller FG, Halpern SD. The dead-donor rule and the future of organ donation. N Engl J Med. 2013;369:1287–9.
18. Kompanje EJO. Prognostication in neurocritical care: just crystal ball gazing? Neurocrit Care. 2013;19:267–8.
19. Kuiper MA. Donation after cardiac death: an ethical balancing act? Neth J Crit Care. 2008;12:31.
20. Kuiper MA, Jansen NE. Legislative amendment legitimises current organ donation practices. Ned Tijdschr Geneeskd. 2013;157(36):A6456.
21. Kuiper MA, Kompanje EJ. Only a very bold man would attempt to define death. Intensive Care Med. 2014;40(6):897–9.
22. ANZICS statement on death and organ donation. http://www.anzics.com.au/death-and-organ-donation

Chapter 21
Ethics in the Neuro-ICU

Ludo J. Vanopdenbosch and Fred Rincon

Introduction

Medical ethics deal with moral issues related to the daily practice of medicine [1]. Questions about the behaviors of physicians and health care providers, the decision-making process, values, rights, and responsibilities, generate ethical reflection that require a thorough understanding of philosophical concepts, religion, and the jurisdictional laws. Most texts in Medical ethics are written from a North American or Western European perspective rooted in Judeo-Christian philosophical traditions. For instance Japanese and Chinese medical ethics may have different accents and priorities, so getting acquainted with the jurisdictional cultural trends and laws is an important step towards becoming proficient at dealing with ethical problems in the Neuro-ICU. In the case of life-threatening or terminal conditions, and when faced with the possibility of significant disability or even death, it is difficult to predict how fears of future outcome will ultimately alter the predefined preferences of an individual patient or surrogate decision making. When addressing issues relating to advance directives and withholding and withdrawing life supportive therapy, clinical prognostic questions require specific answers so care takers should attempt to achieve the highest level of certainty regarding the diagnosis and prognosis with the patient's wishes in mind.

L.J. Vanopdenbosch, MD, FAAN
Department of Neurology, AZ Sint Jan Brugge Oostende, Brugge, Belgium

F. Rincon, MD, MSc, MB Ethics, FCCM, FNCS (✉)
Department of Neurosurgery, Thomas Jefferson University Hospital, Philadelphia, PA, USA
e-mail: fred.rincon@jefferson.edu

© Springer International Publishing Switzerland 2015
K.E. Wartenberg et al. (eds.), *Neurointensive Care: A Clinical Guide to Patient Safety*, DOI 10.1007/978-3-319-17293-4_21

Case Scenario

A 66-year-old woman, retired nurse, had a severe traumatic brain injury (TBI). She ran her bike into an opening door of a stationary car, toppled over her steering wheel, and hit the pavement with her head. She was unconscious for several minutes, had regained consciousness upon arrival of the paramedics, but was somnolent and disoriented afterwards. On arrival to the emergency room her Glasgow Coma Scale (GCS) was 11, she was non-cooperative, but did not show overt lateralization. Cranial computed tomography (CT) showed a fracture of the right frontal bone, a contrecoup hemorrhagic contusion in the left temporal lobe and a 2–3 mm thick subdural hematoma over the left occipital lobe. She was transferred to the Neuro-ICU for care and further observation. At this time, no neurosurgical procedure was performed. Over the next days her consciousness deteriorated and a follow up cranial CT showed a small increase in the left temporal contusion with some oedema, and the subdural hematoma resolved spontaneously over days. Over several weeks, she recovered consciousness, but remained severely aphasic and most likely severely amnestic.

It was noted that she had worked as a nurse in a palliative care unit several years before retiring. She asked her sister many times to promise her that "no matter what, she would not want to live in a dependent state or unable to communicate with her family and friends." However, she had never made a written advance directive. She never married and had no children.

After 2 months in the general hospital, she was discharged home on explicit request of her family and friends, who promised to take care of her 24 h a day at home. She was walking, feeding herself with supervision, taking care of her personal care and clothing with supervision, the speech was severely affected, but she understood simple commands and could speak very simple sentences. She was completely amnestic with disorientation to time and space. The care at home proved to be very difficult, because of nocturnal confusion and incontinence. She was admitted to a long-term rehabilitation hospital where her neurological function deteriorated with increasing gait difficulty and progressive loss of speech. A CT scan of the head showed communicating hydrocephalus.

The sister of the patient initially refused to consent to a neurosurgical procedure to insert a ventriculo-peritoneal shunt (VPS). With several consultations, she gave consent, understanding the procedure could substantially improve her sister's condition and was not a very invasive procedure. However, patient did not improve as expected with VPS. In the following months she remained severely disabled, not able to speak, feeding herself when offered food, and not walking independently. The family continued to stress the patient's previously but not written wishes that this situation was not acceptable.

This case raises several ethical issues that can, as in any other instance, impact on the patient's safety, well-being, and dignity as a whole. In this chapter, we will discuss the ethical framework of consent for treatments, the decision-making process in incapacitated individuals, and end-of life issues related to withdrawal and withholding, and palliative care.

Ethical Principles

The foundations of medical ethics can be found in Hippocratic and Aesclepian philosophical concepts; and in the Platonic and Aristotelian theories of morality [1]. Medical ethics as a field has also recently been influenced by the application of modern moral theories [2]. In addition, the human rights movement, in general, has nurtured the conceptual foundations of medical ethics by landmark contributions such as the Nuremberg Code [3], the Declaration of Helsinki [4], and the Belmont Report [5]. With this in mind, care of critically ill neurological patients, as in any other field, demands the application of basic ethical principles. Ethical principles classically associated with the ethical decision-making process are autonomy, beneficence, nonmaleficence, and distributive justice [2].

But how can we determine what is ethical? In reality, there is no right or wrong answer, and ethical analysis may vary from place to place and every individual is ultimately responsible for making their own ethical decisions and implementing them. In practice, the study of morality pertains to the determination of actions that may be right or wrong and ethics, the study of morality, helps us in informing why. There are several "rational" ways of approaching ethical dilemmas which are characterized by a systematic, reflective use of reason in decision making: Principlism, Deontology, Consequentialism and Utilitarianism, and Virtue Ethics [1, 3].

Principlism

As its name implies, this moral theory uses ethical principles as the basis for making moral decisions. It applies the principles of *autonomy, justice, beneficence, and nonmaleficence* [2] to particular cases to determine what is right or wrong. However, the choice of these principles, and especially the prioritization of patient autonomy over the other principles, may reflect Western liberal philosophies, which may not be widely accepted in other cultures or jurisdictions [6]. Moreover, these principles may clash in particular clinical situations where there is a need for some additional criteria, or thought process (other moral theories), for resolving such ethical conflicts [7].

Deontology

Deontology is moral theory promoted by Immanuel Kant, who preached a theory of "duty." Kant referred to the demands of the moral law as "categorical imperatives." Categorical imperatives are principles that are intrinsically valid; they are good in and of themselves; they must be obeyed by all people in all situations and circumstances if our behavior is to observe the moral law. It is from the categorical imperative that all other moral obligations are generated, and it is by this imperative that all moral obligations can be tested. In other words, deontology involves a search for well-founded rules that can serve as the basis for making moral decisions where the "means justify the end" [2, 6].

Consequentialism and Utilitarianism

Consequentialism is a label affixed to theories holding that actions are right or wrong according to the balance of their good and bad consequences. In other words, it denotes theories that take the promotion of value to determine what is right or wrong. What is right or ethical, therefore, is the act that produces the best overall results determined by a relevant theory of value. One of the best-known forms of consequentialism is utilitarianism. The classic origins of this moral theory are found in the writings of Jeremy Bentham and John Stuart Mill. Utilitarians based their ethical decision making on an analysis of the likely consequences or outcomes of different choices or actions [2, 6]. In consequentialism, the end justifies the means.

Virtue Ethics

This moral theory is rooted in ancient Greek philosophical principles preached by Plato and Aristotle. Virtue ethics focuses less on decision making (rules) and more on the character of the decision makers as reflected in their behavior (virtues). A virtue is a type of moral excellence, such as compassion, honesty, prudence, and dedication. Physicians who possess these virtues are assumed to be more likely to make good decisions and to implement them in a good way [6].

Risks to Patient Safety in the Decision-Making Process and Ethical Safety Barriers

Informed Consent

Treatments in general require an appropriate consent process. The process of informed consent is a dynamic process that requires the application of basic principles of autonomy and self-determination, competence, and voluntariness [4]. Informed consent is defined as "an autonomous authorization of individuals of a medical intervention or of involvement in research" [3]. The concept of informed consent stems from a principle of personal autonomy, which allows for moral self-determination and is based on five important elements: (a) decision-making capacity, (b) disclosure, (c) understanding, (d) voluntary choice, and (e) formal authorization to be treated or included in research [3]. The principle of autonomy implies that rational individuals with decisional capacity, or competency in legal terms, are uniquely qualified to decide what is best for themselves. It also means that people should be allowed to do whatever they want, even if doing so involves considerable risk or would be deemed foolish by others, provided that their decision does not infringe in the autonomy of another. Ethically, the principle of informed consent is also supported by concepts of beneficence related to professional duty to promote well-being, nonmaleficence related to the duty of not inflicting harm, and justice by providing fair and equitable access to health care and research.

Implied Consent

In certain circumstances, like in the setting of life-threatening conditions, the process of obtaining informed consent for clinical care may be waived. In emergency, life-threatening, or time-critical situations, physicians have the duty to preserve life. In very few life-threatening conditions patients may be involved in the consent process. However, physicians often use an "implied consent" principle to perform life-saving interventions in those patients who lack decision-making capacity or surrogates. The emergency doctrine of "implied consent" allows providers to deliver certain interventions that if not performed in a timely basis could potentially lead to increase morbidity and mortality. If the following conditions are met, the physician can use the "implied consent" doctrine: (a) the treatment in question represents the usual and customary standard of care for the condition being treated, (b) it would be clearly harmful to the patient to delay treatment awaiting explicit consent, and (c) patients ordinarily would be expected to consent for the treatment in question if they had the capacity to do so [5].

When a critically ill neurological patient is deemed not to have decision-making capacity, the physician must seek alternate pathways to obtain consent. The options in these cases are to determine if the patient has drafted an advance directive such as a living will or durable power of attorney (for health care); or in the absence of an advance directive, the physician must seek the substituted judgment of a proxy or surrogate authorized by the jurisdictional law (family friends, etc). If the physician is unable to identify an alternative form of consent, the physician must choose to invoke the emergency situation as justification for treatment the emergency doctrine of "implied consent" or "best interest" standard but this may apply only to emergency situations. It is imperative to seek informed consent as soon as the patient is stabilized and treatment priorities might have to be reconsidered.

Advance Directive or Living Will

It is probably a good tool to direct care in the event of incapacity, but usually also helpful in situations related to terminal conditions, futile care, and multi-organ dysfunction. Shortcomings of these documents are (a) that the physician may not find instructions that clearly guide certain treatment decisions and (b) the ethical argument that once cannot predict a person's own reaction when faced with disability [8]. Studies have demonstrated a tendency among the nondisabled to view disability as equivalent to death [9, 10] and historically, investigators frequently dump death with the severe disability group [11]. In this sense, advance directives or living wills, even if legally valid, are suboptimal to find treatment directions in critical illness particularly when goals of self-determination and perceptions that guide one's chosen moral course may change [8].

Substituted Judgment

Obtaining informed consent by an authorized surrogate decision maker is an alternative to direct informed consent. Appointees by advance directive, or living will, or durable power of attorney (for health care decisions), or a family member identified by state law are expected to make the same decisions as the patient would if the patient's capacity were intact. This idea of substituted judgment is widely accepted as a valid means of respecting patient preferences [12]. Shortcomings of the substituted judgment standard are related to the poor accuracy of the proxy's ability to predict the patient's will, which some studies have found to be no better than random chance [6, 12], the inherent difficulty of making therapeutic decisions for other persons which may make proxies reluctant to participate in a consent process and make them more likely to defer to the physician's expertise without even considering the full disclosure of risks and benefits associated with the intervention [7, 10].

Best Interest Standard

A legal exception to the consent process may be invoked in certain clinical settings and particularly in emergency situations, in which case the consent of a reasonable person to appropriate treatment is implied [3], so the *best interest standard* may be applied in these circumstances. The best interests' standard is a widely used ethical, legal, and social basis for policy and decision making involving incompetent persons to determine a wide range of issues relating to their well-being [13]. This principle could also be applicable in those cases when the burden of a therapy outweighs the benefits and the pain of interventions which would make them inhumane

[14]. One of the shortcomings of using the *best interest standard* is the possibility of the physician being judged as paternalistic [15] based on the inherent role of physicians to prevent evil or harm by promoting good and welfare for others (beneficence) [3]. Physicians and health care providers have to realize that they use their own reference frame of what is acceptable. This might be quite different to the patients' perspective e.g. patients with severe congenital cognitive defects. It is important to remain humble and open-minded.

The Principle of "Clear and Convincing Evidence"

In some jurisdictions of the United States, the principle of "clear and convincing evidence" may be used in lieu of the *substituted judgment standard*. This is one of the legal principles used in the US legal system (the other two being beyond the reasonable doubt and preponderance of evidence). This principle can be used by physicians in certain jurisdictions of the United States (Missouri, New York, Florida) to withdraw life support or any other intervention when there is "clear and convincing evidence" of previous patient's statements and in the absence of a "declaration" such as a living will, advance directive, or durable power of attorney (DPA). This principle is valid in many places of the world however the practicalities, the paperwork, whether or not courts of law have to be consulted are rather country specific.

Withdrawal or Withholding

When facing withdrawal or withholding of medical interventions, ethical questions cannot be addressed successfully unless the probability of outcomes is entertained. Health care providers should make every effort to acquire the highest level of certainty regarding the diagnosis, disease severity, and prognosis with the patient's wishes in mind. To attain a balanced view of the impact of therapeutic decisions and the expected disability to the patient, the effort will require a thorough knowledge of the literature and a multidisciplinary team approach. In addressing these issues, clinical prognostic questions that require specific answers include: (a) what is the probability of death during the next month and next year (and what are the confidence intervals around that probability; (b) what are the likely causes of death during the first month and subsequently; (c) if the patient survives, what level of disability and handicap will the patient suffer; and (d) what impact will the intervention have on survival or disability [16]. Advanced directives, the substituted judgment standard, the best interest standard, and the clear and convincing evidence principle (when applicable by the jurisdiction), may be used in these circumstances.

Is There a Difference Between Withdrawing and Withholding?

Generally, the ethical principles of beneficence, nonmaleficence, distributive justice; the legal implications of due care and negligence; and orthodox religious view, form the basis for this question [14]. Patients, family members, physicians, and health care providers may have strong arguments. Some may feel comfortable with both situations, some may feel comfortable only when deciding not to start a therapy, but some may feel uncomfortable deciding when to stop that therapy [14]. The court system in the United States has examined this controversy, and has noted that withholding a therapy can be based on an (a) active or (b) inadvertent omission. However, the moral and legal implications are based on the issue of intent [14]. If one has a duty to treat, but actively or inadvertently omits an effective therapy, then one can be found negligent by the court or legal system; but fundamentally, without moral or legal pre-notions, both acts are similar in the way that the treatment is never started [14].

In practice, when physicians and health care providers encounter these situations, some feel morally responsible for the effects of withdrawing care, others may find that there is no difference, and therefore will feel no moral responsibility for the end results. According to Miller and Truog, "what distinguishes withdrawing from withholding, is that in the former, the agent initiates the fatal consequence, as distinct from merely permitting it to continue without intervention to stop it" [17]. According to Beauchamp and Childress, "feelings of reluctance about withdrawing treatments are understandable, but the distinction between withdrawing and withholding is morally irrelevant and can be dangerous" [3]. In regard to life sustaining therapies, other courts in the United States have upheld the concept that there is no difference between withdrawing and withholding [2, 18]. Both are medical decisions with an obligation to inform the patients and/or his representative and consent has to be sought.

Very frequently in the Neuro-ICU, physicians and health care providers do not know whether a therapy will be effective. In this case, it would be better to attempt a trial of medical therapy, by setting-up "goals" of care, determining whether those goals can be achieved by ongoing re-assessment, and allowing the Neuro-ICU team to find if the therapy is ineffective while maintaining good communication with patient's families, friends, and/or surrogates [14]. This approach would allow the physician or health care team to withdraw an ineffective therapy rather than withhold a potentially beneficial treatment, limiting the chance for under-treatment and avoiding ethical dilemmas.

Health in its broader sense is defined as "a state of complete physical, mental, and social well-being and not merely the absence of disease or infirmity" [19], a sometimes difficult to achieve goal in the Neuro-ICU, that is echoed by the words of Hippocrates: the purpose of medicine is to do away with the sufferings of the sick, to lessen the violence of their diseases, and to refuse to treat those who are overmastered by their diseases, realizing that in such cases, medicine is powerless" [3, 14]. In such cases, treatment may be considered *futile* [20]. According to the

Society of Critical Care Medicine's Ethics Committee, treatments that offer no physiological benefit to the patient and therefore fail to achieve their intended goal may be considered as futile. Additionally, the Ethics Committee advised against treatments that are unlikely to confer any benefit, or possibly beneficial but extremely costly, or treatments that are controversial and of uncertain benefit [20].

Ethical Analysis of the Case and Discussion

Our case illustrates a challenging ethical conundrum. From very early on, we asked the advice of the specialist in palliative care medicine. They helped us in defining treatment goals, figuring out the legal position of the not-written advanced care directive, and the deciding power of the family. They guided us in symptom control and discharge planning. At no time it was felt that the patient was uncomfortable, anxious or in pain. A DNR code was written and the family was informed. This brought some assurance that patient would not be subjected to intensive care treatment which were judged futile. She was never tube-fed; the food offered was never rejected. We felt it not ethical to withdraw this feeding by spoon (nonmaleficence). Psychological and spiritual counseling was offered to the family. We tried to make clear that advance care directives do not protect people from disease or handicap. That despite her wish not be in a dependent state that we could not have avoided present situation and that there is no means to stop. Even in countries with euthanasia laws, this would not be applicable to presented patient-case. An aspect in advance directives but also in this case is a mistrust of the general public in the medicine and doctors. The family took patient home believing they could provide better care at home than was offered in hospital, grossly underestimating the actual care at the hospital. The case illustrates the difficulty in prognostication. Both at first admission and at insertion of VPS, the expectations of recovery were not met.

Dos and Don'ts

Dos

- Know the country specific judicial rules and laws about the process of withholding and withdrawing of medical treatment
- Try to get an honest idea of prognosis and expectations of treatments and interventions
- Be humble and open minded
- Work in a group, discuss with colleagues, nurses, ethicists, palliative care specialists
- Seek early palliative care consultation since they often offer a different view on treatment goals, expectations, patient wishes and symptom control

Don'ts

- Impose your own view on a situation
- Avoid an honest process of informing patients about the present situation and expectations
- Avoid withdrawing or withholding therapies thinking this might save you time or save you from lengthy and personal discussions
- Base your judgment on individual patient experience rather than published and validated data
- Give up too easily

References

1. Medical ethics manual. Ferney-Volaire Cedex: World Medical Association; 2005.
2. The Belmont report: ethical principles and guidelines for the protection of human subjects of research. Accessed 20 July 2011, at http://ohsr.od.nih.gov/guidelines/belmont.html.
3. Beauchamp TL, Childress JF. Principles of biomedical ethics. New York: Oxford University Press; 2009.
4. Silverman HJ. Ethical considerations of ensuring an informed and autonomous consent in research involving critically ill patients. Am J Respir Crit Care Med. 1996;154:582–6.
5. Bernat JL. Ethical practice. Ethical issues in neurology. 3rd ed. Philadelphia: Lippincott Williams & Wilkins; 2008. p. 24–48.
6. Seckler AB, Meier DE, Mulvihill M, Paris BE. Substituted judgment: how accurate are proxy predictions? Ann Intern Med. 1991;115:92–8.
7. Fleck LM, Hayes OW. Ethics and consent to treat issues in acute stroke therapy. Emerg Med Clin North Am. 2002;20:703–15.
8. Stein J. The ethics of advance directives: a rehabilitation perspective. Am J Phys Med Rehabil Assoc Acad Physiatrists. 2003;82:152–7.
9. Ciccone A. Consent to thrombolysis in acute ischaemic stroke: from trial to practice. Lancet Neurol. 2003;2:375–8.
10. Ciccone A, Bonito V. Thrombolysis for acute ischemic stroke: the problem of consent. Neurol Sci Off J Ital Neurol Soc Ital Soc Clin Neurophysiol. 2001;22:339–51.
11. Chiu D, Peterson L, Elkind MS, Rosand J, Gerber LM, Silverstein MD. Comparison of outcomes after intracerebral hemorrhage and ischemic stroke. J Stroke Cerebrovasc Dis Off J Nat Stroke Assoc. 2010;19:225–9.
12. Suhl J, Simons P, Reedy T, Garrick T. Myth of substituted judgment. Surrogate decision making regarding life support is unreliable. Arch Intern Med. 1994;154:90–6.
13. Kopelman LM. The best interests standard for incompetent or incapacitated persons of all ages. J Law Med Ethics J Am Soc Law Med Ethics. 2007;35:187–96.
14. Kummer HB, Thompson DR. Critical care ethics. Mount Prospect: Society of Critical Care Medicine; 2009.
15. Kottow M. The battering of informed consent. J Med Ethics. 2004;30:565–9.
16. Louw SJ, Keeble JA. Stroke medicine-ethical and legal considerations. Age Ageing. 2002; 31 Suppl 3:31–5.
17. Witdrawing life-sustaining therapy. In: Miller FG, Truog RD, editors. Death, dying, and organ transplantation. New York: Oxford Press; 2012. p. 1–25.
18. Brophy v. New England Sinai Hospital, Inc. North East Rep Second Ser. 1986;497:626–46.
19. Constitution of the World Health Organization. Basic documents. 45th ed. Geneva: WHO; 2006.
20. Consensus statement of the Society of Critical Care Medicine's Ethics Committee regarding futile and other possibly inadvisable treatments. Crit Care Med. 1997;25:887–91.

Index

A

Acute spinal cord injury
  acute kidney injury, 263
  airway, 260, 261, 266, 268, 271–273
  analgesia, 262, 267, 271, 275
  anxiety, 264, 269
  aspiration, 261, 263, 266
  Canadian C-spine rule, 260
  decompressive surgery, 274
  deep venous thrombosis, 264
  depression, 264
  dexmedetomidine, 264
  emergency management, 258–262,
      264–266, 268, 271, 273, 274
  etiology, 260, 270
  fluid management, 262, 263
  hyperglycemia, 263
  hypoglycemia, 263
  hypotension, 259, 260, 263, 264, 266, 271
  ileus, 261, 263
  immobilization, 259, 262–264, 266–268,
      271, 272
  neuroimaging, 267
  NEXUS criteria, 260
  pneumonia, 258, 262, 268
  pressure ulcers, 261
  prolonged mechanical ventilation, 264
  propofol, 264
  respiratory insufficiency, 260, 262, 264
  sedation, 258, 260, 262, 267, 271
  spinal cord edema, 259
  spinal fracture, 261
  steroids, 264, 274
  stress gastric ulcer prophylaxis, 268
  traction, 262, 264, 267, 271, 275
  urinary retention, 261, 263

Airway
  airway equipment, 29
  airway humidification, 37, 39
  airway obstruction, 20, 23
  airway protection, 20, 37–39
  airway team, 28–29
  awake intubation, 30, 32
  bag-mask ventilation, 23, 28, 30, 31, 33, 38
  BURP maneuver, 23, 31
  cerebral herniation, 22, 24–25, 27, 39
  cerebral ischemia, 26
  cerebral perfusion pressure (CPP), 24, 26
  cervical spine injury, 26–27
  complications, 27–28
  continuous EEG, 27, 39
  Cormack–Lehane grading system, 23
  cricothyroidotomy, 31
  cuff leak, 32, 34, 37, 39
  difficult airway, 21–23, 28–32, 35, 36,
      38, 39
  dislodgement of tracheostomy tube, 38
  early tracheostomy, 36
  endotracheal tube introducer (bougie), 28,
      32, 35
  end-tidal CO2, capnography, 25, 28, 38
  etomidate, 22, 26
  extraglottic airway, 31, 32
  extubation, 32–39
  extubation failure, 25, 33, 39
  fentanyl, 24
  fiberoptic intubation, 21, 32, 39
  hyperkalemia, 26
  hyperosmolar therapy, 25, 27
  increased ICP, 24–28, 39
  ketamine, 24, 26
  laryngoscope, 21, 23, 29, 32

© Springer International Publishing Switzerland 2015
K.E. Wartenberg et al. (eds.), *Neurointensive Care: A Clinical Guide
to Patient Safety*, DOI 10.1007/978-3-319-17293-4

Airway (*Cont.*)
    lidocaine, 24
    Malampatti score, 22
    neck hematoma, 21, 38
    neurological examination, 19, 27, 38
    neuromuscular blockade, 24
    peak expiratory flow, 36
    post-extubation stridor, 33–35, 39
    RAMP positioning, 23, 31
    rapid sequence intubation, 21, 22, 24, 38
    reintubation, 33–39
    Sellick's maneuver, 31
    steroids, 35
    unplanned extubation, 37–39
    video laryngoscopy, 31

B
Bacterial meningitis
    antibiotics, 187–190, 192, 196–198
    causative organisms, 192
    cerebrospinal fluid, 185
    cerebrospinal fluid leakage, 185, 196
    chemoprophylaxis, 196–197
    clinical presentation, 186, 187, 189, 190,
        193, 194, 198
    complications, 192, 193, 196
    diagnosis, 186–188
    epidemiology, 197
    hyperosmolar therapy, 193
    hyponatremia, 192
    ICP, 187, 188, 190, 192–195
    intraventricular antibiotics, 190, 191
    isolation precautions, 196–197
    lumbar drainage, 193
    meningitis, bacterial, viral,
        tubercular, 188
    Nuchal rigidity, 187
    risk of mortality, 197
    septic shock, 193
    source of infection, 187
    steroids, 192
    treatment, 189–190, 192–198
    vaccination, 197
Brain abscess
    antimicrobial therapy, 201, 205
    cerebellar abscess, 201, 202, 204, 205, 207
    definition, 201
    intraventricular rupture, 203, 205
    prognosis, 203–205
    seizure prophylaxis, 206
    steroids, 206, 207
    surgical treatment, 203, 204, 206, 207

Brain death
    ancillary tests, 318, 322
    apnea test, 315–318, 323, 324
    criteria, 313, 314, 317–323
    dead donor rule, 320, 321
    definition, 313, 314, 319–322
    diagnosis, 315–319, 321, 322
    mimics, 317
    organ donation, 313–316, 320–324

C
Cerebral sinus thrombosis
    anticoagulation, 174, 176–181
    D-Dimer, 174, 175, 181
    definition, 171
    diagnosis, 172–181
    etiology
        coagulopathy, 172, 177, 180
        pregnancy, 172, 177
    follow up imaging, 176
    ICP, 181
    misdiagnosis, 176
    neuroimaging
        computed tomography (CT), 173
        CT venography, 174
        digital subtraction cerebral angiography
          (DSA), 174
        magnetic resonance imaging (MRI),
          173, 174
    seizure prophylaxis, 172–175, 177
    thrombectomy, 179, 181
    thrombolysis, 179–181
    treatment, 174, 177–181
Complications of catastrophic brain injury
    acidosis, respiratory–metabolic, 280, 281,
        285
    acute kidney injury, 284–286
    alkalosis, respiratory–metabolic,
        280, 281
    anemia, 280, 287
    arrhythmias, 290, 291
    catheter-related blood stream infections,
        294
    coagulopathy, 280, 287, 288
    diarrhea, 283, 286, 287
    ECG changes, 290, 291
    external ventricular catheter related
        meningitis, 296
    fluid balance, 280, 282, 284, 285
    hemoglobin level, 287
    hypernatremia, diabetes insipidus–central,
        renal, 283

hyponatremia
 cerebral salt wasting syndrome, 283
 SIADH, 283
myocardial infarction, 290, 291
neurogenic pulmonary edema, 292, 293
neurogenic stunned myocardium/Tako
  Tsubo cardiomyopathy, 289–291
nosocomial infections, 294, 295
oliguria, 285
peptic stress ulcers, 286
pneumonia, 286, 292–295
polyuria, 279, 280, 284–286
pseudomembranous colitis secondary to
 clostridium difficile, 294
urinary tract infections, 294
ventilator-associated pneumonia,
  293, 294
vomiting, 283, 285–287

E
Ethics and end of life
 advanced directives, 333
 autonomy, 329–331
 beneficence, 329, 331, 333, 334
 best interest standard, 331–333
 clear and convincing evidence, 333
 consequentialism, 329, 330
 deontology, 329, 330
 ethical principles, 329, 334
 implied consent, 331
 informed consent, 330–332
 justice, 329, 331, 334
 living will, 331–333
 nonmaleficence, 321, 329, 331, 334, 335
 substituted judgment, 331–333
 utilitarianism, 329, 330
 virtue ethics, 329, 330
 withdrawal of care, 328, 333–335
 withholding of care, 328, 333–335

G
Guillain–Barré syndrome
 autonomic dysfunction, 251, 252, 254
 dysphagia, 4, 7, 65–67, 108, 118, 159–161,
  164, 165
 epidemiology, 251
 immunoglobulins, 249
 monitoring of respiratory function, 252,
  254
 monitoring requirements, 250–254
 plasma exchange, 249

prognosis, 165, 179, 203–205, 219, 227,
  289, 291, 315, 316, 319, 321, 327,
  333, 335
threshold for intubation, 252
treatment, 249, 250, 252
ventilation, 250, 252–255

I
Intracerebral hemorrhage
 blood pressure control, 146, 148, 153
 decompressive surgery, 149, 150
 epidemiology, 148, 149
 etiology, 145
 extraventricular catheter, 149, 153
 hematoma expansion, 146, 149, 150, 153
 hydrocephalus, 149, 150, 153
 hyperosmolar therapy, 149
 ICP, 146, 148–150, 153
 intraventricular hemorrhage, 146, 149
 intraventricular thrombolysis, 146, 149,
  152
 outcome, 145, 146, 148–150
 outcome predictors, 149
 rebleeding, 150
 reversal of coagulopathy, 145, 151, 153
 seizure, 148–150
 seizure prophylaxis, 149
 surgical clot removal, 150, 153
Intracranial pressure monitoring
 CPP, 88, 92
 definition, 87
 extraventricular catheter/ventriculostomy,
  87–91
 intracranial hemorrhage, 88, 91
 intracranial pressure (ICP), 87–93
 malposition, 91
 meningitis,
Ischemic infarction/stroke, 100

M
Mechanical ventilation
 acute respiratory distress syndrome
  (ARDS), 44–48, 50–53
 CPP, 48–52
 ICP, 45–53
 interventional lung assist, 51
 neurogenic pulmonary edema, 45, 50
 neuromonitoring, 52
 neuromuscular blockade, 47, 49
 nitric oxide inhalation, 51
 permissive hypercapnia, 46, 47, 49, 50, 53

Mechanical ventilation (*Cont.*)
  positive end-expiratory pressure, 44, 47–49
  prone positioning, 45, 47, 50, 52, 53
  ventilator-induced lung injury, 46
Monitoring in neurointensive care unit
  brain tissue oxygen tension, 74, 77–78
  cerebral microdialysis, 74, 78–79
  clinical examination, 73, 76–78, 81, 83
  cytochrome c oxidase (CCO), 78
  electrocencephalography (EEG), 79, 80
  evoked potentials, 74, 80
  extraventricular catheter,
  fiberoptic ICP monitor, 74–76, 81
  hydrocephalus, 75, 76
  ICP, 74–77, 79–83
  jugular venous oximetry, 74, 77
  multimodal monitoring, 74, 81, 83
  near infrared spectroscopy, 74, 78
  neuroimaging, CT, MRI, 73–75, 81
  subdural bolt, 76
  transcranial Doppler sonography, 74

N
Neuroimaging
  artifacts, 310, 311
  contrast CT, 300, 301, 308, 309
  contrast induced renal injury, 310
  CT, 299–312
  doppler sonography, 300
  intrahospital transportation, 307
  MRI, 299–301
  portable CT scan, 301, 306–309, 311
  radiation safety precautions, 310
  radiograph, 299, 301, 308
  risk of radiation exposure, 300, 302, 303,
    308
Nutrition
  assessment of nutritional status, 60
  caloric requirement, 61, 67
  dysphagia, 65–67
  enteral nutrition, 57, 58, 63, 64, 67–69
  feeding intolerance, 62–63
  gastric residual volume, 69
  glutamine supplementation, 62
  glycemic control, 63
  hyperglycemia, 57, 58, 63
  hypermetabolic state, 57
  hypoglycemia, 63
  ileus, 66
  micronutrient supplementation, 65
  parenteral nutrition, 58, 64, 69
  prokinetic drugs, 59, 60, 62, 67, 69
  protein requirement, 61–62

  refeeding syndrome, 59, 65, 68
  transpyloric route, 60

P
Patient safety
  advanced practice practitioners, 163
  certification, 1, 4, 9, 10
  clinical nurse specialist, 158, 159
  closed ICU, 161
  dysphagia screening, 160, 161, 165
  education, 162, 164, 165
  environment factors, 161
  health care quality, 162, 165, 166
  health care safety, 161, 165
  leadership, 4, 5, 10
  length of stay, 159
  mortality, 159, 161
  multidisciplinary team, 165
  neurocritical care units, 158, 162
  open ICU,
  organizational culture, 10
  outcome measures, 2, 3, 11–12
  role modeling, 4
  safety standards, 1–14, 157–166
  staffing, 3, 5–8, 10, 12
  system factors, 4
Postoperative care in neurooncology
  alterations of consciousness, 112
  anticoagulation, 112
  blood pressure management, 96
  brain edema, 101, 103–105
  brain tumor, 95
  Burdenko respiratory insufficiency scale
    (BRIS), 108–110
  cerebral salt wasting syndrome, 113
  deep venous thrombosis prophylaxis, 131,
    159, 164, 229, 287
  diencephalon dysfunction syndrome, 112,
    118
  elective neurosurgery, 97
  hydrocephalus, 96, 110, 118
  hyperbaric oxygen therapy, 102
  hyponatremia, 113, 118
  hypothermia, 101, 102
  ICP, 101, 103, 110, 118
  ileus, 114, 115, 118
  intracranial hemorrhage, 99, 101, 103
  ischemic infarction/stroke, 100
  meningitis, 111, 115–116
  organ dysfunction, 112, 114
  pain, 108, 116, 118
  paradoxical venous air embolism, 100,
    101, 104

posterior fossa tumors, 106, 107, 118
postoperative nausea and vomiting
     (PONV), 116, 117
postoperative new neurologic deficit,
     98–99
postoperative recovery, 97–98
postoperative seizures, 106
recovery room, 97
residual neuromuscular blockade (RNMB),
     116, 117
respiratory insufficiency, 96, 108, 109,
     115, 118
seizure prophylaxis, 95, 106, 113, 114
sellar region tumors, 96, 97, 110, 111, 118
SIADH, 113
steroids, 116
venous cerebral infarction, 101, 102
Post stroke complications
     aspiration, 158–160, 164
     decubitus ulcers, 161
     deep venous thrombosis, 159, 164
     delirium, 164
     dysphagia, 159–161, 164, 165
     falls, 159, 160, 164
     pneumonia, 158–161
     pulmonary embolism, 160
     urinary tract infection, 159, 160

Q
Quality improvement initiative, 161

S
Safety bundles, 161, 165
Secondary stroke prevention, 164
Seizures and status epilepticus
     benzodiazepines, 213, 214, 216
     complications, 21, 209, 210, 214–216
     continuous EEG, 211, 216
     definition status epilepticus, 209
     diagnosis, 209–217
     epidemiology,
     etiology, 210, 213
     nonepileptiform seizures, 209–217
     postictal delirium and psychosis, 211, 215,
          216
     propofol, 214
     seizure precautions, 215
     seizure recognition, 210
     sudden unexpected death in epilepsy, 215
     treatment, 210–214
Stroke unit, 161, 162, 165

Subarachnoid hemorrhage
     analgesia, 132
     aneurysm repair, 130–132, 137, 138
     antifibrinolytic therapy, 130, 131
     blood pressure management, 131
     cerebrospinal fluid, 128
     clinical presentation, 127
     CT, 126–129, 132
     deep venous thrombosis, 131
     delayed cerebral ischemia, 130, 133
     diagnosis, 126–130, 137, 138
     endovascular coiling, 130, 131
     extraventricular catheter,
     fever, 127, 132, 133
     fluid balance, 137, 138
     FOUR score, 137
     gastrointestinal bleeding, 130, 135
     Glasgow coma scale, 137
     Hunt and Hess scale, 132, 137
     hydrocephalus, 131, 132, 134
     hyperdynamic therapy, 133, 138
     hyperglycemia, 132
     hypertonic saline, 132, 133, 135
     hyponatremia, 133, 135
     ICP, 132, 138
     levetiracetam, 136
     lindegaard index, 133, 134
     mannitol, 132
     medical complications, 134
     misdiagnosis, 127, 128
     nimodipine, 133, 138
     peptic ulcer prophylaxis, 135
     phenytoin, 136
     pulmonary embolus, 131, 133, 139
     rebleeding, 130–132, 134, 136, 138
     sedation, 132, 133, 136
     seizure prophylaxis, 130, 136
     seizures, 127, 135, 138
     statins, 164
     surgical clipping, 130, 131, 135
     thunderclap headache, 127
     transcranial Doppler sonography, 133
     vasopressor, 134
     WFNS scale, 137
     xantochromia, 128, 129

T
Thrombolysis
     arterial/local, 180
     systemic/intravenous/recombinant
          tissue plasminogen activator,
          162 164, 166

Traumatic brain injury
  acute respiratory distress syndrome, 225
  analgesia, 242
  antiseizure prophylaxis, 220, 237
  barbiturates, 232, 233, 235, 236
  blood pressure/hemodynamics, 220, 221,
        224, 225, 229, 234
  brain tissue oxygen tension, 234, 238
  brain trauma foundation guidelines, 219
  caloric requirement, 61, 67, 236
  CPP, 222, 225, 226, 230, 231, 233–234,
        240
  decompressive hemicraniectomy, 236
  deep venous thrombosis, prophylaxis, 229
  epidemiology,
  erythropoietin, 241
  extraventricular drain/external ventricular
        catheter, 149, 153, 205
  hyperbaric oxygen therapy, 241
  hyperglycemia, 236, 237
  hyperosmolar therapy
        hypertonic saline, 226, 240

  mannitol, 149, 193, 225
  hyperventilation, 220, 225, 226, 232,
        238–240, 243
  hypothermia, 220, 226, 227, 233, 236, 240
  ICP, 222, 225–242
  ICP monitoring, 225, 229–231, 234, 242
  infection prophylaxis, 220, 227, 229
  jugular venous oxygen saturation, 232, 238
  levetiracetam, 237
  neuroprotection, 240, 241
  nutrition, 220, 223, 236, 237, 242
  outcome, 220, 224, 227, 230–242
  oxygenation/ventilator settings, 220,
        224–226, 232–234, 241
  phenytoin, 223, 237
  progesterone, 241
  prognosis, 219, 227
  sedation, 222, 232, 235, 236, 238, 240,
        242, 243
  steroids, 220, 239, 243
  tracheostomy, 223, 228
  valproic acid, 210